Psychoanalysis and the family in twentieth-century France

MANCHESTER
1824
Manchester University Press

Studies in Modern French and Francophone History

Edited by
Máire Cross, David Hopkin and Jennifer Sessions

This series is published in collaboration with the Society for the Study of French History (UK) and the French Colonial Historical Society. It aims to showcase innovative monographs and edited collections on the history of France, its colonies and imperial undertakings, and the francophone world more generally since *c.* 1750. Authors demonstrate how sources and interpretations are being opened to historical investigation in new and interesting ways, and how unfamiliar subjects have the capacity to tell us more about France and the French colonial empire, their relationships in the world, and their legacies in the present. The series is particularly receptive to studies that break down traditional boundaries and conventional disciplinary divisions.

To buy or to find out more about the books currently available in this series, please go to:

https://manchesteruniversitypress.co.uk/series/studies-in-modern-french-and-francophone-history/

The Society for the Study of French History

FCHS SHCF
FRENCH COLONIAL HISTORICAL SOCIETY
SOCIÉTÉ D'HISTOIRE COLONIALE FRANÇAISE

Psychoanalysis and the family in twentieth-century France

Françoise Dolto and her legacy

Richard Bates

Manchester University Press

Published by Manchester University Press
Oxford Road, Manchester M13 9PL

www.manchesteruniversitypress.co.uk

British Library Cataloguing-in-Publication Data
A catalogue record for this book is available from the British Library

ISBN 978 1 5261 5962 5 hardback

First published 2022

Typeset
by Deanta Global Publishing Services, Chennai, India

Contents

Figures

Acknowledgements

This project was made possible by funding awarded by the Arts and Humanities Research Council (AHRC).

I would like to thank Catherine Dolto-Tolitch, for allowing me generous access to the Archives Françoise Dolto before their move to the Archives Nationales. Special thanks also to Iulia, Stéphane and Bérénice Michel for their assistance while working in Dolto's archives, and to Yann Potin and Clotilde Le Calvé at the Archives Nationales.

I am indebted to my mentors at the University of Nottingham, who have helped shape this project, and my career more broadly. Karen Adler supported this project from the outset and constantly pressed me to be more rigorous, nuanced and sophisticated in my thinking and writing. Colin Heywood offered many considered readings of my work and prompted me to think about the bigger historical picture. Anna Greenwood and Paul Crawford supported my development in myriad ways and generously granted me time to work on this book alongside other commitments. Academics from the University of Nottingham Department of History provided much encouragement and support over the years, especially Maiken Umbach, Liz Harvey, Jörg Arnold, David Laven and Spencer Mawby, while Maroula Perisanidi, Amy Calladine, Lucila Mallart, Dan O'Neill and Siobhan Hearne formed the core of an immensely helpful postgraduate community. The Centre for Political Ideologies also encouraged my work and helped me to publish a related article in the *Journal of Political Ideologies* – thanks to Mathew Humphrey, in particular, for this support.

This book has also benefited greatly from the support of the wider French history community. I would particularly like to thank

Siân Reynolds for supporting my work and for many helpful comments, Joan Tumblety for enormously helpful reflections on the book proposal and Sophie Heywood for many helpful suggestions. My thinking also benefited from conversations with, among others, Jonathyne Briggs, Rebecca Scales, Julian Jackson, Kevin Passmore, Jackie Clarke, Chris Millington, Lindsey Dodd, Miranda Sachs, Sam Wilkinson, Sam Matuszewski and Paul Smith.

Thanks to James Harris and Ewa Szypula for assisting with translations, and to James Burrows and Peter Bates for reading the text and making many useful suggestions.

Thanks to Alun Richards and the team at Manchester University Press for championing this project, including to the anonymous reviewers for their invaluable sharp-eyed suggestions.

Thanks also to those who helped make my research stays in Paris productive and enjoyable, especially Eve Judelson, Olivier and Cécile Fouquet, Estelle Murail, Gwen Cariou, Pippa Rimmer and Sebastien Massart. An AHRC Research and Travel Grant facilitated one of my study periods in Paris.

Thanks to my wonderful parents Maureen and Peter for supporting me in innumerable ways; to say that I could not have reached this point without them is a considerable understatement. And thanks finally to Ewa, for the happiness and stability without which undertaking this kind of project would not have been conceivable.

Abbreviations

AFD	Archives Françoise Dolto
CCB	Centre Claude Bernard
CDE	*Les Chemins de l'éducation* (book by Dolto)
CMPP	Centre Médico Psycho-Pédagogique
EDP	École des Parents
EFP	École Freudienne de Paris
EME	*Les Étapes majeures de l'enfance* (book by Dolto)
EP	*L'Évolution psychiatrique*
FFEPH	Fondation Française pour l'Étude des Problèmes Humains (Fondation Carrel)
IPA	International Psychoanalytic Association
LAEP	Lieux d'Accueil Enfants-Parents
MDF	Mouvement Démocratique Féminin
MFPF	Mouvement Français pour le Planning Familial
MRP	Mouvement Républicain Populaire
MV	Maison Verte
ORTF	Office de Radiodiffusion-Télévision Française
PECS	Picture Exchange Communication System
RFP	*Revue française de psychanalyse*
RTF	Radio-Télévision Française
RTL	Radio-Télévision Luxembourg
SFP	Société Française de Psychanalyse
SPP	Société Psychanalytique de Paris
STO	Service du travail obligatoire
TEACHH	Treatment and Education of Autistic and Related Communication Handicapped Children
UFF	Union des Femmes Françaises
UMP	Union pour un Movement Populaire

Introduction: Doltomania

In 1982, a twenty-nine-year-old nurse from a small town near the Swiss-French border wrote a letter to a woman she had never met, but nonetheless considered her 'last thread of hope'. The nurse described herself as a 'frigid and neurotic woman' whose life was in 'psychological chaos', exacerbated by the fact that her therapist had moved away. 'The worst thing is that I have a child', she wrote. 'I'm terribly afraid of making my child psychologically ill as a result of all of this.' But, having chanced across a book written by the woman she was writing to – Françoise Dolto – the nurse was no longer in despair. Reading the book, 'it was as if for the first time, after so many years, someone finally truly spoke to me … To know that you are there, and that you understand so many things, filled me with new hope', she wrote. 'I now cling to you with all my strength.'[1]

The nurse was not the only person to feel this way. From the 1970s until the end of the twentieth century and arguably beyond, Dolto was an important figure in the French cultural landscape. Her numerous books were widely read and studied. Her daily fifteen-minute broadcast on the France Inter radio station was a source of 'hope and love' for thousands of listeners.[2] Dolto appeared all over the media, commenting on a wide range of issues connected to psychology, parenting, education, gender, sexuality, family, bioethics and children's literature, culture and rights. She was seen as a French national treasure. Across France, hundreds of public institutions were named in her honour, from schools, crèches, children's centres and youth clubs to clinics, medical centres and hospital wings.[3] Roads in Paris and other cities bear her name. In the 2008 film *Entre les murs* (*The Class*), Laurent Cantet and François

Bégaudeau's critical examination of the French republican education system, the fictional school is named 'Collège Françoise Dolto': chosen in part because the name was one of the most archetypal, unremarkable names possible for a French school at that time.[4] More than thirty years after her death, her work has continued to be highlighted regularly by media outlets such as the France Culture radio station and *Psychologies* magazine.[5]

Dolto is part of the French cultural and institutional fabric, in ways that may not be immediately obvious to outsiders. Millions of French children born in the last quarter of the twentieth century were raised against the backdrop of her ideas, many by parents who had her books on their shelves. Commentators spoke of a 'Dolto generation'.[6] Her fame took off in 1976, when she commenced her daily *Lorsque l'enfant paraît* broadcasts on the state radio station France Inter. She had already been a public figure for some time, having made occasional appearances in the press and broadcast media since the 1940s, but the new series of broadcasts took her from the fringes of national conversation into the mainstream. By the time Dolto died in 1988, the response reflected a sense that France had been deprived of an important national figure. *Paris Match*'s obituary ran to six pages; messages of condolence came in from political leaders including President François Mitterrand.[7] There was a feeling that Dolto's ideas would not die with her but would remain of lasting relevance.[8] In the 1990s, publishers capitalised by reissuing many of Dolto's books and producing a stream of posthumous publications. Two commemorative conferences were held under the auspices of UNESCO in Paris, in 1999 and on Dolto's centenary in 2008. By 1992, Dolto's influence had become sufficiently prevalent among middle-class French parents that journalist Guy Baret could write a successful book, *Allô maman Dolto*,[9] mocking what he termed '*doltomaniaques*' – defined as mothers who dogmatically attempted to apply Dolto's ideas in all situations, even if it resulted in absurd outcomes.[10] Baret argued that Dolto had become so fashionable that bourgeois mothers were engaging in a form of one-upmanship, seeking to outdo each other in their ostentatiously thorough application of her ideas. A 1994 theatrical adaptation of *Allô maman Dolto* by Sophie Duprès was a nationwide hit, and continued to be staged regularly into the 2010s. Baret followed up with a further book, *Comment rater l'éducation de votre enfant avec Françoise Dolto* (*How to Mess Up Your Parenting with Françoise Dolto*, 2003), deriding some of Dolto's ideas and exploring the anxieties of parents who tried to implement them.[11] Whether as a model to be followed or a target to be shot at, Dolto's approach was an inescapable reference point in late twentieth-century French discussions of parenting.

The phenomenon of Dolto's popularity and pervasive influence requires explanation. Clearly, it has to do with the things that Dolto did, wrote and said. A significant part of this book will examine the development of Dolto's ideas, exploring their roots and contexts in the 1930s and how they played out prior to the emergence of 'Doltomania'. But celebrity and charisma have long been recognised as two-sided phenomena, co-creations between the famous individual and the social collective that assigns significance to their personas, ideas and practices.[12] Why did Dolto, an experienced psychoanalyst of children, become someone from whom a lot of French people wanted to hear in the late 1970s and subsequently? What kinds of demand was she responding to? What were the cultural, social and political conditions that enabled her to succeed?

A key element of Dolto's success was that she became the personal embodiment of a societal transition in parenting techniques and ideals – from a vision based on upholding paternal authority, honour, tradition and deference, to one based on more autonomy, respect and empathy for children. She was not the first person to propose this change, but she crystallised it for her audience, articulating it in ways that confirmed for parents of the 1970s and 1980s that they were on the right track. As a white, wealthy, grandmotherly, Christian woman, with views that were socially conservative in many respects, she was a good messenger for this shift in values, since her persona made clear that no wider upsetting of the social edifice would follow from implementing it. Indeed, if there was one word that Dolto's audience used to describe her more than any other, it was 'reassuring'.

The widespread need for reassurance spoke to the fact that Dolto's emergence took place during a transitional period in French history. In 1975, France had entered its most severe recession since the 1940s, ending the 'thirty glorious years' of postwar boom and commencing 'twenty-five inglorious' ones characterised by stagflation, abrupt economic policy shifts and subsequently austerity and inequality.[13] The high birth rates and full employment of the *trente glorieuses* gave way to years of smaller family sizes and high structural unemployment. Marriage rates fell and divorces increased, as more people lived alone or cohabited without marrying. Cities were continuing to expand, sprouting new housing estates, while rural France, no longer a peasant- and artisan-based economy, sustained fewer (albeit more productive) jobs. Agriculture's share of the workforce fell from 27 per cent in 1954 to under 10 per cent in 1975.[14] Heavy (and heavily unionised) industries such as coal and steel were declining, as were the small proprietor businesses of the traditional middle class, while job opportunities grew in the salaried white-collar and service sectors. France had lost almost all of its remaining formal empire in the 1960s, and was periodically seized by fears of being swamped by non-white immigrants from former colonies, prompting the government to ban new immigration other than for purposes of family reunification.[15]

France in the mid-1970s looked and felt a lot different to twenty years previously. Most people no longer lived or expected to live as their parents and grandparents had: only 22 per cent of the sons of shopkeepers and artisans and 38 per cent of the sons of farmers followed their fathers' professions in 1977, compared to 48 per cent and 60 per cent, respectively, in 1953.[16] Nor did they look to the same sources of reassurance and guidance in the face of these upheavals. The Catholic Church saw sharp drops in church attendance, baptisms and ordinations into the clergy during the 1970s, while readership of daily newspapers also declined. At the same time, more and more French people owned telephones and radio sets, read magazines and watched television. The state-controlled audiovisual sector, as Tamara Chaplin has written, was belatedly recognising a need 'to start acknowledging public opinion, liberalising political coverage, and catering to popular taste'.[17] A new media landscape was emerging: more diverse and attentive to the demands of audiences than in earlier decades, but still top-down in comparison to the later eras of private television channels, Minitel chat forums and eventually online communities.[18]

This new atmosphere created opportunities for a new kind of media personality or expert figure, one who still depended on elite networks to obtain a platform, but who sought increased interaction with audiences. Judith Coffin's recent book on Simone de Beauvoir,

Sex, Love, and Letters, clearly shows the growing and powerful public demand for a kind of intimate communication with celebrity figures.[19] Dolto's career and archive, alongside those of the broadcaster Ménie Grégoire, whose papers now occupy vast swathes of the Archives Départementales in Tours, is further evidence that large numbers of French people were craving guidance on their private problems, and willing to reveal intimate information to strangers in order to obtain it.[20] Dolto encouraged the belief that the radio was a good place to turn for solace, speaking of the possibility of 'wireless transference', while Grégoire described a 'community of hearts' that unified her with her listeners. Both figures adopted a certain informality of style, wanting to appear in close sympathy with their audiences rather than as distant authorities. Yet, in the absence of the kind of genuine peer-to-peer communities that would emerge with the internet, they were still elite personalities, whose opportunities were ultimately provided by what Robert Gildea calls 'a closed group of producers, editors and presenters in Paris who made their decisions in the light of sales and ratings'.[21]

One thing that certainly sold well in the French 1970s was psychoanalysis. This was something of a new phenomenon. For reasons that are explored in Chapter 1, psychoanalysis began relatively late in France, and as late as the 1950s only a very small minority – mostly wealthy Parisians – had undergone analysis, which was commonly viewed as something 'American', aimed at intellectuals, artists and '*les riches*'.[22] However, by the mid-1970s, France had developed a full-blown psychoanalytic culture. Freudian thinking – fundamentally, the idea that explanations and solutions to the psychological and emotional problems of adulthood could be found by exploring, examining and working through early childhood experiences, especially their sexual or phantasmagorical aspects – had penetrated into many areas of French life. Sherry Turkle's contemporary research found that child-raising manuals, vocational counselling, education and social work had all 'gone psychoanalytic', while psychoanalysis had become 'big news in French medicine, psychiatry, and publishing'; psychoanalytic vocabulary had 'invaded French life and language, changing the ways people think about politics, discuss literature, and address their children'.[23] An obvious turning point, Turkle suggested, was the protest and strike movement of May 1968 and the longer-term responses to the events of that month. There were echoes of psychoanalytic language in the protests themselves, with demonstrators speaking in terms of desire and repression, of wanting to access ways of living that were blocked by existing social and political structures. After the demonstrations failed to remove the Right from power, many political radicals turned towards psychoanalysis in the hope of developing a deeper understanding both of themselves and the world around them. Psychoanalysis could serve as a bridge between the politics of social activism that characterised May 1968 and the politics of the person that became more prominent in the 1970s.[24] Whether one supported or opposed the 1968 radicals, a turn to psychoanalysis was widely perceived as necessary to understand what was happening in French society. The early 1970s saw a publishing boom in psychoanalytic texts, and the University of Vincennes, founded as a direct response to the May events, included a Department of Psychoanalysis. Sigmund Freud's work had already been added to the philosophy syllabus for the *baccalauréat* in 1968. Around the same time, the use of psychoanalysis took off within psychiatry, as championed by psychiatrists such as Paul-Claude Racamier, whose *Le Psychanalyste sans divan* (*The Couch-Less Psychoanalyst*, 1970), argued for psychoanalytic thinking to be deployed in reconceptualising mental health institutions.[25]

The increased diffusion of Freudian thinking was reflected in the growth of psychoanalytic organisations. French psychoanalytic associations had a combined total of 243 members in 1964; by 1981, this had risen to 981.[26] The community had split three times by 1969. The reasons for the first two splits (in 1953 and 1964) are explored in Chapter 3, but the common factor to all three was controversy around the methods and personality of Jacques Lacan (1901–81), who had emerged as the movement's dominant personality and its best-known figure, with his *Écrits* (1966) becoming a bestseller. Lacan led the École Freudienne de Paris (EFP), created in 1964, which became by far the largest of the associations, with 609 members by 1980. Lacan's appeal among analysts and trainees resulted from a combination of factors. First was his theoretical orientation: his proposal to re-interpret Sigmund Freud's writings through the prism of Saussurian linguistics and Lévi-Straussian structuralist anthropology, while also relating these to ideas taken from philosophy, literature and art. Lacan proposed a renewal of psychoanalysis, away from its postwar conservative and Catholic-leaning direction, and gained an enthusiastic audience of avant-garde intellectuals. Second were Lacan's practical innovations: his use of short and variable-length sessions, his championing of non-medics becoming analysts and his opposition to hierarchical structures. These innovations helped French psychoanalysis to create distinct organisational and operational tendencies and to preserve its independence from medicine – but they also contributed to internal splits and to Lacanian analysis being cut off from the international psychoanalytic movement, which especially rejected Lacan's use of short sessions. Lacan's rise was further aided by his intense personal magnetism – one anthropologist, observing his seminar, compared his 'radiant influence' to that of a shaman – his erudition and his elite connections.[27] In his later years, this morphed into a religious-style cult of personality – some young psychoanalysts referred to him as 'God the Father' – overseen by his son-in-law Jacques-Alain Miller.[28]

Dolto was an important professional friend and ally of Lacan, supporting him in the psychoanalytic movement's splits. Other than Lacan himself, she was the oldest member of the EFP and the only one to have qualified as an analyst before World War II. She and Lacan have been described as the 'parental couple' of French psychoanalysis, with Dolto's reassuring, maternal presence complementing Lacan's role as the movement's intellectual leader and father figure.[29] Yet Lacan does not in fact feature as prominently in Dolto's story as one might expect. Considering herself his contemporary and professional equal, Dolto avoided the deferential relationship to Lacan that characterised many younger analysts, and seldom worked directly with him. Though their ideas certainly overlapped, Dolto rarely referred to Lacan in her work, and freely admitted to not understanding some of what he wrote – while simultaneously indirectly benefiting from the intellectual credibility that Lacan conferred on the whole French psychoanalytic movement. Dolto did not stand entirely apart from the internal politics of psychoanalytic organisations, but she was nowhere near as invested in them as Lacan, and did not use them as a means of wielding wider influence.

Lacan and Dolto spoke to very different audiences. Where Lacan's was primarily intellectual, Dolto spoke to a mainly female audience of French parents/grandparents and people whose profession involved day-to-day care or supervision of children. Lacan addressed the avant-garde elite, seeking to convince them that psychoanalysis not only held the keys to understanding the human mind but could also connect and illuminate different strands of the twentieth-century social sciences: structuralism, linguistics, Marxist and post-Marxist politics, anthropology. He refused to simplify his ideas to gain a popular audience, making clear, when interviewed for the cultural affairs television programme *Un certain regard* in 1974, that he was 'speaking to those who are savvy, to the non-idiots'.[30] Dolto, by contrast, did not generate theories that international academics found useful, but focused instead on bringing psychoanalysis into the everyday lives of ordinary French people. She used the mass media to speak to parents, grandparents, teachers, childminders and healthcare workers, and impress her views upon politicians and policy makers.

Dolto's reputation was also different in that she was known specifically as a leading *child* psychoanalyst: unlike Lacan and other senior colleagues, her patient base consisted mainly of children, and her pedagogical work focused on training others how to conduct psychoanalysis with children. Child psychoanalysis had existed as a sub-field since the interwar period, having been pioneered in the 1910s and 1920s by the Viennese analyst Hermine Hug-Hellmuth, and subsequently developed by Anna Freud, Melanie Klein and Donald Winnicott in London.[31] Its pioneer in France was Sophie Morgenstern (discussed further in Chapter 1); her death in 1940 left Dolto as the most experienced child analyst in the country. The appeal of analysing children was that it introduced the possibility of pre-empting the kinds of psychological problems that analysts saw in their adult patients, and which they were convinced had their roots in childhood. But psychoanalysing children was not straightforward. Children could not be guided through their unconscious thought processes using the techniques (such as dream analysis) that analysts applied to adults. Instead, the early child analysts developed new methods, such as interpreting children's drawings, modellings or play. Another challenge was convincing parents and/or public institutions to pay for children to be treated in this way. The success or failure of child analysis would thus depend on the wider cultural prestige of psychoanalysis, and the willingness of parents, doctors and government officials to accept the premises of psychoanalytic thinking – especially the idea that adult problems were determined by childhood experiences – and to accord legitimacy to Freudian practitioners.

Specialising in child psychoanalysis placed Dolto in a more stereotypically 'female' sphere, one concerned with children and families, while Lacan laid claim to the historically male domain of abstract philosophy. From a historical standpoint, Dolto's focus on children makes it particularly important to approach her not only through the prism of the history of psychoanalysis, but also through that of family politics. It was not just that Dolto's public profile accorded her the opportunity to contribute to shaping family policy – as she did in the 1980s when taking part in government-commissioned study groups on issues of divorce, child custody and bioethics – but that her advice to the public on child-rearing questions emerged from decades of intense discourse and debate around gender, sexuality and the role of women in society. The history of these questions has been a rich field of historical investigation since the 1990s, and this book accordingly draws on the essential insights provided by the works of, among others, Karen Adler, Sylvie Chaperon, Jackie Clarke, Kelly Ricciardi Colvin, Claire Duchen, Sarah Fishman, Sandrine Garcia, Lisa Greenwald, Francine Muel-Dreyfus, Susan Pedersen, Miranda Pollard, Rebecca Pulju, Siân Reynolds, Kristin Ross and Joan Tumblety.[32] Questions of family/gender roles, sexuality and education were central to Dolto's own life choices – in her early life, determined to have a career in medicine, Dolto pushed at the boundaries of what her family and social milieu deemed acceptable for a woman of her class – and to her relationship with the French public. Despite her reputation as a progressive and liberal voice on child-rearing questions, Dolto's leading message on family structure was that a strong fatherly presence was crucially important for children's psychical health, whereas an over-powerful mother could have potentially devastatingly destructive effects on her children's psyches. It followed that mothers should, ideally, confine themselves to the conventionally feminine virtues of maternal care and subservience to male authority. Such beliefs led Dolto to oppose, for example, reforms to marriage law in 1965 that granted women additional rights, as well as the legalisation of abortion in 1975.

Dolto's views in these areas are related to the (far-)right-wing politics of the 1930s that she encountered through her family and key professional influences, especially René Laforgue, her analyst, and her thesis supervisor Édouard Pichon. It was in the late 1930s that Dolto's ideas took shape, among a circle of right-wing (or even far-right and antisemitic) psychoanalytic thinkers. Laforgue, in particular, emerges from this book as someone whose importance has been hitherto underestimated. In addition to Dolto, a number of other figures who were central in disseminating psychoanalytic thinking in France were his analysands, including Ménie Grégoire, Georges Mauco and André Berge. The key concept that Laforgue developed and communicated was that of the *névrose familiale* (family neurosis – discussed further in Chapter 1): the idea that neuroses developed according to the family environment, tended to run in families and were especially likely to be transmitted by a mother to a child. Pichon, for his part, used psychoanalytic theory to help him develop a libertarian approach to child-rearing, and also to attempt to 'cure' people of non-heteronormative sexuality. Dolto absorbed concepts from this crucible without questioning their scientific provenance or political implications. She did not think of herself as a conservative. On sexual questions, she rejected the intransigent Catholic emphasis on sexual purity and innocence, promoted sex education and dismissed anxieties about the evils of masturbation or of sexual talk and play among children. On education, following Pichon, she was a libertarian, rejecting corporal punishment and resisting state oversight. Bolstered by the pushback that she encountered on such views, notably from traditionalist Christian segments of her audience, she saw herself as a radical liberal challenging established, constricting shibboleths – even as most of her arguments, in practice, tended to reinforce classic heteronormative assumptions and the male-breadwinner family model.

In the post-1968 context, Dolto did not tend to advertise the fact that her ideas had been formed in the interwar period, shaped by right-wing opponents of France's republican tradition. Yet this, too, may have been part of her appeal. Dolto's thinking was inflected with a ruralist nostalgia that crossed political boundaries but was especially prevalent on the 1930s Right, often among its clerical and monarchist extremes.[33] In her 1940s writings she upheld an ideal of a village family doctor who, rather than merely respond with a prescription when something went wrong, would proactively maintain the community's health by adopting a pastoral role, forming deep-rooted and long-term patient relationships. What she offered on the radio – after soliciting listeners to write long letters in which they poured out their family histories as the background to their current suffering – was a kind of mediatised echo of this idealised function. Her focus on the supposedly timeless psychological conflicts at the heart of families served to downplay the impact of history, presenting the family as something eternal, stable, a *repère* for an anxious 1970s populace. The suggestion of nostalgia in her worldview was an important part of her persona, as was her grandmotherly manner. The family, as she presented it, was a self-contained cocoon in which problems could be solved simply by 'by bringing [children] to express themselves and decoding what they say' – without needing to think too hard about the world outside.[34]

To her fans, Dolto was doing something simple and admirable: encouraging family members to communicate better, and providing them with tools to do so. But Dolto's emphasis was underpinned by childhood determinism: the idea that a person's character, psychological makeup and life chances were determined by their experiences in the first years of life. According to this thinking, serious, long-term consequences could flow from apparently innocuous events and actions, such as toilet training occurring too soon, changes to childcare arrangements or children sharing the parental bed.[35] Any childhood psychological or even medical condition could, by this logic, legitimately be blamed on the parents – a stigma that the mothers of autistic children, in particular, had to spend decades fighting off in the wake of Dolto's influence in that field (Chapter 5). Parents with chaotic or unconventional lives could be viewed as potential producers of psychologically disturbed children. The political implications of reading everything through the prism of parental relationships and early childhood are perhaps easier to see in instances when Dolto applied her logic to broader social phenomena. The opening pages of her popular 1987 book *Tout est langage* (*Everything is Language*), for example, discuss juvenile delinquency in France during World War II. Dolto attributed this to the absence of one and a half million men from French society as prisoners of war (POWs) in Germany – the same explanation provided by the Vichy government during the war itself. In Dolto's version, the children of POWs understood that one became a prisoner because one had committed a crime. Therefore, they were disconcerted to see their mothers' relative happiness to discover that their husbands were in prison (since this proved they had survived the battles). The children surmised that committing a crime or delinquent act, as their fathers must have done, would enhance their value in their mother's eyes – and acted accordingly.[36] Dolto's story is neat, recounted with some élan, and narratively plausible. It is, however, untrue: Sarah Fishman has demonstrated that poverty was the major factor in wartime delinquency, and that there was no causal relationship between POW fathers and juvenile delinquency.[37] Dolto had not researched the topic. Instead, she had used a psychoanalytic framework to rationalise and update a Vichyite canard.

Dolto's advice was intended not only to help individuals, but to improve the overall psychological health of the French nation – or, as she revealingly referred to it, the French '*ethnie*' (race or ethnic group). She assumed an overwhelmingly white and culturally Catholic audience. She did not foreground the voices of people on the margins of French society or particularly seek to appeal to immigrant communities; working-class and immigrant areas were underrepresented in her mailbag. Her thinking was shaped in an era and a milieu that took for granted France's status as a colonial power and its right to disseminate its civilisation to colonised peoples. Race and colonialism were, moreover, the kinds of historical factor to which Dolto preferred not to assign much psychological significance. There was a strand of universalism in her thinking which may be compared to that in French republicanism, but perhaps more pertinently to missionary Christianity. In Dolto's mind, psychoanalysis was akin to Christian gospel, a universal truth suitable for missionary diffusion worldwide without the kind of adaptation to local circumstances that more perceptive psychiatric practitioners, such as Frantz Fanon, understood to be necessary.[38] At its extreme, this amounted to a virtual dismissal of the psychological impact even of the Holocaust, as Chapters 3 and 4 show. Only on one brief occasion, highlighted in the Afterword, did Dolto seem to perceive the importance of race as a psychological category, and she found the experience disconcerting.

This book thus approaches Dolto as a thoroughly political figure, placing her ideas in their political context, even when that context appears at a couple of removes from her direct interventions. As communist critics of psychoanalysis pointed out in the 1940s (see Chapter 4), by focusing their attention on the internal dynamics of the family and on the individual psyche as the site of change, psychoanalysts were implicitly aligning themselves with a conservative conception of society as an amalgamation of individuals. It was precisely to avoid such criticisms that Lacan tried to ally psychoanalysis with left-wing philosophy and to borrow the language of structural social critique. Dolto used that language too, but for her, at least, it seems to have been a matter of convenience as much as conviction. Dolto did not share the goal of 1960s and 1970s radicals seeking a fundamental overhaul of France's economic and social order. Her ideal vision for society was nostalgically conservative: small-scale, intimate, artisanal rural communities populated by healthy individuals who spent lots of time outdoors engaged in physical pursuits and crafts rather than intellectual pursuits, and where mothers happily devoted themselves to their children and husbands rather than professional careers. In dispensing advice to patients that was informed by this vision, Dolto blurred the lines between medicine and politics, deploying her medical, psychoanalytic and cultural authority to advance what was ultimately a political agenda.

In seeing Dolto as a political figure, *Psychoanalysis and the family in twentieth-century France* follows a direction set by three important recent works on psychoanalysis, and its relationship to broader social, political and cultural histories, by Dagmar Herzog, Michal Shapira and Camille Robcis, respectively. Herzog's *Cold War Freud* (2017) emphasises the plasticity and multiplicity of Cold War-era psychoanalysis, showing how, while turning inwards and towards sexual conservatism in the postwar United States, it enjoyed a 'second golden age' in Europe, impacting on a range of fields from the German legal approach to Holocaust reparations, to radical politics in France and ethnography in Switzerland. Several of Herzog's central themes recur in this book, including the dialogue and rapprochement between Christianity and psychoanalysis after 1945, the interplay between the history of psychoanalysis and that of sexuality and the significance of the anti-authoritarian strand of psychoanalysis associated in France with Félix Guattari. More broadly, I share

Herzog's sense that, in John Forrester's words, important aspects of the history of psychoanalysis have been 'lost from sight' because 'we have been looking for too long in the wrong places'.[39] In the French context, the 'wrong places' include the extensive attention paid to theoretical debates and internal intrigues around Lacan, at the expense of the everyday experiences of ordinary people. In aiming to help redress this balance, this book draws on Michal Shapira's work on the impacts of psychoanalysis in 1940s Britain, in *The War Inside* (2013), which was pioneering in moving the historical focus, in Shapira's term, 'beyond the couch', considering psychoanalysts as 'social actors in their cultures' and psychoanalysis as 'an immensely influential political discipline'.[40] My work echoes both Shapira's focus on the psychoanalysis of children, and her emphasis on the importance of the 'medico-psychological' institutions that appeared in both countries – in England, the Tavistock Clinic and the Institute for the Scientific Treatment of Delinquency; in France, the so-called Centres Médico-Psycho-Pédagogiques (CMPPs) (Chapter 4), and the Maison Verte (MV) network of children's centres (Chapter 6). Shapira's concept of 'constructed sensitivities' – meaning ideas about what children supposedly naturally do or need, but which are in fact historically constructed and contingent – is also a useful way to think about the shifts in thinking about families and child-rearing that Dolto articulated and epitomised.

Relatively few historical works have addressed psychoanalysis as a factor in French social history. Sherry Turkle's *Psychoanalytic Politics* (1978) took initial steps in this direction, but was written too early to capture the full scope, just missing the Dolto phenomenon.[41] Élisabeth Roudinesco's two-volume work *La Bataille de cent ans* (*The Hundred-Year Battle*, 1982/1986) was essentially an insider history, as was Claudine and Pierre Geissmann's *A History of Child Psychoanalysis* (1992).[42] Annick Ohayon's *L'Impossible Rencontre* (*The Impossible Meeting*, 1999) incorporated psychoanalysis into the wider history of French psychology, while Agnès Desmazières's *L'Inconscient au paradis* (*The Unconscious in Heaven*, 2011) examined the relationship between psychoanalysis and the Catholic Church.[43] The book that most closely shares the aims of the present text is Camille Robcis's *The Law of Kinship* (2013). Robcis emphasises the long-term influence of Lacanian psychoanalysis and Claude Lévi-Strauss's structuralist anthropology on French family policy, and especially the repercussions for 1990s debates over bioethics, same sex parenting and civil partnerships. Robcis's key argument is that the 'structuralist social contract' – the wide acceptance of a 'causal relation between kinship and socialisation [which] posited sexual difference as the necessary condition for all social and psychic organisation' (and thus privileged the maintenance of the heteronormative family as crucial to the constitution of both the self and the state) – was not only used in political and judicial spheres to resist reforms to family policy, but became seen as synonymous with French republicanism. Robcis identifies Dolto as one of a series of 'bridge figures', alongside her colleagues André Berge and Georges Mauco, whose function was to mediate the structuralist social contract for a popular audience. These popularisers, Robcis argues, ignored any caveats in Lévi-Strauss's and Lacan's writings and drew simplified conclusions, 'filling the empty signifiers that structuralism posited with real people, real mothers, fathers and children', collapsing distinctions between the descriptive and the prescriptive or between the normative and the heteronormative.[44]

Robcis's thesis is perceptive and often persuasive, bringing to bear a wealth of material on the history of French family policy and on the deployment of structuralist language by politicians and judges to support heteronormative conclusions. Her analytic framework has some limitations, however, where the 'bridge figures' are concerned. Robcis supposes a unidirectional line of influence – running from the intellectual elite, represented by Lacan and Lévi-Strauss, to ordinary people via second-rate thinkers like Dolto – and assumes that Lacan provided the intellectual foundation for Dolto's work. My study does not support those suppositions. To see Dolto as primarily a conduit for Lacan's structuralist ideas is, I think, to misrepresent her true significance for French culture and to misunderstand the roots of her approach. As will be shown, Dolto's thinking was formed in the 1930s under the influence of Édouard Pichon and René Laforgue, significantly pre-dating Lévi-Strauss's and Lacan's postwar structuralist writings. Indeed it is Laforgue, not Lacan, who most shaped the thinking of all three of Robcis's 'bridge figures', having psychoanalysed each of them. While Lacan was certainly an influential figure, it may ultimately be more helpful to think of him less as the fount of twentieth-century French psychoanalytic thinking, but rather as only one articulation of it – someone whose value lay to some extent in his ability to give old ideas new credibility by recasting them in structuralist vocabulary. As the underappreciated 1993 work of Carolyn Dean, *The Self and Its Pleasures*, also suggested, the real roots of the psychoanalytic ideas that took hold in France from the 1960s onwards need to be sought in the 1930s – i.e. precisely the time when both Lacan and Dolto, separately, began to engage with them.[45]

Aside from Robcis's work, Dolto has been the subject of a 2009 English-language book aimed at psychoanalysts and featuring an introduction by Juliet Mitchell, while Sarah Fishman's 2017 study of gender and family life in postwar France, *From Vichy to the Sexual Revolution*, considered Dolto as part of a chapter on the influence of Freud, Beauvoir and Alfred Kinsey in the 1950s, with little reference to Dolto's subsequent career.[46] In France, a sympathetic biography by Jean-François de Sauverzac, a psychoanalyst who knew Dolto personally, appeared in 1995, and a further uncritical book-length portrayal by a journalist, Daniela Lumbroso, in 2007.[47] Dolto has drawn critical attention from sociologists, such as Dominique Mehl, who assessed Dolto's influence on French media, and Sandrine Garcia, who studied her in the context of the postwar family planning and women's rights movements.[48] Both Mehl and Garcia view Dolto as a purveyor of regressive gender attitudes, with Garcia arguing that she upheld and perpetuated the Vichy-era vision of the '*éternel féminin*' – but this remains some way apart from her popular reputation, with books praising Dolto's ideas and her social impact continuing to appear well into the twenty-first century.[49] (Dolto's contemporary reputation in France will be discussed further in the Afterword.)

Given this limited scholarship, the major source of information on Dolto's life remains her own autobiographical publications, *Enfances* (1986) and *Autoportrait d'une psychanalyste* (1989).[50] These need to be handled with some care, since Dolto's storytelling, as in the example of wartime juvenile delinquency noted above, has a tendency to result in suspiciously neat conclusions that seem designed to validate her psychoanalytic theories. The same year that *Enfances* was published, Pierre Bourdieu put all biographers and autobiographers on the defensive with the concept of the 'biographical illusion' – the coherence artificially accorded to life events by the conventions of narrative writing. Whereas real life trajectories are determined by a myriad of socio-economic and cultural factors, Bourdieu argued that (auto)biographies tend to highlight narratively seductive but ultimately irrelevant details, such as how their authors had 'always loved music' or 'always wanted to perform'.[51] Dolto's autobiographical texts contain numerous examples of just this kind of elision – for example recounting how, aged eight, she told her family that she wished to become a 'doctor of education' (*médecin d'éducation*), seeing this as an early prefiguration of her later vocation.[52] Playing down the contribution of external social, cultural or political factors to her eventual career, Dolto framed her youth as a case study in timeless psychological issues, inviting her readers to do the same when reflecting on their own lives. However, in other ways, Dolto is a good biographical subject. She left behind a wealth of previously unexplored primary source material, now at the Archives Nationales, including voluminous correspondence, clinical case files and various other documents concerning her public work – as well as the thousands of letters sent in by listeners to her radio programmes, examined in Chapter 6. In addition, her life and work were bound up with major events and developments in twentieth-century French history. Her archives, as will be seen, can shed new light on such diverse subjects as the interwar Parisian bourgeoisie, the exodus from Paris of June 1940, women's magazines in the Occupation and Liberation periods and the scandal around autism treatment that emerged in the early twenty-first century. In this sense, this book, to borrow the subtitle of David Looseley's study of Édith Piaf, is intended more as a 'cultural history' of Dolto than as a traditional biography.[53]

That is not to deny the personal fascination of Dolto as a character and cultural phenomenon. At times intellectually open, generous, insightful and empathetic, at others blinkered, vituperative and capable of causing significant suffering, Dolto led a varied career encompassing a number of absorbing episodes, as I hope to show in the chapters that follow. Often maternally reassuring and unifying, on other occasions bitterly polarising, Dolto was an undeniably consequential, if sometimes unsympathetic or even monstrous, figure. Her attempts to guide French people through family life, among the social upheavals of the second half of the twentieth century, have had lasting ramifications.

Chapter structure

The first half of the book examines the origins of Dolto's ideas and her early articulations of them. Chapter 1 explores the history of psychoanalysis in France before 1939, situating it with respect to the politics of science and medicine in the later Third Republic, and the politics of the family in relation to interwar natalism. It shows that while the early French psychoanalytic movement was politically diverse, those who mentored Dolto, notably Édouard Pichon and René Laforgue, were very much from its Catholic, French-nationalist wing. It further explores the 'family neurosis' concept and other ideas that Dolto took from these thinkers. Chapter 2 examines Dolto's family and social environment during her youth, looking especially at her family's cultural and political values and conception of women's roles. It shows how, like her contemporaries Simone de Beauvoir and Élisabeth Lacoin (the 'Zaza' of Beauvoir's memoirs), Dolto struggled to escape the cultural expectations placed on young women from bourgeois families and assert her right to an independent, intellectual vocation. Dolto's eventual hard-won break with her family's right-wing ideological background was less than complete, and less comprehensive than Dolto later suggested. Chapter 3 explores Dolto's early career, which began in the context of war, occupation and liberation. Believing in the potential of holistic medicine and humanist Catholicism to help bring about a French national recovery, Dolto perceived revitalising possibilities in Pétainism, but subsequently found that her holistic-psychoanalytic orientation also sat easily in the political context of the Liberation period. The chapter further examines Dolto's Christianity, especially regarding her approach to the themes of sexuality and guilt in the context of broader developments in French Catholicism and psychoanalysis after 1945. The 1953 split in French psychoanalysis is shown to have had religious and racial undertones, with Catholic analysts more likely than Jewish ones to break away from the original society and support 'lay' (i.e. non-medical) variants of psychoanalysis that drew on other healing traditions.

The second half of the book focuses on Dolto as a public figure. Chapter 4 examines her interactions with the French public via the media and in institutional settings between 1945 and 1968. It centres on the issues of liberal parenting and patriarchal family structures, demonstrating how Dolto advocated the former without calling the latter into question. It places her ideas in these decades in the context of contemporary social change, especially the battle for increased reproductive and civil rights for women, which Dolto opposed. Chapter 5 looks at Dolto's ideas in relation to autism, and the scandal around the relatively poor outcomes for French autistic children that emerged after 2000 – a key negative aspect of Dolto's legacy. The chapter shows that Dolto played a significant and hitherto under-appreciated role in promoting psychoanalytic understandings and treatments of autism in France, specifically the idea of autism as resulting from defective or toxic mothering, as highlighted in her popular book-length case study, *Le Cas Dominique* (1971). It places this aspect of her career in the context of the radical psychiatry movement of the 1960s and 1970s, showing how Dolto's association with radical and progressive currents could coexist with her advocacy of ideas that now appear troubling. The final main chapter looks at Dolto as a national broadcaster and popular child-rearing expert. Drawing notably on archive material from her radio shows *S.O.S. Psychanalyste!* (1968–69) and *Lorsque l'enfant paraît* ('When the Baby Comes' or 'When the Child Appears', 1976–78), it assesses her radio career, while also examining Dolto's interventions regarding education and homosexuality in the context of contemporary political debates. The last section analyses the Maison Verte children's centres – whose creation and ethos were inspired by Dolto – arguing that they constitute one of the most successful penetrations of psychoanalytic thinking into everyday life and institutions in France of all time, and indeed, arguably anywhere in the world.

The concluding Afterword returns to the question of Dolto's twenty-first-century reputation and of what France is to do with her legacy. Can the ongoing desire to celebrate the positive aspects of her interventions withstand an increased awareness – indeed, mockery – of the problematic and outdated aspects of her ideas? This book is written in the hope that the kind of historical contextualisation offered in the pages that follow will, if nothing else, lead to better-informed answers.

Notes

1 Archives Françoise Dolto, Paris (hereafter AFD), LLP Divers, unclassified letter, May 1982. Since I undertook this research, Dolto's archives have been transferred to the Archives Nationales, which has overlaid its own classification system on top of that used by the AFD archivists. In this book I use the AFD referencing system. The *Lorsque l'enfant paraît* archives are held under the Archives Nationales classifications 752AP/150–65.

2 Listener letter dated June 1978. AFD, LLP 14, 39/24. Under French law, the letter writers must remain anonymous to protect their privacy.

3 The number of institutions named for Dolto, according to the AFD's records, reached 230 by 1999. More recent examples include a new secondary school in 2013 and a care unit at Gentilly hospital in 2014.

4 *Entre les murs* (*The Class*), dir. Laurent Cantet, 2008. François Bégaudeau, *Entre les murs* (Paris: Éditions Verticales, 2006).

5 France Culture ran an episode of *Les Nuits de France Culture* focused on Dolto on 12 June 2020, and an episode of *Les Chemins de la philosophie* on her on 23 September 2019. Tessa Ivascu, 'Françoise Dolto, la fervente militante de la cause des enfants', *Psychologies*, 26 December 2019.

6 Didier Pleux, *Génération Dolto* (Paris: Odile Jacob, 2008).

7 *Paris Match*, 2050, September 1988. Politicians' messages: AFD, box labelled 'Obsèques', letters addressed to Catherine Dolto dated 27 August–3 September 1988.

8 'Dolto: She still speaks to our children', was a front-page headline in 1990 in the weekly news magazine *L'Express* ('Dolto parle encore à nos enfants', *L'Express*, 12 January 1990). Dolto similarly appeared on the cover of *Le Nouvel Observateur*, 1452, in September 1992, accompanied by an eleven-page feature, and again on that of *L'Express* on 8 April 1993.

9 The title was an allusion to Alain Souchon's self-pitying 1978 hit song *Allô! Maman bobo* – which roughly translates as 'mummy, it hurts'.

10 Guy Baret, *Allô maman Dolto: Halte à la doltomania!* (Paris: R. Deforges, 1992).

11 Guy Baret, *Comment rater l'éducation de votre enfant avec Françoise Dolto* (Paris: Ramsay, 2003).

12 See e.g. Edward Berenson and Eva Giloi (eds), *Constructing Charisma: Celebrity, Fame, and Power in Nineteenth Century Europe* (New York: Berghahn, 2010); Fred Inglis, *A Short History of Celebrity* (Princeton, NJ: Princeton University Press, 2010); John Potts, *A History of Charisma* (Basingstoke: Palgrave, 2009).

13 Robert Gildea, *France Since 1945* (Oxford: Oxford University Press, 2002), p. 93.
14 *Ibid.*, p. 105.
15 Robert Gildea, *Empires of the Mind: The Colonial Past and the Politics of the Present* (Cambridge: Cambridge University Press, 2019), pp. 132–4; Rod Kedward, *La Vie en bleu: France and the French Since 1900* (London: Allen Lane, 2005), Ch. 17.
16 Gildea, *France Since 1945*, p. 115.
17 Tamara Chaplin, *Turning on the Mind: French Philosophers on Television* (Chicago: University of Chicago Press, 2007), p. 129.
18 On Minitel communities see Tamara Chaplin, 'Lesbians Online: Queer Identity and Community Formation on the French Minitel', *Journal of the History of Sexuality*, 23:3 (2014), 451–72.
19 Judith Coffin, *Sex, Love, and Letters: Writing Simone de Beauvoir* (Ithaca, NY: Cornell University Press, 2020).
20 Coffin has written on Grégoire in 'From Interiority to Intimacy: Psychoanalysis and Radio in Twentieth-Century France', *Cultural Critique*, 91 (2015), 114–49. For further references on Grégoire, see Chapter 6, n. 42.
21 Gildea, *France Since 1945*, p. 190.
22 Serge Moscovici, *La Psychanalyse: son image et son public. Étude sur la représentation sociale de la psychanalyse* (Paris: Presses universitaires de France, 1961), pp. 146, 222.
23 Sherry Turkle, *Psychoanalytic Politics: Freud's French Revolution* (New York: Guilford Press, 1992 (1978)), p. 6.
24 *Ibid.*, p. 10.
25 Paul-Claude Racamier (ed.), *Le Psychanalyste sans divan: La psychanalyse et les institutions de soins psychiatriques* (Paris: Payot, 1970).
26 Élisabeth Roudinesco, *Jacques Lacan & Co.: A History of Psychoanalysis in France, 1925–1985*, trans. Jeffrey Mehlman (London: Free Association, 1990), pp. 706–7.
27 Quoted in *ibid.*, p. 362.
28 Quoted in *ibid.*, p. 424.
29 Françoise Hivernel, '"The Parental Couple": Françoise Dolto and Jacques Lacan: Contributions to the Mirror Stage', *British Journal of Psychotherapy*, 29:4 (2013), 505–18.
30 Quoted in Chaplin, *Turning on the Mind*, p. 124.
31 Claudine and Pierre Geissmann, *Histoire de la psychanalyse de l'enfant. Mouvements, idées, perspectives* (Paris: Bayard, 1992), translated by the Melanie Klein Trust as *A History of Child Psychoanalysis* (London: Routledge, 1998), see pp. 40–60 (in the English translation) on Hug-Hellmuth.

32 Karen Adler, *Jews and Gender in Liberation France* (Cambridge: Cambridge University Press, 2003); Sylvie Chaperon, *Les Années Beauvoir (1945–1970)* (Paris: Fayard, 2000); Jackie Clarke, *France in the Age of Organization: Factory, Home and Nation from the 1920s to Vichy* (New York: Berghahn, 2011); Kelly Ricciardi Colvin, *Gender and French Identity after the Second World War, 1944–1954: Engendering Frenchness* (London: Bloomsbury, 2017); Claire Duchen, *Women's Rights and Women's Lives in France, 1944–1968* (London: Routledge, 1994); Sarah Fishman, *From Vichy to the Sexual Revolution: Gender and Family Life in Postwar France* (Oxford: Oxford University Press, 2017); Sandrine Garcia, *Mères sous influence: de la cause des femmes à la cause des enfants* (Paris: La Découverte, 2011); Lisa Greenwald, *Daughters of 1968: Redefining French Feminism and the Women's Liberation Movement* (Lincoln, NE: University of Nebraska Press, 2018); Francine Muel-Dreyfus, *Vichy et l'éternel féminin. Contribution à une sociologie politique de l'ordre des corps* (Paris: Seuil, 1996); Susan Pedersen, *Family, Dependence, and the Origins of the Welfare State: Britain and France, 1914–1945* (Cambridge: Cambridge University Press, 1993); Miranda Pollard, *Reign of Virtue: Mobilizing Gender in Vichy France* (Chicago: University of Chicago Press, 1998); Rebecca Pulju, *Women and Mass Consumer Society in Postwar France* (Cambridge: Cambridge University Press, 2011); Siân Reynolds, *France between the Wars: Gender and Politics* (London: Routledge, 1996); Kristin Ross, *Fast Cars, Clean Bodies: Decolonization and the Reordering of French Culture* (Cambridge, MA: MIT Press, 1995); Joan Tumblety, *Remaking the Male Body: Masculinity and the Uses of Physical Culture in Interwar and Vichy France* (Oxford: Oxford University Press, 2012).

33 Kedward, *La Vie en bleu*, loc. 4100.

34 Françoise Dolto, *L'Image inconsciente du corps* (Paris: Seuil, 1984), p. 327.

35 See e.g. Françoise Dolto, *Tout est langage* (Paris: Carrère, 1987), pp. 23–4; *L'Image inconsciente*, pp. 238–43, 296.

36 Dolto, *Tout est langage*, pp. 21–3.

37 Sarah Fishman, *The Battle for Children: World War II, Youth Crime, and Juvenile Justice in Twentieth-Century France* (Cambridge, MA: Harvard University Press, 2002).

38 Camille Robcis, 'Frantz Fanon, Institutional Psychotherapy, and the Decolonization of Psychiatry', *Journal of the History of Ideas*, 81:2 (2020), 303–25.

39 Dagmar Herzog, *Cold War Freud: Psychoanalysis in an Age of Catastrophes* (Cambridge: Cambridge University Press, 2017), p. 9; John Forrester, 'Editorial', *Psychoanalysis and History*, 16:1 (2014), 1–2.

40 Michal Shapira, *The War Inside: Psychoanalysis, Total War, and the Making of the Democratic Self in Postwar Britain* (Cambridge: Cambridge University Press, 2013), pp. 1–2, 236–7.
41 Turkle, *Psychoanalytic Politics.*
42 Élisabeth Roudinesco, *La Bataille de cent ans: Histoire de la psychanalyse en France* (Paris: Ramsay, 1982/Paris: Seuil, 1986). The second volume appeared in English as *Jacques Lacan & Co.: A History of Psychoanalysis in France, 1925–1985*, trans. Jeffrey Mehlman (London: Free Association, 1990). Geissmann and Geissmann, *A History of Child Psychoanalysis.*
43 Annick Ohayon, *L'Impossible Rencontre: psychologie et psychanalyse en France, 1919–1969* (Paris: La Découverte, 2006 (1999)); Agnès Desmazières, *L'Inconscient au paradis: comment les catholiques ont reçu la psychanalyse, 1920–1965* (Paris: Payot, 2011).
44 Camille Robcis, *The Law of Kinship: Anthropology, Psychoanalysis, and the Family in France* (Ithaca, NY: Cornell University Press, 2013), pp. 4, 139, 104.
45 Carolyn Dean, *The Self and Its Pleasures: Bataille, Lacan, and the History of the Decentered Subject* (Ithaca, NY: Cornell University Press, 1992).
46 Guy Hall, Françoise Hivernel, and Siân Morgan (eds), *Theory and Practice in Child Psychoanalysis: An Introduction to the Work of Francoise Dolto* (London: Karnac, 2009); Fishman, *Vichy to the Sexual Revolution*, p. 45.
47 Jean-François de Sauverzac, *Françoise Dolto: Itinéraire d'une psychanalyste: essai* (Paris; Flammarion, 1995); Daniela Lumbroso, *Françoise Dolto, la vie d'une femme libre* (Paris: Plon, 2007).
48 Dominique Mehl, *La Bonne Parole: Quand les psys plaident dans les médias* (Paris: La Martinière, 2003).
49 E.g. Sophie Chérer, *Ma Dolto* (Paris: Stock, 2008); Claude Schauder (ed.), *Lire Dolto aujourd'hui* (Ramonville Saint-Agne: Érès, 2004).
50 Françoise Dolto, *Enfances* (Paris: Seuil, 1986); *Autoportrait d'une psychanalyste: 1934–1988* (Paris: Seuil, 1989).
51 Pierre Bourdieu, 'L'Illusion biographique', *Actes de la recherche en sciences sociales*, 62–3 (1986), 69–72.
52 Dolto, *Autoportrait*, pp. 52–4.
53 David Looseley, *Édith Piaf: A Cultural History* (Liverpool: Liverpool University Press, 2015).

1

Family neuroses: psychoanalysis in interwar France

Psychoanalysis in 1934 was no longer a particularly young discipline. Sigmund Freud had published *The Interpretation of Dreams*, with its new theory of the unconscious mind and an early version of the Oedipus complex, some thirty-five years earlier in 1899 (dating it 1900 to emphasise its novelty and modernity). The Vienna Psychoanalytic Society was founded in 1902, and the International Psychoanalytic Association (IPA) in 1910. By the mid-1930s, Freud was in his late seventies with most of his major publications behind him, and psychoanalysis had grown far beyond the stage at which it depended on any one individual. Younger cohorts of analysts were spreading it across Europe and the United States and disseminating psychoanalytic thinking into the wider culture. From 1934 Ernest Jones headed the IPA from London, where Melanie Klein's work on child analysis and object relations was providing theoretical impetus. Psychoanalysis was also taking off in the United States, where a number of German analysts had fled from the Nazis. On Freud's death in 1939, the Anglo-American poet W. H. Auden wrote of him having created 'a whole climate of opinion under [which] we conduct our different lives'.[1]

In France, however, the psychoanalytic movement was still in its relative infancy. In 1914, by which time psychoanalytic associations existed in Budapest, London, Berlin, Munich, Zurich and New York – but not Paris – Freud wrote that 'among European countries France has hitherto shown itself the least disposed to welcome psycho-analysis'.[2] French translations of Freud's works appeared only from the early 1920s, a decade later than equivalent English versions. The Société Psychanalytique de Paris (SPP) was eventually founded in 1926 with a dozen members, followed by a journal, the *Revue française de psychanalyse* (*RFP*), in 1927. The SPP grew slowly for most of its first decade. Only in 1934 – the year that Dolto began her personal psychoanalysis – did it begin to formalise its standing, creating a professional organisation and a training institute, whereas the London Institute of Psychoanalysis had been founded in 1919. By 1939 the SPP had grown to twenty-four titular and twenty adhering members, but was still small by international standards.

Historians have been puzzled by these slow beginnings. Sherry Turkle attributed it to the 'stability and security' of French bourgeois society around 1900, contending that unlike its American or Viennese equivalents, 'French bourgeois society was more secure than ever about its sense of itself … the Gallic version of "civilised" morality was not in crisis at the turn of the century.'[3] Yet it can more plausibly be argued that French bourgeois society at the time of the Dreyfus Affair was riven with *in*security: preoccupied by culture wars and deep anxieties regarding industrialisation, urbanisation, national and colonial rivalries, immigration, crime, degeneration and morality. Mark Micale and Élisabeth Roudinesco have accordingly proposed more or less the opposite explanation: that French society around 1900, disconcerted by the scale and pace of social change, responded by 'constitut[ing] the change itself as pathological, that is, formulat[ing] the very idea of psychological traumatics'.[4] From the 1880s, interest in psychical phenomena and depth psychology became widespread among French scientists, novelists, philosophers and popular writers, including Pierre Janet, Jean-Martin Charcot, Charles Richet, Hippolyte Bernheim, Émile Zola, Henri Bergson and Gustave Le Bon. Since such writers produced a plethora of works exploring the psyche and its unconscious workings, Freud appeared to be saying little that was new or different, other than perhaps his particular insistence on sexuality as the cause of neurological disturbances.[5] His work did not capture the intellectual imagination. Those pre-1914 French scholars who did find Freud interesting, such as Bergson, Marcel Foucault or Théodule Ribot, used his ideas to develop their own concepts, rather than becoming practitioners of or evangelisers for Freudian analysis.[6]

The late beginnings of French psychoanalysis had consequences for its eventual intellectual and social composition, and thus for its ideological orientation at the time of Dolto's arrival in the group. The Third Republic's pre-1914 intellectual culture had valorised science as a central aspect of its programme to contest German hegemony, develop imperial power and modernise economically.[7] Republican intellectuals attributed France's defeat in 1870–71 to its scientific and technological shortcomings, and considered empirical science (representing rational masculinity) as a weapon in struggles against the Republic's (implicitly feminised) Catholic and monarchical opponents.[8] Doctors were prominent in these conflicts and a vital part of the republican polity, overrepresented on municipal councils and in the National Assembly.[9] Empiricism mattered for them too, in their localised battles for influence with priests and faith healers in rural areas. Notably, much early French criticism of Freud's ideas took place on empirical grounds, questioning their anatomical and physiological basis and the level of proof provided for the efficacy of the talking cure.[10] Biologist Yves Delage equated Freud's 'half-proofs' to those of esoteric fields 'such as telepathy, action at a distance, levitation, materialisation etc.' whose woolly thinking needed to be resisted for both scientific and political reasons.[11]

This background helps to explain why the earliest members of the SPP, when it was founded in 1926, were not generally drawn from the ranks of French republican medicine or academic psychology. The prestige and confidence of these fields had in any case been shaken by World War I, during which doctors who refused to acknowledge the reality and scale of shell shock had been challenged in public and in court.[12] The death toll from the war and the 1918–20 influenza pandemic led to a surge of interest in spiritualism and other esoteric fields, as people sought to reconnect with the dead and missing. Intellectuals, artists and surrealists now argued that the positivist quest for objectivity had ignored whole areas of human behaviour and experience. Freud's ideas found new appeal in this changed context. In 1922 a play with Freudian themes, Henri-René Lenormand's *Le Mangeur de rêves*, was staged in Geneva and Paris.[13] *La Nouvelle Revue française* ran articles on Freud and reviewed the 1923 French translation of his *Three Essays on the Theory of Sexuality*.[14] The new interest was led by literary intellectuals such as Romain Rolland, André Gide and Jacques Rivière, and the surrealists Louis Aragon and André Breton; French doctors and scientists, trained in the pre-1914 context, were slower to respond.[15]

Six of the SPP's founders had not been born in France. Three – Eugénie Sokolnicka, Sophie Morgenstern and Rudolph Loewenstein – were Jews born in Poland. Raymond de Saussure and Charles Odier were Swiss. René Laforgue, from Alsace, had for much of his life been a German citizen, and during World War I had been a doctor in the Kaiser's army on the Eastern Front. There were four women in the early group: Sokolnicka, Morgenstern, Françoise Minkowska and Marie Bonaparte – the latter a writer and socialite who, despite her imperial surname and marriage to a Greek prince, was republican in her French politics. The rest of the founders were French-born male doctors, but they were not from the pre-1914 anti-clerical, republican, positivist mould. Rather, this group – Édouard Pichon, Adrien Borel, René Allendy, Georges Parcheminey, Henri Codet and Angelo Hesnard – sympathised politically with the nationalist and anti-republican Right, Pichon emphatically so as a member of the far-right monarchist group Action Française. Several of them were interested in esoteric or mystical forms of knowledge – homeopathy, theosophy, paracelsianism, even alchemy.

Along with Laforgue, these doctors set up a journal, *L'Évolution psychiatrique* (*EP*), in 1925. Aware of the scepticism towards psychoanalysis in orthodox French medical circles, the *EP* group adopted a defensive posture, admitting that doubts persisted about the empirical validity of Freud's work but hoping that submitting psychoanalysis to 'our French spirit of sincerity and moderation' would lead to its 'perfecting'.[16] They downplayed Freud's grand hopes of establishing psychoanalysis as a common foundation underpinning all of the human sciences, instead emphasising its limited applications.[17] Pichon made clear that psychoanalysis could not 'tackle [*entamer*] the moral problem, nor the religious problem, nor the aesthetic problem ... [in other words] psychoanalysis in no way claims to resolve the threefold problem of philosophy, that of the Good, the True, and the Beautiful'.[18] Psychoanalysis was merely a useful technique, 'a serious benefit to psychological medicine ... [but] destined to become dissolved into psychiatry and medicine'.[19] The group courted medical patrons, with a view to getting psychoanalytic methods accepted as legitimate within state-managed scientific and medical institutions.

The most significant patron was Georges Heuyer (1884–1977), a psychiatrist and director of the child neuropsychiatry clinic at the

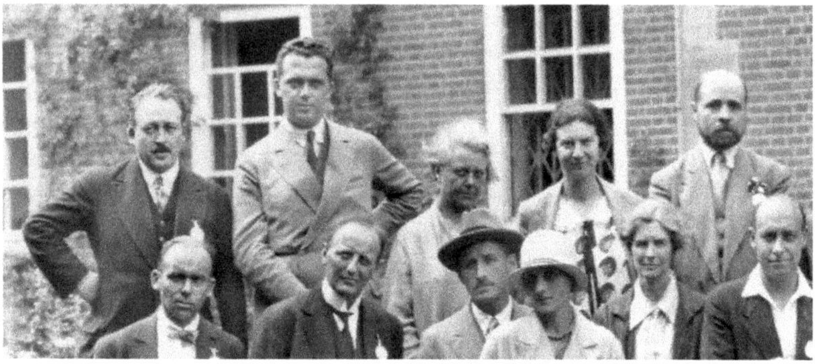

Figure 1.1 Early members of the Société Psychanalytique de Paris at the Eleventh Congress of the International Psycho-Analytical Association, Oxford, England, July 1929. Back row l–r: René Laforgue, Raymond de Saussure, Sophie Morgenstern, Yvonne Allendy, René Allendy

Salpêtrière from 1925. Child psychiatry had arisen as a medical sub-field out of the broader nineteenth-century interest in criminality and heredity, linked to fears about a degenerating population in the face of such scourges as alcoholism, tuberculosis and venereal disease.[20] It largely focused on children labelled abnormal, deviant, delinquent or backward. Alfred Binet had driven the development of psychometric intelligence testing as a way to identify so-called abnormal children, defined as those likely to encounter severe difficulties at school.[21] Heuyer, who like many contemporary French scientists believed in the Lamarckian inheritance of acquired characteristics, defined abnormal children as those who, 'under the influence of morbid defects, most often hereditary, present with constitutional deficiencies of an intellectual or moral nature which prevent them from spontaneously adapting to their familial or social environment'.[22] Heuyer wrote or oversaw numerous studies which claimed to demonstrate that such children were disproportionately responsible for crime and delinquency, concluding that all children should undergo psychiatric screening to identify potential future delinquents.[23] This approach was not uncontested within psychology: Swiss psychologist Jean Piaget proposed a psychological development model built around 'the study of normality' rather than its opposite, while the left-wing French psychologist Henri Wallon argued that the causes of children's mental 'turbulence' lay in the material, family and social environment rather than the 'constitutional' factors Heuyer emphasised.[24] Nonetheless, Heuyer, especially after his 1925 appointment at the Salpêtrière, exerted significant influence over the field.[25]

Early psychoanalysts were able to use Heuyer's patronage to gain valuable entry points into French academic medicine.[26] The first psychoanalyst to practise in France, having been trained by Sigmund Freud personally, was Eugénie Sokolnicka, a Polish-born Jewish woman with a science degree from the Sorbonne. Heuyer brought Sokolnicka into his clinic at Hôpital Sainte-Anne in 1922–23. He subsequently awarded posts to other psychoanalysts including Pierre Mâle, Jean Dublineau and Jenny Aubry.[27] At the Salpêtrière from 1925, he engaged as his (seemingly unpaid) assistant Sophie Morgenstern, also of Polish-Jewish origin, who co-wrote several publications with Heuyer and became France's first dedicated child psychoanalyst.[28] Morgenstern developed analytic techniques based on the analysis of children's drawings – which she encouraged them to produce during their consultations with her – as a way to analyse their unconscious thoughts. Morgenstern detailed her methods in a 1937 book supervised by Heuyer, *La Psychanalyse infantile*.[29]

Much of this background would have a direct effect on Dolto, who commenced her own analysis in 1934 and began seriously considering training as an analyst herself in around 1936. Morgenstern's technique, to which Dolto added modelling clay as well as drawing materials, became a cornerstone of Dolto's clinical methodology. When she undertook a period of training in child psychiatry in 1938, Dolto's first patients were at a clinic for 'abnormal and backward children' at the Hôpital Bretonneau near Montmartre.[30] By that time, she had already completed a medical externship at Heuyer's child psychiatry clinic at the Vaugirard hospital in 1936–37, as part of her training in paediatrics.[31] She was not impressed, later speaking of her 'horrified' disapproval of Heuyer's methods:

> For me, paediatricians owed it to themselves to have empathy with the child they were treating – instead of saying [as Heuyer did]: 'You ran away from home and you're not even sorry! You can see it almost drove your mother mad and you don't care!' And, since this approach made the young adolescent angry, Heuyer added: 'Unfrightenable!' [*inintimidable*] Then he wrote in the file: "Child unfrightenable. Mother: massive idiot [*grosse débile*]. Correction facility." I thought it horrendous.[32]

A similar portrait was given by another of Heuyer's future-psychoanalyst pupils, Serge Leclaire, who described Heuyer's consultations as peremptory to the point of caricature.[33] Heuyer's position in relation to psychoanalysis seems curious: he clearly considered it valuable enough to hire and encourage people who practised it, yet he did not allow the humanistic aspects of psychoanalytic theory to influence his own methods, hereditist outlook or tendency to regard children primarily as specimens. To him, it would appear, 'Freud' meant a limited set of discrete techniques, not a broader ethos. Though Dolto was appalled at Heuyer's disposition towards children, some elements of her later thinking about the psyche nonetheless retained Heuyerian echoes. Heuyer, with his Lamarckian belief in the inheritance of acquired characteristics, believed that, since people's life experiences and behaviours shaped their biological legacy, it made most sense to use psychoanalytic techniques with people of or below child-bearing age (especially children) in the hope of shaping their future behaviour and therefore their genetic material. Without subscribing to Heuyer's physical Lamarckianism, Dolto believed in another form of heredity, that of psychic inheritances transmitted via the unconscious. She wrote in the 1980s of her belief in a 'genetic solidarity' and a 'transgenerational unconscious', arguing that 'the events which occur in a human being's family before they're born, while they are a foetus ... are capable of inducing a psychosis in that gestating being'.[34] Rather than an outright rejection of Heuyer's constitutionalist orientation, this reads like an adaptation of it to the metaphysical level of the unconscious.

A second prominent patron of psychoanalysis within French medicine was the psychiatrist Henri Claude, who ran the mental illness clinic (*Clinique des maladies mentales*) at Hôpital Sainte-Anne from 1922. Like Heuyer, Claude was open to employing psychoanalysts in his clinic and adopting some of their techniques, without himself becoming an analyst or adopting Freudian theory wholesale. Claude was adamant that psychoanalysis could only be practised by qualified doctors, preferably neuropsychiatrists.[35] He offered internships to budding psychoanalysts, including Jacques Lacan and Daniel Lagache. Under his auspices, a special issue of the *Journal médical français* was devoted to psychoanalysis in 1933, with several articles written by *L'Évolution psychiatrique* members, allowing them to reach a much larger medical audience than they could through their own journal, as well as to benefit from the prestige of featuring in the better-known publication.

Though the advantages of patronage from figures like Claude were clear, *EP*'s stress on the limitations of psychoanalysis and its ultimate subservience to medicine created a long-lasting faultline within the SPP over the validity of lay (i.e. non-medical) analysis, and the applicability of psychoanalytic concepts in domains beyond medicine. Marie Bonaparte, who was not a doctor, led the arguments in favour of lay analysis and of applying Freud's thought to such fields as criminology, literature and anthropology. When in 1927 the SPP created the *RFP*, with the aim of targeting a broader audience than *EP*, several *EP* members objected to Bonaparte's proposal to feature Freud's name on its cover.[36] Bonaparte, who was part-funding the venture, won out, but conceded a division of the *RFP* into 'medical' and 'non-medical' sections. The *EP* members Angelo Hesnard and Édouard Pichon publicly criticised the *RFP* in 1930 for acting 'as a magnifying lens for the defects of the Freudian theories', and attacked Bonaparte for 'finding excuses to quote Freudian texts' rather than carrying out 'research of a positive nature'.[37] Some *EP* members cited Pierre Janet at least as frequently and positively as they cited Freud – especially Pichon, who had married Janet's daughter in 1927.[38]

Despite these tensions, the two tendencies coexisted successfully as the SPP expanded from its original twelve members in 1926 to forty-four in 1939. They organised conferences together and collaborated on translations of psychoanalytic texts. Their efforts could be complementary: while the *EP* group focused on winning over medical leaders, Bonaparte concentrated on developing French psychoanalysis as an independent lay discipline. In 1934, at Pichon's suggestion, the SPP set up the Association Professionnelle des Psychanalystes, an organisation intended to provide support and professional accreditation for non-medical analysts.[39] The same year, thanks largely to the efforts and financial resources of Bonaparte, the society also created a training institute for new analysts, which offered 'psychoanalytic scholarships' to selected candidates.[40] When Dolto entered analysis with Laforgue in 1934, therefore, she was coming into the orbit of a psychoanalytic society that, while still small by international standards and containing internal tensions, was in a phase of growth and optimism. It was also sufficiently well-resourced to be able to provide financial support to promising trainees – as Dolto would soon prove herself to be.

The gender politics of family neuroses

Its relatively late beginnings meant that this early expansion phase for French psychoanalysis took place in the distinct political atmosphere of the 1930s. By that time, the medical profession was no longer the bastion of republican political and intellectual values that it had been in the 1880s. As state intervention in healthcare increased, doctors became more protective of their profession's autonomy, privileges and social composition. Medical unions sought to restrict the numbers of medical students by raising the educational requirements. In the 1930s, measures were taken to exclude recent immigrants from practising law and medicine until they had held citizenship for ten years. As Julie Fette has written, foreigners (especially Jewish ones) and women 'were especially singled out as scapegoats whose legitimate presence in French medicine could be challenged when professional survival seemed to be at stake'.[41] Concern about the consequences of 'democratising' medicine contributed to a substantial rightward shift in the profession's political composition: 45 per cent of doctors elected to the National Assembly in 1936 sat on the extreme Right.[42]

Discussion about women, gender and the family that took place within the SPP after 1926 were influenced by this context, but also by the larger debates over these questions taking place within French society and, separately, in the international psychoanalytic movement. The perceived imperative to increase the birth rate had been a commonplace of French political culture since the mid-nineteenth century, with renewed impetus provided in the 1920s by France's World War I losses. (When Dolto's brother Jacques was born in 1922, her mother, who had hoped for a girl, commented that a boy was at least 'very useful for the country'.[43]) The social dislocations provoked by the war, including the increased employment of women, fuelled debates about the future of families. Some Frenchmen conflated changes in women's social position with a generalised sense of cultural malaise.[44] So-called female deviance, as manifested through the 1920s figures of the New Woman and the cross-dressing *garçonne*, was frequently equated with a loss of national power and virility that could only be restored if women reassumed the roles of wife and mother. Belief in the need to increase the birth rate was shared across the political spectrum, but Right and Left approached it in different ways. The right-wing Bloc National administrations (1919–23) took symbolic steps to promote procreation, including instituting Mothers' Day, awarding medals to mothers of five or more children and imposing punitive restrictions on contraception and abortion. Conservative Catholic familialists like Fernand Boverat, leader of the Alliance Nationale Contre la Dépopulation (National Alliance Against Depopulation), argued for wealth redistribution from childless citizens to large families, and for married women to be given a state allowance so that they need not work for money.[45] Radicals and socialists preferred measures to promote children's welfare, support working mothers and reduce infant mortality. Their vision resulted in the introduction of maternity pay in 1930, family allowances in 1932 and some workplace crèches. These policies to some extent undermined the familialist position, by facilitating women's paid employment and reducing their dependence on the male breadwinner wage, but could also discursively reinforce it.[46] For example, new attention was focused on the health and education of young children by Adolphe Pinard, an obstetrician, eugenicist and Radical Party politician, who successfully promoted the concept of *puériculture*, the science of child-rearing.[47] From 1923, fortnightly lessons for schoolgirls in feeding, bathing and changing infants became a mandatory part of the school curriculum. Presented as a scientific attempt to improve the health, hygiene and quality of the population, *puériculture* stimulated governmental focus on resources for mothers and children – and was accordingly welcomed by some feminists – but ultimately emphasised that girls should first and foremost be prepared for futures revolving around motherhood.

In the 1930s, especially following the Nazi rise to power which rekindled fears of France being demographically and militarily outcompeted by an aggressive Germany, nationalist politicians renewed the pressure on working women to give up their jobs. In 1935, married women were excluded from certain civil service positions, while the 1939 Code de la Famille (Family Code) replaced child benefits with the *allocation de mère au foyer*, an allowance provided to mothers who were not in paid employment. Couples were offered rewards for having children within two years of marriage; punishments for promoting contraception and abortion were further reinforced.[48] However, these measures proved ineffective in raising the birth rate. One-child families remained common among the working and lower-middle classes, especially in cities where the prevalence of small, poor-quality housing made large families impractical.[49] Parents found that concentrating financial and educational resources on a single child maximised the potential for social mobility, while many women refused to settle for a housewife's estate and continued to seek entry into public life. Though the vote remained denied to them, feminists obtained some significant victories, including the granting of full civil capacity for married women in the 1938 Civil Code.

Meanwhile, the way that psychoanalysis as an international movement thought about the family and women's roles had evolved considerably by the 1930s. Marxist historian Eli Zaretsky has posited that the 'original historical telos [of psychoanalysis] was *defamilialisation*, the freeing of individuals from unconscious images of authority originally rooted in the family'.[50] Much of Freud's pre-1914 thinking on these subjects certainly seemed to emphasise individual freedom from the constraints of family duty and social morality: Freud argued that sexual satisfaction was an important element of the mental health of both sexes, and that nervous illness was often traceable to the restrictions of Victorian-era 'civilised sexual morality'.[51] Against the grain of much contemporary medical opinion, he also contended that if women undertook fulfilling intellectual work then this would help prevent, rather than provoke, nervous illnesses.[52] Mari Jo Buhle has shown that, for these reasons, at least some pre-World War I feminists considered psychoanalysis to be a potential 'handmaiden to women's sexual emancipation'.[53]

However, in the prevailing anti-feminist atmosphere after 1918, the connection between psychoanalysis and women's liberation became strained. Freud now made the concept of penis envy central to his understanding of women's sexuality, while other analysts posited a link between feminism and aberrant psychosexual development. Karl Abraham, in 'Manifestations of the Female Castration Complex', a text written in the early 1920s and praised by Freud, argued that the resentment towards men allegedly exhibited by feminists (or other women who did not restrict themselves to domestic roles) resulted from unresolved jealousy about their anatomical 'inferiority' to men.[54] From such assumptions, it followed that women and men required different approaches when in psychotherapy: men should be encouraged to develop their sexual and professional capacities, women to resign themselves to their natural inferiority. This position was inevitably challenged, notably by Karen Horney, giving rise to what Buhle calls 'the great debate' over female sexuality within psychoanalysis.[55] As with the interwar discussion of childhood abnormality and delinquency, this was in large part a nature/nurture debate with political ramifications. Either women's inferiority was innate – a conclusion that buttressed the views of conservative familialists – or, as Horney suggested, it was culturally produced, and thus remediable through a combination of individual psychotherapy and collective political action.[56] The debate went to the heart of the bigger and longer-term question of what psychoanalysis existed to achieve – should it seek to reconcile individuals to social structures, or to transform those structures in pursuit of a psychologically healthier society?

This was the intellectual context in which the SPP was formed, and this background helps to make sense of early French analysts' theorising around the family and women's sexuality. Of particular importance for Dolto's story is René Laforgue's concept of the *névrose familiale* (family neurosis): the idea that neuroses could be passed around a family almost like viruses, and specifically the belief that children's neuroses often resembled or derived from the neuroses of other family members. Abraham's 1920 paper on the 'female castration complex' had ended by warning of the complex's potential to damage the next generation: 'Women whose ideas and feelings are influenced and governed by the castration complex to an important degree … transplant [the effects] of this complex onto their children.'[57] Since mothers had more influence on children's early development than fathers, their castration complex could be 'a dangerous enemy' of their children's development. Therefore, 'if we succeed in freeing [a mother] from … the burdens of her castration complex, then we obviate the neuroses of children, to a great extent'.[58] With the notion of the *névrose familiale*, Laforgue broadened out this idea, writing in the first edition of the *RFP* that 'a neurosis can be passed on by family tradition, in exactly the same manner as civilisation'.[59]

Returning to the subject in a longer article in 1936, Laforgue stated that children's neuroses could sometimes be solved by treating the psychological problems of one or both parents, without it being necessary to work with the child at all.[60] In general, though, the responsibility for a 'family complex' lay with (or could be traced back to) the 'influence that an unbalanced mother has on her child'.[61] The definition of 'unbalanced' women, for Laforgue as for Abraham, included feminists, and any women who were not comfortable with the role of wife and mother. In 1935, Laforgue argued that 'the origin of many familial neurotic symptoms must be looked for in frigidity'.[62] In his conception, frigidity, defined as the lack of appropriate release of women's sexual energies, could lead to those energies being expressed either in 'a certain virility' – seeking to compete with men in a professional or intellectual setting, for example – or in an overly strong attachment to a child.[63] Alternatively, such women might unconsciously seek out and marry effeminate-intellectual or repressed-homosexual men, risking confusion in their children as to what constituted gender-appropriate behaviour.[64] For an analyst faced with frigid women, Laforgue argued, 'the only way to act is to cure [them] of the need to flee from normal sexuality: you will then see, in certain favourable cases, all the complications disappear as if by magic'.[65] 'Normal' sexuality had miraculous powers to make all kinds of symptoms disappear.

Édouard Pichon, Laforgue's *EP* colleague, was likewise drawn to psychoanalysis partly because of its supposed ability to cure deviant sexuality. Pichon argued in 1934 that an attraction of psychoanalysis was its ability to facilitate treatment of certain conditions that had previously appeared intractable – for example, homosexuality.[66] Drawing on his other career as a grammarian, Pichon claimed that the existence of linguistic genders constituted evidence that polarisation into binary sexual roles was a fundamental aspect of human society.[67] Unlike Abraham, Pichon did not ascribe gender inequalities to anatomy, but rather saw them as deeply rooted in ancient civilisational patterns.[68] Nonetheless, the conclusion was the same. Those who were 'in revolt' against such structures – feminists, *garçonnes*, homosexuals – 'are in reality uncomfortable in themselves; they are neurotic. In returning them to the [normal] conceptions [of love], *we heal them*.'[69] Pichon's ideas were linked to his Catholic-nationalist politics. He once described himself, in a letter to the Action Française leader Charles Maurras, as 'entirely Catholic, insofar as Catholicism, as a bastion of the social, familial, and national order, stands opposed to the Jewish or Protestant spirit'.[70] He founded an association, Les Michelots, whose aims included the Francisation of Jewish names – Pichon insisted on referring to Sigmund Freud, for example, as 'Sigismond'.[71] Rudolph Loewenstein had Pichon in mind when, describing the welcome he received in Paris as a Polish Jew in 1925, he encountered 'xenophobia, antisemitism and jingoism, pronounced among certain people'.[72]

The stridency of Pichon's politics was attenuated by his personal charm – and on other subjects, such as educational theory, Pichon could sound innovative and progressive.[73] His bestselling 1936 child-rearing manual *Le Développement psychique de l'enfant et de l'adolescent*, which remained popular well into the 1950s (a third edition was published in 1953), was an eclectic mix.[74] It combined ideas from a number of fields and thinkers, including Sigmund and Anna Freud, psychologists including Binet, Janet, Wallon and Piaget, and the educational philosophies of Maria Montessori, John Dewey and Jean-Jacques Rousseau. Filtering this mixture through the prism of his own linguistic expertise and religious and political principles, Pichon produced a series of practical recommendations concerning individual parenting and societal approaches to children and education. Drawing on Dewey, Pichon proposed treating children as fully human from the youngest age: 'the child is, in himself and for himself, a complete being ... a being absolutely vibrating with life and experiencing joys and sorrows'.[75] He advocated tenderness in child-rearing and condemned 'systematically rigorous paternal authoritarianism, slaps and smacks, education without tenderness, unnecessary exiles to boarding schools'.[76] Parents should be taught to value their children and see child-rearing as a serious subject that required study and training along the lines of Pinard's *puériculture*. He stressed the importance of linguistic communication between parents and young children: 'It is extremely dangerous to treat babies like little unconscious things ... Young children must be *talked to a lot*, to make them understand the nature of language.'[77] He cited Sophie Morgenstern as a pioneer in using children's drawings and play in psychotherapy as ways to access their non-verbal language.

Pichon's tone hardened, however, when he broached the topics of gender relations and family structure. He appealed to the public authorities 'to renounce their systematic undermining of the dignity, strength and practical value of marriage, as they have been doing in France since the start of the Third Republic'.[78] He asserted that parental separation, widowhood, divorce, remarriage and illegitimacy were all dangerous for the psychic equilibrium and happiness of the children involved:

> A child's psychical development can only proceed perfectly within a legitimate household united by a solid love, forming an indivisible unit in relation to its offspring, and whose two foundational elements have the good fortune to live until the child can be considered to have become an adult. In addition, it is desirable for it not to be an only child.[79]

Pichon condemned the idea of married women working outside of the home, praised the scouting movement and advised parents to shave the heads of young boys to ensure they did not look feminine. A clear separation between genders and gender roles was psychologically healthy for individuals and for the nation as a whole. Fathers should not intervene too much in day-to-day child rearing, lest they 'thereby usurp … a maternal role … such an error could disturb the development of the Oedipus complex in their children'.[80]

Many of these ideas of Pichon's became cornerstones of Dolto's later thinking. Indeed, the resemblances between Pichon's 1936 statements and those for which Dolto was hailed as radical and innovative in the 1960s and 1970s are striking. Though Laforgue was her analyst and provided Dolto with an important new social circle (see Chapter 2), Pichon was probably her foremost intellectual influence. The distinct combination of a liberal approach to education and an insistence on the essential psychological importance of a strict separation of gender roles – rooted in Catholic, right-wing, racist politics – was more pronounced in Dolto and Pichon than in any of their colleagues. By 1938, following the end of her analysis with Laforgue, Dolto had become something of a Pichon protégé. She worked under him at the Bretonneau hospital while writing her thesis, *Psychanalyse et pédiatrie*, which he supervised. Most of the children whose cases Dolto discussed in that work had been referred to her by Pichon, who also wrote a preface for the published version.[81] Pichon's death in January 1940 meant that his relationship with Dolto did not last beyond this formative stage of her life, but Dolto occasionally referred in correspondence to Pichon as her '*maître*' ('master'), implying that she saw herself as his intellectual disciple.[82] However, perhaps mindful of his far-right associations, she rarely talked publicly about the extent to which his ideas had shaped hers. Her 1980s autobiographies did not mention Pichon at all, and discussed Laforgue only in the context of her personal analysis with him, rather than in terms of the theoretical orientation that she learned from him.

Dolto would likely have been aware, however, that Laforgue and Pichon's theories represented the extreme anti-feminist end of the psychoanalytic spectrum in the 1930s. Looking at the broader picture, it is clear that there were elements of ambivalence and paradox to the relationship between feminism and psychoanalysis in the interwar period. Psychoanalysis continued to provide individual women with tools to contest and free themselves from a family environment that they found oppressive or constraining, and offered them a slowly increasing number of professional opportunities. By one count, the global number of practising psychoanalysts went from 221 men and thirty-nine women in 1919, to 219 men and ninety-two women in 1929 – women thus accounting for all of the growth. Psychoanalysis was far more open to women than other professions: 40 per cent of psychoanalysts in Germany were women in 1933, compared to 1.3 per cent of lawyers, for example.[83] In France, many of the leading male psychoanalysts had been analysed by women, including Laforgue and Pichon, who were both analysands of Eugénie Sokolnicka. Women such as Marie Bonaparte, Melanie Klein, Sabina Spielrein, Karen Horney and Helene Deutsch were able to wield considerable influence within the international movement. They pushed Freud to explain female sexuality further, but finding his efforts lacking in explanatory power, led psychoanalysis as a whole into exploring pre-Oedipal child-mother relations, edging fathers out of the picture. The anti-feminist thrust of psychoanalytic theory in the 1920s and 1930s, with its insistence on women's anatomical inferiority and pathologisation of their desire for a professional career, was thus not overtly reflected in the movement itself. The paradox of Laforgue, Pichon and their colleagues was that they sought to diagnose feminism or simple deviance from patriarchal norms as a medical condition, at the same time as they contributed to providing individual women with professional opportunities.

It might be argued that psychoanalysis in this sense acted as a microcosm of broader French society, where in the interwar period the predominant discursive emphasis on domesticity and the birth rate was in practice accompanied by an overall expansion of educational and professional opportunities for women. Nonetheless, those opportunities, in this transitional period, remained relatively rare and constrained. Women accounted for only around 600 out of a total of 25,000 French doctors in 1934, under 3 per cent (though by 1939, 10 per cent of interns and 25 per cent of externs in the Paris hospital system were women).[84] Those who qualified were more likely to go on to positions in paediatrics – since the care of children was coded as feminine – or gynaecology and obstetrics, rather than other specialisms. Within psychoanalysis, similarly, women had a disproportionate tendency to specialise in child analysis or 'applied analysis' (i.e. education or social work), again because these fitted better with stereotypes of roles that were more appropriate for women.[85] This was also the direction in which Dolto, as the protégée of anti-feminist doctor-psychoanalysts, took her career. It was as if her response to working with such figures was to embrace everything that was on offer – the professional opportunities that they provided and the anti-feminist theories that went with them. She did this despite the fact that the circumstances of her upbringing, as the next chapter describes, gave her more reason than most to question theories which advocated women's confinement to the domestic sphere.

Notes

1 W. H. Auden, 'In Memory of Sigmund Freud', first published in *Another Time* (London: Random House, 1940).

2 Sigmund Freud, 'On the History of the Psycho-Analytic Movement' (1914), in James Strachey (ed.), *The Standard Edition of the Complete Psychological Works of Sigmund Freud Vol. 14 (1914–1916): On the History of the Psycho-Analytic Movement, Papers on Meta-Psychology and Other Works* (London: Hogarth, 1957), pp. 7–66, 31.

3 Turkle, *Psychoanalytic Politics*, pp. 31–4.
4 Mark S. Micale, 'Jean-Martin Charcot and Les Névroses Traumatiques: From Medicine to Culture in French Trauma Theory of the Late Nineteenth Century', in Mark S. Micale and Paul Frederick Lerner (eds), *Traumatic Pasts: History, Psychiatry, and Trauma in the Modern Age, 1870–1930* (Cambridge: Cambridge University Press, 2001), pp. 115–39.
5 Roudinesco, *Bataille*, 1, pp. 213–21. Two early French reviews of Freud in this vein are A. Cullère, 'De l'excitation sexuelle dans les psychopathies anxieuses', *Archives de neurologie*, 19 (1905) 81–99; Évariste Marandon de Montyel, 'Obsessions et vie sexuelle', *Archives de neurologie*, 18 (1904), 289–304.
6 See Jacqueline Carroy, Annick Ohayon and Régine Plas, *Histoire de la psychologie en France XIXe–XXe siècles* (Paris: La Découverte, 2006), pp. 110–11.
7 Robert Fox, *The Savant and the State: Science and Cultural Politics in Nineteenth-Century France* (Baltimore: Johns Hopkins University Press, 2012).
8 M. Brady Brower, 'Science, Seduction, and the Lure of Reality in Third Republic France', *History of the Present*, 1 (2011), 170–93; Philip G. Nord, *The Republican Moment: Struggles for Democracy in Nineteenth-Century France* (Cambridge, MA: Harvard University Press, 1995); Judith Surkis, *Sexing the Citizen: Morality and Masculinity in France, 1870–1920* (Ithaca, NY: Cornell University Press, 2006).
9 Jack D. Ellis, *The Physician-Legislators of France: Medicine and Politics in the Early Third Republic, 1870–1914* (Cambridge: Cambridge University Press, 1990).
10 See Ohayon, *L'Impossible Rencontre*, p. 18.
11 Yves Delage, 'La Psychanalyse: le système de Freud et de son école,' *L'Année biologique*, 19 (1914), xxxi.
12 Marc Roudebush, 'A Patient Fights Back: Neurology in the Court of Public Opinion in France during the First World War', *Journal of Contemporary History*, 35 (2000), 29–38; Mark S. Micale, 'On the "Disappearance" of Hysteria: A Study in the Clinical Deconstruction of a Diagnosis', *Isis*, 84 (1993), 496–526, 517.
13 A playbill can be viewed at www.tce-archives.fr/document/73-le-mangeur-de-reves, accessed 29 January 2021.
14 Ramon Fernandez, 'Trois essais sur la théorie de la sexualité, par Sigmund Freud', *La Nouvelle Revue française*, 120 (1923), 91–5.
15 David Steel, 'Les débuts de la psychanalyse dans les lettres françaises: 1914–1922. Apollinaire, Cendrars, "Le Mercure de France", "La Revue de l'époque", Morand, Bourget, Lenormand', *Revue d'histoire littéraire de la France*, 79:1 (1979), 62–89.

16 'Avant propos', *L'Évolution psychiatrique*, 1 (1925), 7–9 – unsigned editorial, probably written by Laforgue and Hesnard.
17 On Freud's ambition in this area see Sarah Winter, *Freud and the Institution of Psychoanalytic Knowledge* (Stanford, CA: Stanford University Press, 1999).
18 Édouard Pichon, 'Extension du domaine de la psychanalyse', *L'Évolution psychiatrique*, 2 (1927), 217–28.
19 Édouard Pichon, 'La Psychanalyse dans l'art médical', *L'Évolution psychiatrique*, 3 (1932), 77–103, 103.
20 William H. Schneider, *Quality and Quantity: The Quest for Biological Regeneration in Twentieth-Century France* (Cambridge: Cambridge University Press, 1990), pp. 3–11.
21 Alfred Binet and Théodore Simon, *Les Enfants anormaux: guide pour l'admission des enfants anormaux dans les classes de perfectionnement* (Paris: Colin, 1907).
22 Georges Heuyer, *Enfants anormaux et délinquants juvéniles. Nécessité de l'examen psychiatrique des écoliers* (Paris: G. Steinheil, 1914). See Ohayon, *L'Impossible Rencontre*, p. 178, also Fishman, *Battle for Children*, p. 136.
23 E.g. Guy Néron, *L'Enfant vagabond* (1928 thesis supervised by Heuyer); Georges Heuyer and Paul Vervaeck, *Délinquance et criminalité de l'enfance* (Paris: Masson, 1935). See Fishman, *Battle for Children*, on the sampling biases and inference errors affecting these studies.
24 Richard I. Evans, *Jean Piaget: The Man and his Ideas*, trans. Eleanor Duckworth (New York: E. P. Dutton, 1973), p. 106; Henri Wallon, *L'Enfant turbulent. Étude sur les retards et les anomalies du développement moteur et mental* (Paris: Alcan, 1925).
25 On Heuyer's influence, see Didier-Jacques Duché, *Histoire de la psychiatrie de l'enfant* (Paris: Presses universitaires de France, 1990), pp. 339–42.
26 A 1927 editorial in *EP* went out of its way to praise the help already provided by Heuyer: 'À propos de l'historique du mouvement psychanalytique en France', *L'Évolution psychiatrique*, 2 (1927), 245–6.
27 Ohayon, *L'Impossible Rencontre*, p. 174.
28 Geissmann and Geissmann, *A History of Child Psychoanalysis*, p. 150.
29 Sophie Morgenstern, *La Psychanalyse infantile: symbolisme et valeur clinique des créations imaginatives chez l'enfant* (Paris: Denoël, 1937).
30 Geissmann and Geissmann, *A History of Child Psychoanalysis*, p. 292.
31 As Siân Reynolds noted, externships were easier to find than internships, which 'were long jealously guarded by closing them to women. A disproportionate number of women doctors were obliged to seek posts in the expanding public health sector between the wars: in local

clinics, or working for the Assistance Publique. They needed strength of purpose to persevere in the profession, whereas male medical students, following a family tradition, might be no more vocation-driven than Charles Bovary.' *France between the Wars*, p. 96.

32 Dolto, *Autoportrait*, p. 142.

33 Ohayon, *L'Impossible Rencontre*, p. 184.

34 Françoise Dolto, *La Cause des enfants* (Paris: Robert Laffont, 1985), pp. 373–4.

35 Henri Claude, 'Quelques considérations sur la psychanalyse', *Journal médical français*, 22:4 (1933), 107–8.

36 On Marie Bonaparte's place in the SPP, see Roudinesco, *Bataille*, 1, p. 328; Célia Bertin, *Marie Bonaparte, A Life* (New York: Harcourt, 1982), Chs 7 and 8.

37 Angelo Hesnard, Édouard Pichon and Georges Politzer, 'Psychoanalysis in France: Preliminary Note on the Historical Survey of the French Psychoanalytic Movement', *Psychoanalytic Review*, 17 (1930), 426–8.

38 See Annick Ohayon, 'Édouard Pichon, psychanalyste français', in Michel Arrivé, Valelia Muni Toke and Claudine Normand (eds), *De la grammaire à l'inconscient: Dans les traces de Damourette et Pichon: actes du colloque de Cerisy-la-Salle du 1er au 11 août 2009* (Limoges: Lambert-Lucas, 2009), pp. 141–8.

39 See Alain de Mijolla, *Freud et la France: 1885–1945* (Paris: Presses universitaires de France, 2010), pp. 608, 614.

40 *Ibid.*, p. 607; Roudinesco, *Bataille*, 1, p. 361.

41 Julie Fette, *Exclusions: Practicing Prejudice in French Law and Medicine, 1920–1945* (New York: Cornell University Press, 2012), p. 70.

42 See Donna Evleth, 'The Ordre des Médecins and the Jews in Vichy France, 1940–1944', *French History*, 20:2 (2006), pp. 204–24.

43 Suzanne Marette to Françoise Marette, 23 September 1922, in Colette Percheminier (ed.), *Françoise Dolto: Lettres de jeunesse* (Paris: Gallimard, 2003), p. 128.

44 Mary Louise Roberts, *Civilization without Sexes: Reconstructing Gender in Postwar France, 1917–1927* (Chicago: University of Chicago Press, 1994), pp. 9, 214.

45 Fernand Boverat, 'Il faut faire naître', *Revue de l'Alliance nationale pour l'accroissement de la population française*, 143 (1924), 163–71.

46 Pedersen, *Family, Dependence, and the Origins of the Welfare State*, pp. 17–18, 357–68; Kristen Stromberg Childers, *Fathers, Families, and the State in France, 1914–1945* (Ithaca, NY: Cornell University Press, 2003), pp. 7, 19; Reynolds, *France between the Wars*, pp. 32–6.

47 On *puériculture*, see Linda Clark, *Schooling the Daughters of Marianne: Textbooks and the Socialization of Girls on Modern French Primary*

Schools (New York: State University of New York Press, 1984), Ch. 5. For the longer-term background, see Karen Offen, *Debating the Woman Question in the French Third Republic, 1870–1920* (Cambridge: Cambridge University Press, 2018), Ch. 2.

48 See Paul Smith, *Feminism and the Third Republic: Women's Political and Civil Rights in France 1918–1945* (Oxford: Clarendon, 1996), pp. 246–50.

49 See Sarah Maza, *Violette Nozière: A Story of Murder in 1930s Paris* (Berkeley, CA: University of California Press, 2011), for an example of how living conditions and gender relations shaped lives in 1930s Paris.

50 Eli Zaretsky, *Secrets of the Soul: A Social and Cultural History of Psychoanalysis* (New York: Vintage, 2005), p. 5. Zaretsky's emphasis.

51 Sigmund Freud, '"Civilized" Sexual Morality and Modern Nervous Illness' (1908), in James Strachey (ed.), *The Standard Edition of the Complete Psychological Works of Sigmund Freud, Vol. 9 (1906–1908): Jensen's 'Gradiva' and Other Works* (London: Hogarth, 1959), pp. 181–204.

52 Sigmund Freud, 'Sexuality in the Aetiology of the Neuroses' (1898), in James Strachey (ed.), *The Standard Edition of the Complete Psychological Works of Sigmund Freud, Vol. 3 (1893–1899): Early Psycho-Analytic Publications* (London: Hogarth, 1962), pp. 263–86, here p. 272.

53 Mari Jo Buhle, *Feminism and its Discontents: A Century of Struggle with Psychoanalysis* (Cambridge, MA: Harvard University Press, 1998), p. 22.

54 Karl Abraham, 'Manifestations of the Female Castration Complex', *International Journal of Psycho-Analysis*, 3:1 (1922), 1–29. See Buhle, *Feminism*, pp. 66ff.

55 Buhle, *Feminism*, p. 74; Susan Quinn, *A Mind of Her Own: The Life of Karen Horney* (London: Macmillan, 1988), pp. 206–10.

56 Zaretsky, *Secrets*, p. 208.

57 Abraham, 'Manifestations', 27.

58 *Ibid.*, 28–9.

59 René Laforgue, 'Schizophrénie et schizonoïa', *Revue française de psychanalyse* (hereafter *RFP*), 1:1 (1927), 6–23.

60 René Laforgue, 'La Névrose familiale', *RFP*, 9:3 (1936), 327–60, 328.

61 Laforgue, 'Schizophrénie et schizonoïa', 11.

62 René Laforgue, 'À propos de la frigidité de la femme', *RFP*, 8:2 (1935), 217–26, 222. This *RFP* volume was devoted to female sexuality; there was no companion volume on male sexuality.

63 Laforgue, 'La Névrose familiale', 344.

64 *Ibid.*, 328–9, 344.

65 *Ibid.*, 341.
66 Speech by Pichon quoted in 'Comptes rendus', *RFP*, 7:1 (1934), 141.
67 Édouard Pichon, 'La Polarisation masculin-féminin', *L'Évolution psychiatrique*, 4:3 (1934), 59–96. Pichon co-authored with Jacques Damourette a seven-volume treatise on French grammar, *Des Mots à la pensée: essai de grammaire de la langue française* (Paris, 1911–40).
68 Édouard Pichon, 'Le Rôle du sexe dans la civilisation occidentale', *RFP*, 10:1 (1938), 23–37.
69 *Ibid.*, 26. Pichon's emphasis.
70 Cited in Roudinesco, *Bataille*, 1, p. 299.
71 See Ohayon, 'Édouard Pichon', p. 145.
72 *Ibid.*, p. 143.
73 *Ibid.*, p. 144.
74 Édouard Pichon, *Le Développement psychique de l'enfant et de l'adolescent. Évolution normale, pathologie, traitement. Manuel d'étude* (Paris: Masson, 1936).
75 *Ibid.*, p. 25.
76 *Ibid.*, pp. 260–1.
77 *Ibid.*, pp. 63–8, 277–9. Pichon's emphasis.
78 *Ibid.*, p. 34.
79 *Ibid.*, p. 33.
80 *Ibid.*, p. 309.
81 Édouard Pichon, preface to Françoise Marette, *Psychanalyse et pédiatrie: le complexe de castration étude générale – cas cliniques* (Paris, 1940).
82 E.g. Françoise Dolto to Jenny Roudinesco et al., 27 May 1953, in Muriel Djéribi-Valentin (ed.), *Françoise Dolto: Une vie de correspondances (1938–1988)* (Paris: Gallimard, 2005), p. 228.
83 Zaretsky, *Secrets*, p. 195.
84 Fette, *Exclusions*, p. 84.
85 Zaretsky, *Secrets*, p. 196.

2

Dutiful daughters: Françoise breaks free?

The social and political values of Dolto's birth family – the Marettes – were essentially those of the anti-Dreyfusard upper classes of the late nineteenth century and *belle époque*. With wealth derived from the metals industry, the Marettes were a six-child family living in a well-to-do Parisian neighbourhood. Supportive of monarchist (far-) right political currents, they were Catholic, but in a performative or social sense, rather than being especially pious or devout. Somewhat snobbish and suspicious of social deviance, they valued art, classical learning and musical ability highly. They were connected to France's military and to the French Empire: one of Dolto's uncles fought in the Tonkin campaign in Vietnam in 1884, while her eldest brother served in Marshal Lyautey's colonial army in Morocco in the 1920s. The family sought to perpetuate its social and economic status by directing male children into the army and commerce, while requiring daughters to learn a mixture of marriageability-enhancing decorative and practical skills and demeanours.

In the interwar years, the social groups that upheld these values came under various kinds of pressure: economic pressure from inflation and market crises, social pressure as a result of changing economic structures and social mores and political pressure during periods of Radical Party or socialist ascendancy. Nonetheless, for young women from such families, to break with them remained very difficult. Though more opportunities became available for bourgeois women to pursue careers and take part in public life in the interwar period, formidable cultural barriers remained in their way. Dolto's early life is a case study in a transitional moment – much like that of her contemporary, the writer Simone de Beauvoir

(1908–86), who was born in the same year and into a similar social setting, which she described in her first autobiographical volume, *Mémoires d'une jeune fille rangée* (*Memoirs of a Dutiful Daughter*, 1958).[1] Like Beauvoir, Dolto avoided the quasi-aristocratic way of life that her family imagined for her, but her later views, on gender politics especially, were shaped to a far greater extent by those of her family milieu. Questions of gender and feminine identity were central to Dolto's initial encounter with psychoanalysis, and the psychoanalysts who facilitated Dolto's breach with her family largely shared her parents' views on these issues.[2] Though undergoing psychoanalysis and training to become an analyst helped Dolto to gain professional qualifications and personal independence, it also confronted her with new arguments as to why it was not a good idea for most women to do likewise – arguments which, as will be seen, she mostly accepted, and integrated into her own early theorising and professional practice.

The Marettes' family values

Dolto's mother, Suzanne Marette, *née* Demmler (1879–1962), came from a southern German Protestant family that had moved to France in the 1850s. Suzanne's father, Arthur Demmler (1844–1912), grew up speaking German, but fought for France in 1870. After attending the École Polytechnique engineering school, Arthur founded the Métal Déployé (Deployed Metal) factory in the metallurgy centre of Montbard, Burgundy, in 1902. The factory flourished during the industrial expansion of the late nineteenth century, and his marriage to Henriette Secrétan (1860–1938) – daughter of the copper magnate and art collector Eugène, who famously supplied the copper for New York's Statue of Liberty – further elevated Arthur's social station. Suzanne was the Demmlers' eldest child. Her younger brother (Dolto's uncle), Pierre, to whom the young Françoise[3] would become close, died of war wounds in 1916. In her teenage years, Suzanne worked as her father's secretary. The job required her to sit silent and unseen behind a screen, taking notes on Arthur's meetings with other men.[4]

Dolto's father, Henry Marette, born in 1874, was the son of an architect. After his father's death in a railway fire in 1880, Henry boarded at the Lycée Michelet on the outskirts of Paris before progressing to the École Polytechnique and qualifying as an engineer. After graduating, he was hired by Arthur Demmler to work for Métal Déployé. Arthur and Henry developed a close relationship following an incident in a hotel room in which a wardrobe fell onto Demmler, pinning and crushing his leg. Henry rescued his stricken boss and made himself indispensable to the factory's operation during his convalescence.[5] Arthur came to see Henry as a natural successor, regularly inviting him to dinner at his home. The subsequent marriage of Henry Marette and Suzanne Demmler in 1901 thus appears as a sealing of the relationship between the two men, Henry and Arthur, rather than a love match between Henry and Suzanne. Suzanne, indeed, was reluctant. She had envisioned her future husband as a blond, blue-eyed, artistic Protestant.[6] Henry was a brown-haired, brown-eyed, Catholic engineer with a head for figures. Nevertheless, Suzanne acquiesced in her father's plan, and went along with what ultimately proved a generally happy marriage.[7] Her first child, Jacqueline Marette, was born in 1902, when she was twenty-three. Five more children followed by 1915 – four boys plus Françoise, born in 1908. Suzanne's story, which illustrates the lack of agency accorded to bourgeois women in this period, puts into context her later approach to raising her own daughters. Having renounced her personal ambitions in favour of duty to her father, forbearance and family interest, she expected her daughters to make the same sacrifice. When Jacqueline died from cancer in 1920, leaving Françoise as the sole surviving girl, all of this pressure, all of the expectations that the Marettes had for their daughters, fell onto her.

In 1913, Henry, Suzanne and their children moved to a ten-room apartment in a new building at 2 rue Colonel Bonnet, Passy, in the sixteenth arrondissement of Paris. The large fifth-floor apartment offered views of Sacré-Coeur and the Seine.[8] Passy was a wealthy neighbourhood. Its newer buildings, unlike most in the city at the time, had electric lighting, central heating, lifts and hot running water. Above the Marettes lived the CEO of a clothing company with a store on Avenue de l'Opéra; the flat below was occupied by a countess who Dolto later described as 'a haughty woman ... dressed like a princess ... in lace and pearls'.[9] Every summer the family decamped to Deauville, one of the channel coast resorts favoured by the aristocratic, industrial and cultural elite, whose atmosphere of studied casualness and careful attention to social distinctions was described by Marcel Proust in *À l'ombre des jeunes filles en fleurs* (*Within a Budding Grove/In the Shadow of Young Girls in Flower*, 1919).

With their six children (a seventh, Jacques, was born in 1922 after Jacqueline's death), the Marettes were part of a minority of around one in thirteen French families – the *familles nombreuses* – which took on political significance in the interwar pronatalist climate.[10] Given the generally cramped housing on offer in interwar Paris, having a large family was in practice a symbol of wealth. It also tended to correlate with adherence to a certain worldview. Catholic families had higher birth rates than Protestant ones, and birth rates were consequently higher in strongly Catholic areas. Among the upper classes, religious families averaged 6.19 children, compared to 2.73 for non-believers.[11] In other words, while large families were rare in French society overall, they were the expected norm in wealthy Catholic circles.

Despite Suzanne's Protestant background, the Marettes identified as Catholic – but in a way that indicates that, for them, religion, or rather being seen to be religious, was first and foremost a social gambit. According to Dolto, her maternal grandfather Arthur Demmler saw marriage to a Catholic woman as an essential step towards being accepted as fully French. 'In his mind, to be French meant being in favour of the 1789 Declaration of the Rights of Man and being Catholic. Otherwise, you're not French!'[12] Demmler was seeking not only to become French but to be accepted into a particular strand of society. The pattern of the later nineteenth century was for emerging industrial elites gradually to fuse with the aristocracy, adopting its values, and practices such as philanthropy, in order to confer social legitimacy on their recently acquired wealth.[13] In the France of the *belle époque* – polarised around questions of secularisation and clerical influence – outward adherence to Catholicism and anti-Dreyfusard politics underlined one's alignment with aristocratic values.[14] Dolto's memoirs suggest that the Marettes saw their weekly attendance at mass, at Passy's Notre-Dame-de-Grâce church, as the enactment of a social obligation rather than an act of deep piety: 'It was a principle. You had to go to mass on Sunday. We did the bare minimum of worshipping … We'd arrive at 12:10

and leave at 12:20, all together and at full speed [*en famille et en trombe*].'[15]

The family's identification with aristocratic social practices, and especially monarchist politics, was more committed. In particular, Suzanne and her mother Henriette Demmler sympathised with the far-right Action Française movement.[16] Henry Marette had a more liberal-conservative outlook on social questions, which Dolto later attributed to his more modest social origins (he had a socialist brother-in-law, which caused some family friction), but he too identified as a monarchist.[17] The family's preferred newspaper was the conservative and patriotic society daily, *L'Écho de Paris*.[18] As for servants, Dolto's maternal grandparents Henriette and Arthur Demmler employed '*un vrai valet de chambre*' – a convention which distinguished the aristocracy, who did not deign to be served at table by a female servant, from the bourgeoisie who could only afford a *bonne* (maid).[19] The level of formality in the Demmler household may be gauged from the fact that their *valet de chambre* and *cuisinière* (cook) successfully concealed their relationship from their employers for their entire thirty years' service, marrying only upon their retirement.[20] The Marettes themselves employed four full-time staff: a *cuisinière*, a *valet de chambre*, a nanny for the youngest children and a live-in *institutrice* (governess) for the older children. Part-time employees included a *lingère* (washlady) and various private tutors.

Upper-class families exercised considerable control and surveillance over their children, carefully vetting the people and ideas to which they were exposed. One man born in 1921 told the sociologist Eric Mension-Rigau that 'as soon as we talked about inviting someone over, even a child who was with us at the Sisters of the Assumption … we were asked: "What's this? Who is he? What do his parents do?"'[21] Before Simone de Beauvoir was allowed to be friends with 'Zaza' (Élisabeth Lacoin, named in Beauvoir's memoirs as Mabille), 'my father and mother had long discussions about the different branches of various families they had heard of called Mabille'.[22] The Marettes were possibly even more extreme. The young Françoise had few childhood friends, though she did have a close relationship with her German governess Élisabeth Weilandt – complicity between children and live-in servants was common since both groups struggled with the imposed rhythms of upper-class life.[23] Dolto later claimed that she did not so much as eat a meal outside her mother's or grandmother's presence before the age of twenty-five.[24] To visit a friend's house for tea was 'an extraordinary thing'. All social activities had to take place within the family confines:

> We weren't allowed to have friends, moreover, on the pretext that there were already enough of us in the family. On the beach, we weren't allowed to play with other children … As for gymnastics, there was a teacher, man or woman, who came to the house once a week. [25]

Any unsupervised activity was potentially suspect. Unaccompanied journeys were to be avoided: 'My mother fretted about possible encounters on public transport.'[26] Dolto hardly ever travelled alone before the age of twenty-one.

During periods of separation from her parents – almost always spent with her grandmother or another close family member – the young Françoise was required to write regular letters to her parents, reporting on more or less every aspect of her activity and following strict formal and tonal constraints. In this social milieu, letter-writing was a highly performative activity, and correspondence with family was a tool of remote surveillance.[27] Letters from daughters were closely scrutinised for any evidence of departure from expected behaviours. They were not treated as private, but were instead passed around the family and discussed. Mothers might open letters addressed to their daughters, especially if they came from correspondents of whom they disapproved.[28] Though many of Françoise's letters do appear to contain authentic expressions of feeling – some will be quoted as such below – they were also calibrated attempts to manage relationships with people anxious to monitor and police her behaviour.

School was no escape from watchful eyes. From 1914 until 1924 Dolto attended the Cours Sainte-Clotilde, a private, Catholic establishment close to the family apartment in Passy. She was an *élève libre* ('free pupil'), meaning not that the classes were unpaid but rather that she was only required to attend for a few hours per week, with the rest of the work to be done at home. Mothers and governesses sat in on the in-school classes, sewing at the back while the lesson proceeded. The main in-class activity was summarising the week's lessons to prove that the pupils had worked hard at home.[29]

The centre of learning was thus the home, not the school. Upper-class girls' education emphasised subjects such as art and music, which conferred cultural capital and were seen as enhancing their decorative value to potential suitors, over the academic subjects prioritised by the republican state education system established in the 1880s.[30] The Marette children were all expected to learn an instrument, and their parents encouraged further extra-curricular activities such as reading, learning foreign languages and attending lectures, exhibitions, theatrical productions and concerts.[31] Suzanne encouraged Françoise to take an interest in music, painting, ceramics and sewing, and nurtured any signs of aptitude in an approved art or skill: 'Thus I learned how to sew [and] one day, I asked for a real teacher to teach me how to cut fabric. Straight away, my mother found a teacher, who came to the house once a fortnight.'[32] Suzanne's encouraging attitude towards skills she viewed as appropriate for her daughters contrasted sharply with that which she displayed towards formal schooling and Françoise's desire to pursue medical studies, as will be seen below.

Henry Marette's interest in scientific subjects and intellectual culture helped his daughters to broaden their learning beyond the decorative arts. Dolto later wrote that Henry bought twenty books a week – 'everything that came out'.[33] His library featured numerous popular science works from the Bibliothèque Orange, a new forward-thinking reading club.[34] He took his children to public lectures at the Trocadéro Palace, which Dolto recalled as notable for their 'popularisation of fields previously restricted to elites [such as] physics and chemistry. There were also lectures on the seabed, on earthquakes, and so on.'[35] The young Françoise was particularly struck by a demonstration of wireless telegraphy given by radio pioneer Édouard Branly. Helped by her father and illustrated publications with titles like *Le Sans-fil*, she participated in the contemporary craze for building crystal set radios.[36] Suzanne, presumably not wanting these scientific interests to develop too far, encouraged Françoise also to read the novels of Colette Yver, such as *Princesses de science* (1907) which showed intellectual women ('*cervelines*') ending up dried and withered, incapable of love.[37] But unlike the Beauvoirs, who carefully scrutinised and censored their daughters' reading material, Dolto's parents 'never limited my reading', and her father 'allowed me to read everything in his library'.[38] There was one notable exception – '"Zola is absolute piddle"' (*du pot de chambre*) – but otherwise, 'I could read anything my father bought.'[39] She even read his copy of Victor Margueritte's *La Garçonne* (1922), a scandalous work owing to the sexual promiscuity and relative gender nonconformity of its lead character, though she 'didn't understand it at all'.[40] Henry's library opened Dolto's horizons to a wider world of knowledge, and indicated the direction of social, scientific and technological change. By 1924 it included books on and by Freud, probably translations of his 1909 Clark Lectures and *The Psychopathology of Everyday Life*, plus a 1924 explainer by Angelo Hesnard.[41] Françoise encountered these books as a teenager and used them in a school presentation.[42] Her father's middle-class engineering background and strong interest in fashionable scientific developments help explain why, despite being closely wedded to conservative norms, the family was also – relatively unusually – open to sending its children to a psychoanalyst in the 1930s.

The overriding concern affecting Dolto's upbringing was her parents' resolve that their children should advance or at least maintain the family's social status. This required internalising behaviours and ideas appropriate to their station and rejecting outside influences. Key terms in the Marettes' vocabulary acted to enforce this. Correct demeanours were signalled by words such as *poli*, *propre*, *élégant* and *chic* (polite, clean, elegant, smart) – the latter is particularly in evidence in the young Dolto's correspondence. These terms emphasised self-control, refinement and class boundaries: one had to be '*chic*' to distinguish oneself from those who were '*ordinaire*' or, worse, '*vulgaire*'.[43] Such terms also served to police gender norms. Simone de Beauvoir recalled that

> a real 'lady' [*une dame 'comme il faut'*] ought not to show too much bosom, or wear short skirts, or dye her hair, or have it bobbed, or make up, or sprawl on a divan, or kiss her husband in the underground passages of the metro: if she transgressed these rules, she was 'not a lady' [*elle avait mauvais genre*].[44]

The most egregious marker of transgression was divorce. Dolto recalled that her parents referred to divorced women as 'not quite as they should be' (*pas tout à fait comme il faut*):

> Among my parents' friends was a woman whose husband had been cheating on her, and left her. She had two sons at the same school as

> my brothers and she was terribly bored. She came to see my parents, who were kind to her, but they only received her after ten o'clock in the evening. They didn't want people to know that we were receiving a single woman ... They would see her, but all the same they had to be careful that this association didn't lead to them being thought of as 'bad' people [*des gens 'pas bien'*]. [45]

This vignette illustrates the powerful shame attached to divorce – so strong that the Marettes feared reputational contamination from mere association with a divorced woman, on whom the shame was invariably pinned regardless of fault. These short, cutting phrases – *comme il faut*, *pas bien*, *mauvais genre*, *chic* – communicated an implicit but ever-present threat of social ostracism or loss of standing.

This enormous concern with status conditioned Henry and Suzanne's attitude to their children's careers. Their eldest son, Pierre (b. 1903) was encouraged towards an army career from an early age. His success at the prestigious Saint-Cyr military academy delighted Suzanne, who wrote of him affectionately as 'my officer' in her letters.[46] Pierre was posted to Morocco in 1927, where French forces under Hubert Lyautey were consolidating colonial control following the Franco-Spanish suppression of Abd el-Krim's insurgency in the 1925–26 Rif War. In Morocco Pierre met, and subsequently married, a colonel's daughter. This was a good career move, but, as he wrote to Françoise, a decision also taken with the family's interests in mind: 'I thought about it for a long time, seeing if the young person fitted in with my ideas, my way of thinking and especially with our family.'[47] Sympathies with Action Française were widespread in the colonial officer class.[48] Pierre's political opinions at this time can be gauged from a 1927 letter to his sister in which he joked casually about torturing republican politicians:

> It's a shame we can't play a dirty joke on Poinca. [Raymond Poincaré, Prime Minister], Bartho. [Louis Barthou, Minister of Justice] and others, a little Chinese torture ... For example: a forced bath in the Seine with the help of a rubbish chute, or putting them out in the blazing sun and making them drink saltwater. How good that would be![49]

The second son, Jean Marette (b. 1906), was groomed for a business career. He attended the École Centrale Paris engineering school with a view to him subsequently assuming the technical direction of

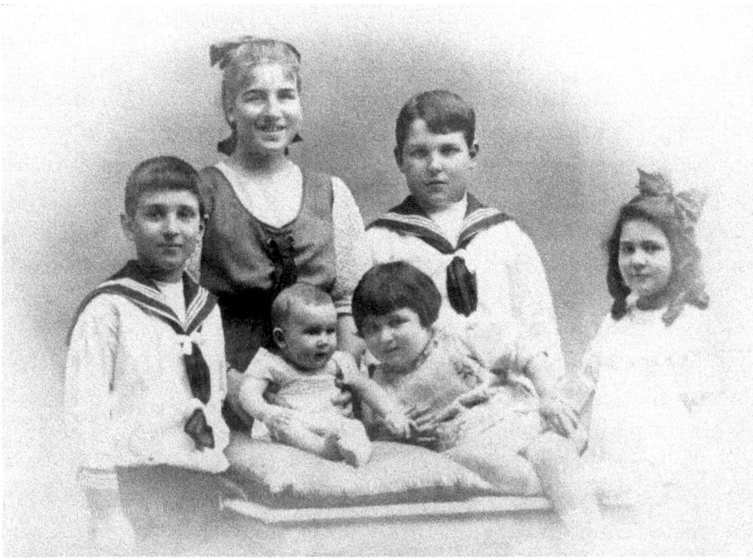

Figure 2.1 The Marette '*famille nombreuse*': Dolto (aged 7–8, far right) with her siblings in 1916. L–r: Jean, Jacqueline, André, Philippe, Pierre and Françoise

the family firm. The third son, Philippe (b. 1913), was pushed into attending the École des Hautes Études Commerciales, which would qualify him to manage the company administration. Dolto's eldest three brothers thus apparently had their destinies predetermined by their parents: the first son to the army – fulfilling the duty of *familles nombreuses* to furnish the nation with soldiers, and bringing prestige on the family – and the second and third sons shepherded into the family business. The younger sons, André (b. 1915) and Jacques (b. 1922), were given more freedom to determine their own destiny. André became a lawyer and manager, while Jacques went into politics, becoming a minister under De Gaulle in the 1960s and a member of Parliament until the 1980s.

As for their daughters – Françoise wrote the following to her mother in September 1922, aged thirteen:

> I'll marry and stay with you, I'll give you lots of grandchildren ... I'll choose a husband who wants lots of children and won't want to be far away from you. On the contrary, you are going to have a very pleasant future, or better yet, the most familial possible.

> Now I am nearly 14. Only two more years of studies and then I'll stay with you.[50]

The central elements of a daughter's education, as far as Suzanne and her peers were concerned, were the strict maintenance of sexual innocence and purity; internalising the rituals and behaviours of upper-class family and social life; learning about childcare in preparation for motherhood; undertaking a limited amount of academic education, but being willing and prepared to swiftly set this aside in favour of extracurricular decorative talents. Suzanne instructed Françoise to 'continue to love me, to apply yourself to schoolwork so as to be rid of it quickly, [which you should do] for me as I'm not keen on that, and get better at sewing, at tennis, and at gentleness – for glassware and newborns are both fragile'.[51]

Preserving sexual purity was particularly essential. In the early twentieth century, even more than the nineteenth, aristocratic families erected a taboo over any and all discussion of sexuality. Colin Heywood has described the period as 'a high point for stories about babies being born under a cabbage-patch leaf or brought by a stork'.[52] Suzanne required her daughter to be 'an honest girl, upright and pure'.[53] She strongly warned the thirteen-year-old Françoise against discussing anything connected with sexuality with her male cousin – or indeed anyone else:

> When you are grown up, about to get married and have children, I will explain some things that you have no need to know now and that you shouldn't try to find out about ... It's not *chic*, not clean [*propre*], and I want to have a clean, orderly girl, a real *maiden* [*jeune fille*] who can be proud of her good white character [*son âme bien blanche*], and guard it jealously, that is to say, not allow anyone to sully it.[54]

Such insistence tended to alienate girls from their sexuality and transmit a large degree of anxiety regarding it. Beauvoir's friend Zaza 'had a precocious understanding of why Madame Mabille had hated the first night of her marriage and had loathed her husband's embraces ever since'.[55] Beauvoir wrote of her own sense during her upbringing that 'the body was by reason of its own nature a dangerous object, [such that] any allusion to its existence, whether serious or frivolous, seemed fraught with peril'.[56]

An important social custom for women in these families were *jours de réception*: regular 'days' on which one received guests. As a young child, Dolto was initiated into the practice by her maternal grandmother, Henriette Demmler, who gave her grandchildren a practice 'day' each.[57] Since hosting one was essential to upholding aristocratic pretensions – Beauvoir's memoirs detail her mother's determination to continue holding them despite the family's straitened circumstances – there were naturally many of them. Dolto recalled that at one stage 'my life was regulated by the fact of these "days" ... So much so that the days were marked by "It's X's day today"'.[58] For her own mother's 'days', 'you had to dress up in something *chic* for four or five hours and go and curtsy in front of each lady'.[59]

Upper-class women were always busy, with days organised into minutely planned blocks; laziness and idleness were equated to degeneracy.[60] All time was to be spent either in society or in structured, useful activity – 'no unemployment allowed', as Françoise wrote to a friend.[61] By the age of seven, Zaza could iron neatly, play piano and violin and make cakes; at age eleven, she apologised in a letter to her parents for her laziness in staying in bed until 7.45 a.m.[62] Madame de Beauvoir never wasted a second, always reading, or knitting, or preparing the next social event. Such incessant activity and the constant social obligations more or less eliminated free time and private life. When Simone complained that 'outside my bed, there wasn't a single corner I could call my own ... I found it painful never to be on my own', it was only partly a comment on the small size of her family's new apartment.[63] Her sister Hélène later commented that 'we weren't allowed the minimum of personal life to which every being is entitled'.[64] Zaza once went so far as to gash her own foot with an axe so as to have an excuse to escape the constant rounds of social events and excursions.[65]

Summertime sojourns at Deauville brought different obligations. As Suzanne made clear in letters to Françoise, the frequent family games of tennis served a serious purpose, not only for improving Françoise's physique ('make the most of [the chance to play] tennis as much as you can, and come back to me thin and supple') but also for the social possibilities:

> I would be glad if you could manage to play well ... Jean [Françoise's brother] would like to play with you, and later on, it would be nice for the two of you to play mixed doubles ... It makes for a different kind of meeting for young people, a lot more familial ... In that sense,

> you can help me ... You'd be very happy later on if Jean married a nice girl who would be about your age ... and who would be a friend for you.[66]

Throughout the 1920s, Françoise's letters from Deauville describe in some detail her progress both in tennis and in controlling her weight; both were clearly important elements in readying her for future marriage, and thus important subjects of family discussion. Tennis represented a rare approved opportunity to meet the opposite sex, albeit in a public, controlled setting. Isabelle Grellet and Caroline Kruse describe how in this period tennis had turned into a 'leisure sport as a form of etiquette, or a kind of communication practised in high society'.[67] It was playing tennis in Morocco in 1929 that Pierre Marette met his future fiancée Yvonne, the colonel's daughter, which can only have underlined its importance to Françoise. Zaza, too, excelled at tennis, and wrote similar letters to her parents charting her progress; Madame Lacoin likewise saw it as a source of potential suitors, but could not tolerate Zaza playing 'with young people from the Sorbonne whose families she doesn't even know'.[68]

Dolto, Beauvoir and Zaza thus had in common their attempts to navigate the almost impossibly codified, confusing social world of upper-class childhood in this period. They also resembled one another in each experiencing an event that effectively brought their childhood to a premature end, eventually prompting them to question and challenge that world to a greater extent than most of their contemporaries. For Beauvoir, this was her family's move to a smaller, cheaper apartment; for Zaza, an enforced breakup with her teenage boyfriend, André. For Dolto, this event was the death from cancer in 1920 of her eighteen-year-old sister Jacqueline, and the effect this had on her mother Suzanne. It was not just the fact of the death itself, but what Jacqueline represented. Tall, blonde, sociable and with little taste for academic study, Jacqueline was very different to the short, stocky, studious Françoise, and exactly the kind of daughter Suzanne wanted. Dolto later wrote how Jacqueline 'liked to laugh, dance, adorn herself' and 'had lots of success with men'.[69] Her parents had already received several marriage proposals. Jacqueline's death threw Suzanne into a violent depression, with knock-on effects for the whole family. On the advice of a doctor, Henry and Suzanne decided to have another child to replace Jacqueline – but rather than a replacement daughter this resulted in the birth of a boy, Jacques, in September 1922.

This context lies behind Françoise's September 1922 letter quoted above, assuring her mother that she intended to marry, have lots of children and stay close to her mother. As the only remaining girl, Françoise felt under enormous pressure to compensate for the loss and live up to the model of the ideal daughter. Suzanne had placed responsibility for the death on her shoulders, telling Françoise, who had been preparing for her first communion at the time, 'you see, you didn't pray right'.[70] Suzanne's grief can also be seen in the reactions of her sons. 'I promise you I'll be just like a daughter to you. I will try to replace Jacqueline for you as much as I can', wrote the sixteen-year-old Jean after the baby's birth.[71] When Pierre married in 1929, he told Françoise that 'my dearest wish is that [my fiancée] should replace our poor Jacq. at home as much as possible'.[72] If the brothers felt the effects of Suzanne's grief strongly, the impact on Françoise, as the sole surviving daughter, was more profound. As her adolescence progressed, Françoise felt an increasing sense of dislocation between her wishes and aptitudes and her mother's demands, albeit one she could not yet articulate. An awareness of her inability to live up to the required ideal, plus a lingering feeling of responsibility for not preventing Jacqueline's death, provoked a strong sense of guilt that she would not be able to address until her psychoanalysis.

The fight for a career

A crucial difference between Dolto and Beauvoir in their teenage years was that the Beauvoirs, not having the financial means to assure dowries for their daughters, decided that they should continue with their studies. Simone could thus take the *baccalauréat* and progress onto a degree programme at the Sorbonne. The Marettes, being wealthier, did not accord Françoise the same opportunity. For her, obtaining the right to take the final part of the *baccalauréat* in 1925 was a hard-won concession. It was only possible in the first place because of a very recent (1924) reform allowing girls to sit for the *baccalauréat* and *agrégation* on more or less equal terms with boys.[73] It required Françoise to leave Sainte-Clotilde, which did not teach the second half of the *baccalauréat* needed for university entry. She enrolled instead at the state-run Lycée Molière. Though the classes were single sex, and the *lycée* was within walking distance of the family apartment, this was still a significant departure. The *lycée*'s routines and methods were a shock and left a lasting imprint on Dolto's views on education (discussed in Chapter 6).[74] Taking the *baccalauréat* was Françoise's first step beyond the limits set down for a young woman of her background. Her mother found it alarming, declaring that 'a girl who has her baccalaureate is no longer marriageable', supported by Pierre who declared that 'I would never marry a girl who has the baccalaureate'.[75] Dolto later claimed that her mother tried at the last minute to collude with the *lycée* management to prevent her *baccalauréat* dossier from being correctly submitted, only to be thwarted by Henry, who supported his daughter's right to obtain the qualification.[76] However, Henry would not push his support for his daughter's studies any further. In her memoirs Dolto suggested that while Henry felt it was a good idea for Françoise to take the 'bac' as an insurance policy – i.e. so that she could get teaching work if she later fell on hard times – he did not think the same way about higher education, or at least did not think it sufficiently valuable to be worth provoking a family conflict.[77] When Françoise expressed a desire to train as a doctor, Henry's response was 'later, later, don't talk about it, you can see it makes your mother angry'.[78] Medicine, in particular, was off-limits for various reasons. It was still very much seen as a male career, and the idea of entrusting their daughters to the company of a cohort of rowdy medical students for several years scandalised most bourgeois parents. The most famous female French doctor to that point was Madeleine Pelletier, a cross-dressing feminist – hardly an acceptable role model from the Marettes' perspective.[79]

In the face of Françoise's unbending desire nonetheless to study medicine, a compromise was agreed: she would be allowed to commence medical studies, but only when she reached the age of twenty-five. Her parents certainly hoped and supposed she would marry before then – but in the meantime, she was obliged to spend a number of somewhat aimless years stuck within the world of the family, denied a purposeful outlet for her academic ability. She occupied her time doing housework, looking after her young brother

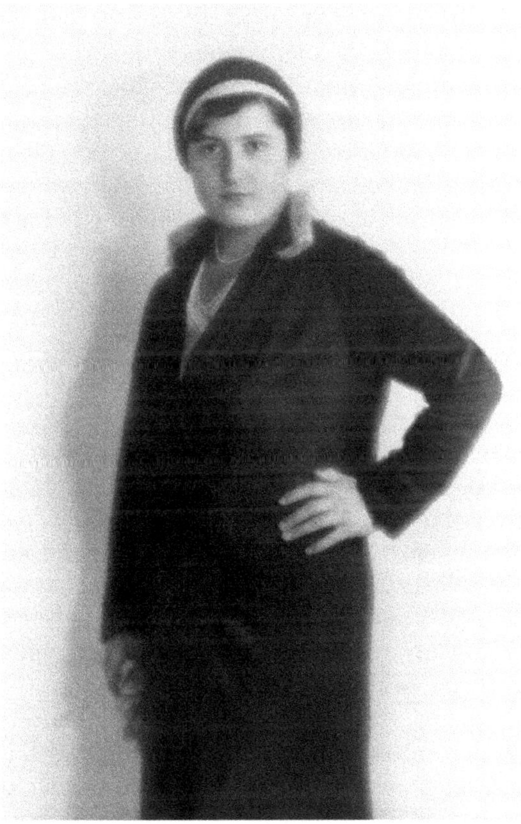

Figure 2.2 Françoise Marette in 1926

Jacques and developing her skills in art, crafts, ceramics, music and reading. In the summers she played tennis in Deauville and took trips with her grandmother to Lourdes, Alsace and the World War I battlefields.

Dolto also appears to have become more passionately religious during these years. She read books on the saints and corresponded at length about religious experience with a childhood friend, Agnès Dognin, who was in the process of becoming a nun.[80] Aged twenty, Françoise wrote to her former governess that 'my heart is so full of God that I really don't know if any man will ever manage to take first place even for an instant'.[81] In one sense, her religiosity was conventional, accepted, approved – notably by her maternal grandmother – but it was also implicated in her standoff with her parents over her future. As many women of earlier centuries had found, a demonstrative commitment to religion or a religious order could be a way of avoiding the marriage trap and opening the door to philanthropic or other roles that would not otherwise be open to women.[82] Since Françoise was determined to keep open the possibility of an independent career, and marriage was the most likely means of preventing this, making God the centre of her emotional life to the exclusion of all men was a form of defence. This seems also to have been part of Dognin's calculations. Initially sent to the convent by her parents to gain experience, in preparation for life as a devoted housewife, Dognin subsequently returned there for good, against her parents' will. She wrote to Françoise of finding in the convent 'a precious solitude ... we don't see *anyone*', a statement which should be read in the context of the extreme lack of privacy and free time accorded to young women of her class.[83]

Despite the pressure placed on her, Françoise did not waver in her pursuit of a career. While her sights remained set on medicine, she also explored potential practical applications for her artistic abilities, learning how to design advertising posters, and attempting to take a certificate of professional aptitude in sewing – only to be rebuffed by Suzanne, who thought that her daughter should pursue these only as decorative attributes, not professional skills.[84] Dolto later imputed her persistence in seeking paths to employability to having observed widowed women during and after World War I:

> I had seen the decrepitude of bourgeois widows who had no profession, unlike manual workers or shopkeepers who were not obliged to change their way of life ... it was awful to see women dressed like my mother, in these beautiful neighbourhoods, begging ... It really affected me, and I thought: 'I must get myself a trade [*métier*]'. [85]

If the war taught Dolto that women could never take financial security for granted so long as they depended on men to provide it, her determination was likely bolstered by a sense that social attitudes were starting to change. Despite all the obstacles in their path, Dolto and Beauvoir grew up at a time when it was becoming conceivable, if still very difficult, for women to enter the liberal professions. It was certainly easier for them than for earlier pioneers such as Madeleine Brès, who became the first French woman to obtain a medical degree in 1875. The proportion of women earning the *baccalauréat* jumped from 6 per cent in 1914 to 36 per cent in 1939.[86] Numbers of women in higher education increased rather more slowly: Beauvoir was only the ninth woman to receive a degree from the Sorbonne, while Dolto, despite the family-imposed delay, was probably among the first thousand French women to obtain a medical degree.[87]

World War I also provided the young Dolto with a model of women taking on important, albeit gendered, healthcare roles. In 1914, her mother played a significant part in the voluntary effort to care for casualties sent for treatment in Deauville. Assisted by the family governess, Suzanne Marette took charge of a forty-bed ward in the Hôtel Royal, where, as Dolto later wrote, 'many ladies had offered their services as volunteer nurses. It was very nice, all these society ladies disguised as nurses.'[88] Nursing in France, long dominated by religious orders, was slowly secularising and coming under greater state control.[89] In the run-up to World War I, volunteering as a nurse became a way for bourgeois women to demonstrate their commitment to the national cause. By 1912–13, the Red Cross and similar organisations were 'all the rage' in women's Catholic Social Action groups.[90] After war broke out, nursing offered an alternative mission to women dissatisfied with the idea of patriotic motherhood as a wartime ideal. There was a wave of volunteering for the Red Cross in July–August 1914, when 'the memoirs and journals of well-to-do women and girls express[ed] an almost universal desire to found hospitals or to nurse war wounded'.[91] For many, this was conceived as a further extension to the charitable work they regularly conducted in their communities – an important aspect of upper-class life which provided opportunities for women to display wealth and status, develop social networks and feel useful.[92]

Suzanne Marette's participation in voluntary nursing efforts in Deauville would therefore be expected given her social status – but it became something more. Most Deauville nursing volunteers had returned to Paris by October 1914. After the initial excitement waned, they lacked the serious commitment required to continue in a role that was more challenging and less glamorous than they had imagined.[93] Yet Suzanne stayed on, leaving in 1915 only because of a pregnancy, suggesting that the work gave her a sense of professional fulfilment. Dolto later commented that 'she most likely wanted to do medicine in her youth'.[94] Dolto's ambition to pursue a medical career thus did not come from nowhere; her mother had, in fact, legitimised it through her own actions. Indeed, during her psychoanalysis, Dolto considered abandoning her medical degree on the grounds that 'my appetite for it had come to me from my mother … When she was a young girl it didn't yet seem acceptable and that was her big regret in life.'[95] At that point Dolto began to doubt whether her desire to study medicine, and the resulting battles with her mother, were not simply a vicarious reflection of Suzanne's inner conflicts rather than an authentic expression of her own wishes.

By the later 1920s, though the secularisation and professionalisation of nursing had progressed, it remained an acceptable temporary occupation for unmarried upper-class women. Retaining associations with charity, self-sacrifice and religious devotion, nursing was seen as good preparation for marriage and motherhood. Nurses were portrayed much more positively in the press and in popular imagery than for example women schoolteachers, who were depicted as likely to end up sad and celibate.[96] Suzanne considered it respectable: 'a woman's profession, free from danger: nursing kept women off the streets and earned them a living!', was how Dolto later summarised her attitude.[97] While still discouraging her daughter from training as a doctor, Suzanne was happy for her to take a Red Cross nursing qualification in 1929–30. Dolto found that she took pride in her ability to make bandages strong enough to give manual workers the confidence to return to work rather than being forced to stay home and lose pay.[98] After completing the course, she continued to administer bandages on a voluntary basis in the evenings.

In November 1931, Françoise won her waiting game. Her parents now allowed her, earlier than agreed, to begin studying for a medical degree, starting with a foundation year. This was because her brother Philippe, having shown little aptitude or interest in the career in business administration laid out for him, had won his parents' permission to switch to medicine. He could thus act as his sister's chaperone in medical school – despite being five years her junior.[99] The fact that Philippe was able to begin immediately, rather than having to wait as his sister had done, underlined the gendered nature of the barriers she faced – but it also acted to Philippe's disadvantage. Having been mentally preparing for her medical studies for years, Françoise soon proved to be noticeably academically superior to her brother. Philippe, brought up to assume inherent male superiority and feeling intimidated by his father, lost confidence. He became plagued by acne, which the Marettes' homeopathic family doctor attributed to his unhappiness at his career direction.[100] Philippe entered psychotherapy – with René Laforgue – in November 1932.

By the time her medical studies began, however, Françoise faced other complications. In summer 1931, aged twenty-two, she had spent two weeks in Provence, staying at the country residence of the Marettes' family friends, the Delebecque family. The Delebecques had connections at the highest levels of Action Française – during Dolto's stay with them, Léon Daudet came to lunch and Charles Maurras sent flowers.[101] They had two daughters close in age to Françoise, and a son, Édouard, two years her junior. The children shared interests in music, literature and art. One daughter, Christiane, was about to begin a degree in Italian at the Sorbonne; Édouard was taking the *agrégation* in classics. Françoise, given her social isolation, was delighted to have made such friends and keen to continue the new relationships. She briefly enrolled with Christiane at the Sorbonne (dropping out when the opportunity to begin medicine unexpectedly arose) and attended museums and concerts with the Delebecques on Sundays. She became particularly close to Édouard, with whom she developed what she later described as 'a loving friendship … affectionate in the manner of comrades, or a brother and sister'.[102] According to Dolto's memoirs (no relevant correspondence survives), what happened next was that 'the mothers had talked amongst themselves. Such that one day my mother said to me, "In any case, I won't let you go back to the D's unless it's clear between the two of you." I said, "Unless what's clear?" – "That you're engaged."'[103]

Dolto later claimed to have agreed to this without taking it entirely seriously, seeing it as preferable to having the friendship abruptly ended – 'as long as we get to see each other, we can call ourselves engaged!'[104] She quickly disabused Édouard of any misconceptions of what this implied: 'We're engaged, we've got time. I want to go to medical school first, we'll get married afterwards. So there's no reason for us to kiss.'[105] She suggested an arrangement in which marriage became a decidedly distant prospect, to take place only after her medical degree and Delebecque's *agrégation* and military service. This was not what the two families had in mind – nor, ultimately, Édouard, who asked her to abandon medicine and marry him. She refused. The uneasy arrangement persisted for two years, coming to a crisis only in February 1934 when relations were decisively, acrimoniously broken off. There were major family arguments: Dolto says she was accused by both families of being a 'bitch' (*salope*) and '*inhumaine*'.[106] Not fully understanding what she had done wrong, Françoise fell into a deep depression. Within a week, she had her first session with Laforgue.

Analysing femininity

In her memoirs, Dolto does not explain the choice of Laforgue as her analyst other than to say that he had already treated her brother Philippe, on the recommendation of their mutual acquaintance Marc Schlumberger. It is worth, however, pausing on who chose Laforgue as Dolto's analyst, and what they were hoping to achieve by doing so.

A July 1934 letter from Françoise to her father Henry clearly suggests that the initiative was his: 'if I hadn't had you to force me to get treatment ... I would never have had the courage to undertake the slightest thing (even less so Psychoanalysis) to get myself out of my distress', she wrote.[107] It was also Henry who was paying. Laforgue, as head of the SPP and the best-known psychoanalyst in France, charged the highest fees of any analyst in Paris, though he offered a 50 per cent discount to medical students.[108] What was Henry paying for, exactly? He likely suspected that Françoise's difficulties had a lot to do with her relationship to Suzanne, and the latter's depression and grief at the death of Jacqueline. Laforgue, as shown in Chapter 1, specialised in 'family neuroses', which in practice often meant assigning responsibility for 'family complexes' to women and especially to 'unbalanced mothers'. But Laforgue also believed that women who attempted to succeed professionally were doing so because, insufficiently reconciled to the natural inferiority of their sex, they were seeking compensation in 'masculine' activity. His treatment thus held out the possibility of 'curing' Françoise of her unnatural desires and bringing her back to a 'healthy' conception of femininity. In July 1934, Françoise wrote to her father in terms suggesting that she had internalised this aim: 'My greatest desire right now is to see this very painful treatment through to the end, because I know that the best way to thank you will be my becoming a woman – in the full sense of the word – of whom you can be proud.'[109] Henry agreed that the treatment 'will help you to transform your nature and become, as you say, a real woman'.[110] Suzanne, for her part, hoped that it would lead to a reconciliation with Delebecque.[111] Henry and Suzanne thus did not see Laforgue as someone who might put dangerous ideas into their daughter's head, but as someone who could reconcile her to her 'true' femininity.

As time went on, however, the 'family neurosis' interpretation became more dominant, and the analysis transformed Françoise in ways that her parents had not foreseen. Laforgue was able, as Dolto later wrote, to 'release me from my guilt, at least enough for me to get out of my visibly depressive state'.[112] She spent early sessions 'crying out all the tears in my body from the guilt I was feeling'.[113] With Laforgue's help she came to the understanding that her mother was the real neurotic and that 'my own neurosis was entirely founded on my mother's'.[114] She realised that 'I had first and foremost to free myself from my mother'.[115] After a year in analysis, her depression and lassitude had lifted. She continued to see Laforgue, by now less out of necessity but rather 'because it interested me' and because the idea had taken root that she might become an analyst herself.[116] Psychoanalysis was providing her with a toolkit for thinking beyond the concepts inculcated by her upbringing, and a new vocabulary for interpreting social relationships. Once this shift became clear to Henry and Suzanne, in 1936, they stopped paying, and Françoise accordingly cut her sessions from three to one per week.[117] She moved out of the family home in November 1936, initially to the Latin Quarter, but moved back to Passy in 1937, renting an apartment close to Laforgue's, in Square Henry-Paté. Laforgue also provided Françoise with a new social circle. He brought his analysands together in a 'crazies' club' (*club des piqués*) and invited a group of them to his residence at La Roquebrussanne in Provence. Françoise went along in September 1935 – aged twenty-six, it was her first truly independent trip. Among those she met was Alain Cuny, later a well-known actor, who became a lifelong friend. Laforgue also introduced her to his training analysands André Berge and Georges Mauco, with whom Dolto would work closely in the future (Chapter 4). It was an exhilarating and formative time for her. She later claimed that when she first left home, she was left with only 'the bare minimum' and that life 'really was very hard'.[118] Any such hardship did not last long, for an accounting note of her father's in her archive shows that he transferred her a lump sum of 150,000 francs in late 1936 or early 1937 (equivalent to six times an average contemporary worker's salary) and provided regular subsidies thereafter.[119] Perhaps it was more the memory of the shock of sudden independence that stuck with her.

As well as gaining new friends and freedoms, Françoise became gradually integrated into the SPP group and absorbed its theoretical positions. The concept of the family neurosis having proved effective for her own treatment, she was happy to run with the idea that 'unbalanced' mothers were a major cause of children's psychological distress, and that the intervention of strong-willed fathers – as her own father had intervened to bring her to psychoanalysis and facilitate her physical separation from the family – was needed to prevent their children's neuroses from developing further. Dolto went on to (over-)apply this idea throughout her career, notably with regard to autism (Chapter 5). The theory of penis envy, the idea that women sought unhealthy compensation in intellectual or professional activity for their innate biological inferiority to men, had not proved as useful in her own analysis. But by the time she wrote up her thesis in 1938–39 – publishing it as a book, *Psychanalyse et pédiatrie* (*Psychoanalysis and Paediatrics*), in 1940 with a preface by Pichon – she had adopted this idea too. Discovering her lack of a penis, she wrote, a girl 'feels deprived and attributes this to sexual mutilation by the mother'.[120] To begin with, 'She starts by trying to deny her inferiority by concentrating on the "thingy"' (*le bouton*, i.e. the clitoris) – but is continually reminded of the fact of her 'phallic castration'.[121] In so-called normal development, this occurrence is helpful, as it gives the girl a feeling of security and enables the transfer of libido towards the vagina, whereas the boy continues to fear future castration. The girl can now abandon clitoral masturbation, but 'the withdrawal of the libido from the phallic erogenous zone cannot be done without compensation'.[122] The young girl therefore takes an interest in hairstyles, clothes, ribbons, jewellery – 'unconsciously compensating for the conscious abandonment of the phallus'. She begins to find herself beautiful, regains self-confidence and manages to 'invest' the vagina with libido (instead of the clitoris). In this case, all is well: 'we see well-adjusted emotional and cultural development'.[123]

However, Dolto wrote, such development is conditional on the mother's psychological health. 'If the mother is sufficiently feminine, she lets the child acquire all the skills which gradually make the child her equal.' But if the mother 'undermines the confidence in herself that her daughter needs to have by preventing her from dressing as she chooses, doing as she likes, engaging in pursuits of her social group [...] then feelings of unconscious guilt towards her mother will cause the little girl to present a pathological *vaginal castration complex*'.[124] This may lead in turn to a 'masculinity complex' as outlined by Freud: a 'character neurosis' featuring 'an aggressive envy towards those who "have more"'– i.e. men – and a 'head-long rush into an ambitious struggle, rivalling boys even in sports, in the same activities, in the same studies'.[125] Such girls are drawn by 'libidinal regression' towards 'masculine' careers and/or lesbianism. If they marry, they become 'frigid, vociferous victims [and] castrating mothers, breeders of family neurosis'.[126] They may well end up in psychoanalysis but will make bad analysands, since they continue to blame their problems on men and view their treatment as 'a new means of acquiring phallic power'.[127]

These passages illustrate the paradoxes of Dolto's liberation in these years. She had broken free of her family – thanks to substantial financial support from her father. She had successfully 'rivalled boys' and pursued a 'masculine' career in medicine and psychoanalysis – and to help her do so, she had adopted a discourse which argued that these things were unhealthy and markers of incomplete psychical development. She chose paediatrics as her medical specialism – seen as more acceptable for a woman than other specialisms because of its perceived proximity to traditionally female caring roles. She did not enter the competitive *concours* for more prestigious medical positions, because 'I didn't want to take someone else's place'.[128] In other words she accepted the codification of the highest and most prestigious medical roles as male, and agreed that it would be undermining of the natural order, even a manifestation of neurosis, for her to seek a position customarily reserved for men. It was as if psychoanalysis had offered her a trade-off: helping her overcome her family's resistance to her professional career, at the price of guiding that career down more acceptably 'feminine' paths. Dolto never broached the further question, tackled by Beauvoir in *The Second Sex* (1949), of the gendered assumptions built into Freudian theory. She never asked whether the psychoanalytic concept of 'normal' sexual development might not represent a recuperation or updating of gendered bourgeois morality into a new scientific-sounding vocabulary – whether penis envy and associated concepts might not simply be, as Beauvoir termed them, 'an *Ersatz*, a substitute for morality'.[129] Nor did Dolto revise her views in later decades. When republishing *Psychanalyse et pédiatrie* with Éditions du Seuil in 1971, she left the text more or less unaltered from its original 1930s form.

The sexual development sections of *Psychanalyse et pédiatrie* can be read alongside a lengthy letter Dolto wrote to her father in 1938, asserting her independence in the aftermath of another family argument. By summer 1938, her psychoanalysis was over. Having respected Laforgue's injunction against commencing an intimate romantic or sexual relationship during her analysis (though she became close to Charles Odier, a founder of the SPP, in 1936), she began to experiment in that direction. Not yet qualified as a doctor or psychoanalyst, she remained financially dependent on Henry, who sought to smooth the ongoing tensions between his wife and daughter. In June, Henry wrote to Françoise reproaching her for having slammed a door on her mother, labelling her attitude 'strange' (*insolite*) and 'deeply cruel'.[130] Françoise's reply showed her definitive psychological separation from the ideological environment of her upbringing, and her new understanding of her childhood years. Aged thirty, she now wanted her father to recognise her as a worthy adult: 'if I am "your" child, I'm no longer "a" child … I'm a woman who does you credit (*une femme qui te fait honneur*)'.[131] Contrary to her mother's insinuations, 'There's nothing in my life that does not honour my parents, my friends, my background (*milieu*), and there never has been.' She had persisted with medicine because 'I had to continue my studies in order to get out of that heavy atmosphere in which people read things into every word said and every gesture made.'[132]

She also reflected on her unusual status as an unmarried, professionally qualified woman:

> there's nothing people like less than not knowing which box to put someone in. Single woman? An easy woman who sleeps with whoever she wants. A maiden? then no experience, no maturity of mind and even less responsibility. I am neither one nor the other ... living alone without being wild ... a doctor without being a feminist, nor an apostle, nor an emancipated woman, intellectual, or rebel, but simply a woman, and, what's more – without even renouncing my milieu, the bourgeoisie, to which I feel naturally connected.[133]

Françoise was attempting to work out how to be the kind of woman she wanted to be – professional, independent, bourgeois – without thereby allowing herself to be placed in one of the categories ('easy woman', 'maiden', 'feminist') that came readily to hand for women who did not conform to prevailing values. Elsewhere in the letter, she applied penis envy theory to herself. In asserting her right to study medicine, 'the key goal I was unconsciously aiming for was to be equal with boys by taking a man's job ... As I discover the woman in me, and renounce these masculine internal demands, my interest in diplomas and exam triumphs is disappearing.'[134] This did not mean that she was about to abandon her career ambitions or refrain from completing her degree. After her experience with Delebecque, she would only consider marrying a man who respected her independent professional vocation. She had, however, consented to feminise her career path, and not to push for the highest levels of professional recognition, in the name of her psychological health.

A compromised freedom?

Young women like Dolto, Beauvoir and Zaza were part of a transitional generation, in Dolto's words 'born too soon in a world that was too old'.[135] They were growing up just as the republican education system was being more fully opened up to girls, part of the first cohorts of young women to have a realistic chance of obtaining the *baccalauréat* and *agrégation* and becoming what Juliette Rennes terms 'agents and protagonists' in French public institutions.[136] But these new openings were not easily pursued. In the 1920s, the girls-only École Normale Supérieure de Jeunes Filles at Sèvres still referred to its pupils as 'virgins, future mothers of men'.[137] Dolto, Beauvoir and their contemporaries grew up in a polity that was starting to offer them new opportunities, while simultaneously embedding them in discourses that asserted that to accept such opportunities ran counter to social expectations. For those from high-society families, pursuing professional qualifications implied the refusal of an entire way of life, one built around the idea of young women's decorative and social roles proceeding seamlessly into maternal and familial ones. As Grellet and Kruse put it, 'if they were no longer to fulfil their role, a whole way of living would be called into question'.[138] The visceral determination of Suzanne Marette and Madame Lacoin to retain their daughters within a constrained social bubble was connected to their awareness of themselves as guardians of a society under threat.

While sensing that the world beyond the family enclosure was beginning to change, Dolto, Beauvoir and Zaza were still unusual in resisting family pressures and pushing at the boundaries of what they could achieve. They did so despite lacking role models to follow or clarity as to the kinds of life they might build, and notwithstanding dire warnings about forfeiting their social status and reputation. They passed through periods of lassitude, depression and uncertainty, when neither following the family-approved model, nor pursuing an ill-defined alternative, seemed possible. Those who managed to emerge with successful careers were exceptional by definition, and aware of themselves as such. As Siân Reynolds notes, they tended to put their success down to 'their own perseverance and merit, rather than change in public perception of the need for more gender balance, let alone feminism'.[139] This was certainly true for Dolto, who saw her completion of her thesis as a heroic act.[140]

Ultimately, Dolto found a point of compromise between her career ambitions and her family's desire – backed by leading psychoanalytic theorists – to temper them. Just as she and her father had wanted back in 1934, she had discovered 'the woman in me'. Or rather, having intuited along with Beauvoir that a woman was not something one was born but rather something one became, she finally, unlike Beauvoir, made a conscious decision to embrace the fate of becoming a bourgeois woman. From this point on, her relationship with her parents became warmer, less conflictual, more mutually accepting. She had finally yielded to their contention that she needed to moderate her ambitions in the name of her femininity and family harmony. To be sure, she did this only after having sufficiently established herself professionally and ensured that there was no longer any prospect of her becoming a conventional housewife. Whereas Suzanne's dreams of becoming a doctor in 1900 were never realistically attainable, Françoise would have the career she wanted. However, the concessions she made in the name of femininity were significant. For all that Dolto later claimed that her ambition all along had been to become a '*médecin d'éducation*', the truth was that choosing paediatrics as her specialism was the path of least resistance in a society obsessed with *puériculture*, birth rates and limiting women's professional domains. It was what was left once she had renounced any ambition of taking the competitive examinations for academic or senior hospital positions so as not to take a man's place. As well as taking the decision to limit the scope of her career, she adopted theoretical ideas which justified such limitations on women as a social or even biological necessity, and defended them until the end of her life.

She did not, however, admit to herself that this was what she had done. As she understood things, psychoanalysis, and the wider social and intellectual benefits of entering the psychoanalytic milieu, had brought her freedom, both catalysing and crystallising her rupture with her youthful life. This experience meant that she thereafter understood psychoanalytic ideas as radical more or less by definition. She never considered that they might also be infused with conservative, anti-feminist assumptions that held her and other women back – or if she did, then she considered this an attraction, one which facilitated her reconciliation with the bourgeois society to which she wished to remain attached. Rather than seeing her own example, of successfully forging a career in the face of social resistance, as undermining of Freudian anti-feminist concepts, she decided, in effect, to build her career on them. Just as she was about to begin, however, World War II intervened.

Notes

1 The comparison between Dolto, Beauvoir and Beauvoir's friend 'Zaza' (Élisabeth Lacoin) has been drawn by Isabelle Grellet and Caroline Kruse in *Des jeunes filles exemplaires: Dolto, Beauvoir et Zaza*

(Paris: Hachette, 2004). Beauvoir told the story of her upbringing in *Mémoires d'une jeune fille rangée* (1958). Quotes are taken from the English translation: *Memoirs of a Dutiful Daughter* (1958), trans. James Kirkup (London: Penguin, 2001).
2 Dolto, *Enfances*, p. 70.
3 As this chapter covers the period prior to her marriage, it occasionally refers to Dolto as 'Françoise' where to use her married surname may lead to anachronism or confusion.
4 Dolto, *Autoportrait*, p. 83.
5 *Ibid.*, p. 84.
6 *Ibid.*, pp. 83–5.
7 *Ibid.*, p. 85.
8 *Ibid.*, p. 59.
9 *Ibid.*, pp. 66–8.
10 Martine Sevegrand, *Les Enfants du bon Dieu: Les catholiques français et la procréation au XX siècle* (Paris: Albin Michel, 1995), p. 20.
11 According to a 1914 study of 1,200 families cited in Sevegrand, *Les Enfants*, p. 20.
12 Dolto, *Autoportrait*, pp. 44–5.
13 Arno Mayer, *The Persistence of the Old Regime: Europe to the Great War* (London: Croom Helm, 1981). On philanthropy, see Elisabeth Macknight, 'Faiths, Fortunes and Feminine Duty: Charity in Parisian High Society 1880–1914', *Journal of Ecclesiastical History*, 58 (2007), 482–506.
14 Eric Mension-Rigau, *L'Enfance au château: L'Éducation familiale des élites françaises au vingtième siècle* (Paris: Rivages, 1990), p. 187.
15 Dolto, *Enfances*, pp. 43–4.
16 See Françoise Marette to Henriette Demmler, 3 April 1926, in Dolto, *Lettres de jeunesse*, p. 165, praising an article by Charles Maurras on the death of the Orléanist pretender, Prince Philippe.
17 Dolto, *Autoportrait*, pp. 88–9.
18 Dolto, *Enfances*, p. 73.
19 *Ibid.*, p. 44; Mension-Rigau, *L'Enfance au château*, p. 101.
20 Dolto, *Enfances*, p. 45.
21 Mension-Rigau, *L'Enfance au château*, p. 78.
22 Beauvoir, *Dutiful Daughter*, p. 92.
23 Mension-Rigau, *L'Enfance au château*, pp. 110–11, on complicity between children and servants.
24 Dolto, *Enfances*, p. 70.
25 *Ibid.*, p. 72.
26 *Ibid.*
27 See Grellet and Kruse, *Des jeunes filles*, pp. 19–20, 40–2.

28 *Ibid.*, pp. 45–6.
29 Dolto, *Enfances*, p. 70.
30 See Mension-Rigau, *L'Enfance au château*, pp. 143ff.
31 Dolto, *Enfances*, p. 76.
32 *Ibid.*, p. 77.
33 Dolto, *Autoportrait*, p. 119.
34 *Ibid.*
35 *Ibid.*, p. 50.
36 *Ibid.*; also *Enfances*, pp. 73–4. For examples of the kind of publication she used, see http://postagalene.free.fr/fichiers/Le_Sans-Filiste_Debrouillard.pdf, accessed 29 January 2021.
37 Dolto, *Autoportrait*, p. 128; Grellet and Kruse, *Des jeunes filles*, p. 23. Colette Yver, *Princesses de science* (Paris: Calmann-Levy, 1907).
38 Dolto, *Enfances*, pp. 80–1.
39 Dolto, *Autoportrait*, p. 76; *Enfances*, pp. 80–1.
40 Dolto, *Enfances*, pp. 80–1.
41 Angelo Hesnard, *La Psychanalyse: Théorie sexuelle de Freud* (Paris: Stock, 1924).
42 Dolto, *Autoportrait*, pp. 120–1.
43 *Ibid.*, p. 58.
44 Beauvoir, *Dutiful Daughter*, p. 82.
45 Dolto, *Enfances*, p. 53.
46 Suzanne Marette to Françoise, 5 August 1925, *Lettres de jeunesse*, pp. 156–7.
47 Pierre Marette to Françoise, 31 December 1929, *Lettres de jeunesse*, p. 228.
48 Eugen Weber, *Action Française: Royalism and Reaction in Twentieth-Century France* (Stanford, CA: Stanford University Press, 1962), p. 193.
49 Pierre Marette to Françoise, 22 July 1927, *Lettres de jeunesse*, p. 182.
50 Françoise to Suzanne, 26 September 1922, *Lettres de jeunesse*, p. 130.
51 Suzanne to Françoise, 27 September 1922, *Lettres de jeunesse*, p. 132.
52 Mension-Rigau, *L'Enfance au château*, pp. 251–2; Colin Heywood, *Growing Up in France: From the Ancien Régime to the Third Republic* (Cambridge: Cambridge University Press, 2007), p. 269; See also Heywood's article 'Innocence and Experience: Sexuality among Young People in Modern France, c. 1750–1950', *French History*, 21 (2007), 44–64.
53 Suzanne to Françoise, 20 September 1922, *Lettres de jeunesse*, pp. 124–5.
54 *Ibid.* Suzanne's emphasis.
55 Beauvoir, *Dutifiul Daughter*, p. 115.

56 *Ibid.*, p. 88.
57 Dolto, *Enfances*, p. 43.
58 *Ibid.*
59 *Ibid.*
60 Mension-Rigau, *L'Enfance au château*, p. 251; Grellet and Kruse, *Des jeunes filles*, pp. 32–3.
61 Agnès Dognin to Françoise Marette, 19 April 1931, quoting a previous letter from Françoise. *Lettres de jeunesse*, p. 262.
62 Grellet and Kruse, *Des jeunes filles*, p. 33, citing Zaza's correspondence.
63 Beauvoir, *Dutiful Daughter*, p. 97.
64 Hélène de Beauvoir, *Souvenirs*, ed. Marcelle Routier (Paris: Séguier, 1987), cited in Grellet and Kruse, *Des jeunes filles*, p. 65.
65 Beauvoir, *Dutiful Daughter*, p. 253.
66 Suzanne to Françoise, 15 September 1922 and 19 September 1922, *Lettres de jeunesse*, pp. 121–3.
67 Grellet and Kruse, *Des jeunes filles*, p. 122.
68 Letter from Zaza to Simone de Beauvoir, 1928, cited in *ibid.*, p. 123.
69 Dolto, *Enfances*, p. 106.
70 *Ibid.*, p. 52.
71 Jean Marette to Suzanne, 26 September 1922, *Lettres de jeunesse*, p. 131.
72 Pierre Marette to Françoise, 31 December 1929, *Lettres de jeunesse*, p. 228.
73 See Reynolds, *France between the Wars*, pp. 48–9.
74 See Dolto, *Cause des enfants*, pp. 399–400.
75 Dolto, *Autoportrait*, pp. 124–5.
76 *Ibid.*, and 'Traversée du siècle', in Yann Potin (ed.), *Françoise Dolto, archives de l'intime* (Paris: Gallimard, 2008), p. 118. The fee-paying *lycée*'s collusion is possibly explained by a desire to retain their pupil, and thus her fees, for another year.
77 Dolto, *Enfances*, p. 78.
78 Dolto, 'Traversée du siècle', p. 118.
79 On Pelletier, see Joan Wallach Scott, *Only Paradoxes to Offer: French Feminists and the Rights of Man* (Cambridge, MA: Harvard University Press, 1996).
80 Agnès Dognin to Françoise Marette, e.g. 14 September 1929, *Lettres de jeunesse*, pp. 224–6. Dolto's side of the correspondence is lost.
81 Françoise Marette to Élisabeth Weilandt, 11 November 1928, *Lettres de jeunesse*, pp. 205–6.
82 On women's work in nineteenth-century religious orders, see Matthieu Brejon de Lavergnée, *Le Temps des cornettes: Histoire des Filles de la Charité XIX-XXe siècle* (Paris: Fayard, 2018).

83 Agnès Dognin to Françoise, 30 August 1928, *Lettres de jeunesse*, p. 203. Original emphasis.
84 Dolto, *Enfances*, pp. 77–9; 'Traversée du siècle', pp. 120–1.
85 Dolto, *Autoportrait*, pp. 54–5.
86 Sandrine Sanos, *Simone de Beauvoir: Creating a Feminist Existence in the World* (New York: Oxford University Press, 2016), p. 12.
87 Based on figures from Antoine Prost, *Histoire de l'enseignement en France, 1800–1967* (Paris: Colin, 1968), p. 243, and Juliette Rennes, 'The French Republic and Women's Access to Professional Work: Issues and Controversies in France from the 1870s to the 1930s', *Gender & History*, 23 (2011), 341–66.
88 Dolto, *Enfances*, p. 29. On Deauville in World War I, see Yves Aublet, *Dans la tourmente de la Grande guerre: 1914–1918: Deauville, Trouville et le canton* (Cabourg: Cahiers du Temps, 2001).
89 Katrin Schultheiss, *Bodies and Souls: Politics and the Professionalization of Nursing in France, 1880–1922* (Cambridge, MA: Harvard University Press, 2001).
90 Margaret Darrow, *French Women and the First World War: War Stories of the Home Front* (Oxford: Berg, 2000), p. 40.
91 *Ibid.*, pp. 71–2.
92 Macknight, 'Faiths, Fortunes and Feminine Duty', 489.
93 Darrow, *French Women*, p. 72.
94 Dolto, *Autoportrait*, p. 127.
95 Françoise to Henry Marette, 15 June 1938, *Lettres de jeunesse*, p. 535.
96 Grellet and Kruse, *Des jeunes filles*, p. 184.
97 Dolto, *Autoportrait*, p. 115.
98 *Ibid.*, pp. 115–8.
99 Dolto, 'Traversée du siècle', p. 122; *Enfances*, p. 92.
100 Dolto, *Autoportrait*, p. 114.
101 Françoise to Suzanne, 22 September 1931, *Lettres de jeunesse*, pp. 279–80.
102 Dolto, *Enfances*, p. 89.
103 Dolto, *Autoportrait*, p. 111.
104 *Ibid.*
105 *Ibid.*
106 Dolto, *Enfances*, pp. 89–90.
107 Françoise to Henry, 22 July 1934, *Lettres de jeunesse*, p. 382.
108 Dolto, *Autoportrait*, pp. 312–13, n. 54. According to Philippe Marette, Laforgue charged 300 francs per hour in the 1930s. Adjusted for inflation, this is equivalent to the notoriously high prices – 500–600 francs per session – charged by Jacques Lacan in the 1970s.
109 Françoise to Henry, 22 July 1934, *Lettres de jeunesse*, p. 382.

110 Henry to Françoise, 24 July 1934, *Lettres de jeunesse*, p. 384.
111 Dolto, *Enfances*, p. 95.
112 *Ibid.*
113 *Ibid.*, p. 94.
114 Françoise to Henry, 15 June 1938, *Lettres de jeunesse*, p. 534.
115 Dolto, *Enfances*, p. 95.
116 *Ibid.*, p. 96.
117 Dolto, *Autoportrait*, p. 312, n. 54.
118 Dolto, *Enfances*, p. 98.
119 Potin (ed.), *Archives de l'intime*, p. 122.
120 Françoise Dolto, *Psychanalyse et pédiatrie* (Paris: Seuil, 1971 (1940)), published in English as *Psychoanalysis and Paediatrics: Key Psychoanalytical Concepts with Sixteen Clinical Observations of Children*, trans. Françoise Hivernel and Fiona Sinclair (London: Karnac, 2013), p. 75.
121 Dolto, *Psychoanalysis and Paediatrics*, p. 76.
122 *Ibid.*, p. 77.
123 *Ibid.*, p. 79.
124 *Ibid.*, pp. 79, 81, original emphasis.
125 *Ibid.*, p. 85.
126 *Ibid.*, p. 86.
127 *Ibid.*, p. 89.
128 Dolto, *Autoportrait*, p. 153.
129 Simone de Beauvoir, *The Second Sex*, trans. Constance Borde and Sheila Malovany Chevallier (New York: Vintage, 2010 (1949)), p. 76. Italics in original.
130 Henry to Françoise, 3 June 1938. *Lettres de jeunesse*, p. 526.
131 Françoise to Henry, 15 June 1938. *Lettres de jeunesse*, pp. 528–39, 530.
132 *Ibid.*, pp. 530, 535.
133 *Ibid.*, p. 537.
134 *Ibid.*, p. 535.
135 Dolto, *Autoportrait*, p. 54.
136 Rennes, 'The French Republic', 344–6.
137 Grellet and Kruse, *Des jeunes filles*, p. 68.
138 *Ibid.*, pp. 15–16.
139 Reynolds, *France between the Wars*, p. 98.
140 Dolto, 'Traversée du siècle', p. 124.

3

Humanism, holism and guilt: Dolto, psychoanalysis and Catholicism from Occupation to Liberation

The years between 1939 and 1953 were ones of enormous upheaval in France. Following the destructive and divisive experience of war, occupation and liberation, by the early 1950s the country was rapidly modernising its economy, while caught up in Cold War geopolitics and fighting to retain its empire. Women had become full citizens, a baby boom was under way and the defeat and moral debasement of the Vichy regime had left the extreme Right discredited. While the 1950s remained an age of social conservatism, signs of changes in attitudes to families, children and gender were appearing. As Sarah Fishman has shown, Sigmund Freud, Simone de Beauvoir and Alfred Kinsey were becoming reference points for incipient changes in social attitudes around sexuality and the self, and France was becoming an ever more 'psychologised' society.[1]

These developments followed a war and occupation in which 600,000 French soldiers and civilians died, 1.6 million soldiers became prisoners of war and 650,000 people undertook forced labour (Service du travail obligatoire – STO) in Germany. Some 75,000 French-resident Jews were murdered in the Holocaust; thousands more spent time in concentration camps or in hiding. The postwar recovery was initially slow to filter through to households, with hardships and cold winters persisting into the later 1940s. Against this backdrop, the Communist Party, imbued with the moral authority of the Resistance, became a major political force. The war meanwhile disrupted France's institutions, including all of those with significance for Dolto. The French psychoanalytic movement largely dissolved, with many members forced into exile. Vichy promoted a strongly patriarchal vision of the family and gender roles, further excluding women from the professions. Its corporatist policies led to the formation of the Ordre des Médecins and increased state oversight of doctors. The Catholic Church assumed greater public prominence, promoting the themes of guilt, expiation and internal renewal.

The first fifteen years of Dolto's career were thus transitional and disruptive – for her, for the psychoanalytic movement and for France in general. Themes of guilt and renewal conditioned her thinking in these years – which, on a personal level, were not unhappy ones. In the 1940s, she began to re-evaluate the foundations of her faith, prompted by her marriage in 1942 to Boris Dolto, an adherent of the Orthodox Christian Church. During the Occupation, Dolto was one of a handful of psychoanalysts to remain in Paris. She continued to see patients in her capacity as a general practitioner, and to incorporate Freudian ideas into her practice. Beyond this, she looked for ways to take her psychoanalytically informed, holistic brand of medicine into the public realm. Between 1940 and 1944, this meant working with organisations sympathetic to Vichy and its ideology, notably the Fondation Française pour l'Étude des Problèmes Humains (French Foundation for the Study of Human Problems – also known as the FFEPH or the Fondation Carrel) and the Pétainist magazine *Vrai*. In the very different political climate of the Liberation, Dolto explored cooperation with figures on the Left, and at one point even referred to herself as a Trotskyist.[2] However, the hardening of Cold War dividing lines in 1947–48 found Dolto and her closest colleagues very much on the side of capitalism and Christianity. Psychoanalysis came under strong attack from French communists in 1949, and in the 1950s was widely perceived as a bourgeois discipline. By 1953, the French psychoanalytic movement had become divided, as its practitioners' very different experiences of the war compounded their disagreements about who should practise psychoanalysis and what exactly it was for. The resulting split in the movement had complex causes, but this chapter contends that underlying politico-religious tensions, linked to choices made under the Occupation, were a factor. The desire of Catholic thinkers grouped around the journals *Psyché* and *Études carmélitaines* to reconcile Catholicism and psychoanalysis, specifically by focusing on the theme of guilt, created tensions with some Jewish analysts that were connected to contrasting wartime loyalties. Dolto was a central figure in the split, and clashed in particular with Sacha Nacht, a Jewish analyst and former resister – revealing antisemitic prejudices in the process. Dolto's role can be related both to her upbringing, and to her response to the difficult moral questions involved in responding to defeat, occupation, collaboration and the Holocaust. The split resulted in Dolto being excluded from the IPA, and thereafter becoming closely allied with her fellow outcast from the international movement, Jacques Lacan.

Humanism and holism, 1935–45

Influential French intellectuals of the 1930s approached humans – or rather, 'Man' – holistically, as a complex physical, psychological and spiritual being. This thinking, drawn from philosophy, psychology, theology and the wider social Catholic movement, spread to scientists, engineers, technocrats, politicians and industrialists, a number of whom inclined to right-wing political sympathies. Such thinkers attempted to instrumentalise holism to develop solutions to so-called human problems that would take the psychological, biological and social complexity of 'Man' – the masculine term that was very frequently used – into account. The essential idea was that humane treatment of workers that understood them not as mere cogs in an industrial machine but in terms of their whole being – albeit within the parameters of a paternalist framework defined and controlled by scientifically educated elites – would both be beneficial for its own sake and help to optimise corporate organisation and efficiency. Combining a scientific disposition with a spiritual (usually Catholic) outlook, 1930s technocrats were thus open to scientific psychology and sociology, but also to esoteric disciplines on the fringes of established science and medicine, such as graphology, characterology or acupuncture, that might conceivably make some contribution to understanding 'Man' in his totality.[3]

Alexis Carrel, the 1912 Nobel laureate for medicine, argued in his bestselling *L'Homme, cet inconnu* (*Man, The Unknown*, 1935) that 'Man is an indivisible whole of extreme complexity. No simple representation of him can be obtained ... Man, as known to the specialists, is far from being the concrete man, the real man.'[4] Like the engineer Jean Coutrot in his influential work *De quoi vivre* (*The Stuff of Living*, 1935), Carrel approached the psychology of labour by taking into account all aspects of workers' lives, in contrast to the discrete, task-based psychology of work associated with Frederick Winslow Taylor and his French popularisers in the 1910s.[5] Carrel proposed a mixture of eugenics, pronatalism and education as the solution to endemic social problems, which, he argued, had caused a 'decrease in the intellectual and moral calibre of those who carry the responsibility of public affairs'.[6] Though opposed to the Nazis, Carrel admired far-right leaders such as Jacques Doriot and Colonel de la Rocque, and expressed hostility to the Third Republic. He converted to Catholicism in 1938.

The interwar drive for technical organisation and modernisation arose first in engineering, but it soon extended to topics such as household management, as Jackie Clarke has shown in her discussion of Paulette Bernège's housewives' manuals.[7] In a medical context, holism meant conceiving of the human body and mind as a single, complex, interrelated system. The logic of such thinking – which arose against a backdrop of increasing specialisation among French doctors, incentivised by the higher fees that specialists could attract within the medical welfare system – implied that over-specialisation of the profession into niche sub-fields should be resisted.[8] Medical holists were interested in homeopathy, esoterism and eugenics, fields which promised a more complete understanding of mind-body interactions.[9] Joan Tumblety has shown that similar holistic thinking underpinned the 'physical culture' movement of the interwar period: physical culturists believed themselves to be pushing at the limitations of empirical medicine, and invoked spiritual and psychic ideas in their quest to 'regenerate the race' by understanding the 'whole man'.[10] This example suggests an undercurrent of racial and colonial anxiety in the entire holistic tendency – a sense that France might not be able to maintain its empire if it did not make use of all available tools to maximise the physical and mental quality of its white population.

Freudian psychoanalysis had some natural affinities with these holistic approaches, and indeed helped to inform them. Freud's writings suggested that the whole of a person's history and the entirety of their psychical life were relevant to their current state of health; psychoanalysis taught that physical symptoms were conditioned by mental processes and often explicable in terms of them. Coutrot and his 'cercle de réflexion' of former *polytechniciens* at X-Crise read

Freud along with Henri Bergson and other theorists of unconscious and irrational thought. 'Man is not made of reason alone', Coutrot argued. 'All that he has within him in terms of sensibility also profoundly conditions his existence and obeys quite different laws.'[11] Holistic thinkers were often also Catholics. Holism resonated with, and existed in the context of, moves to bring Catholicism into greater dialogue with the human sciences. Coutrot, for example, read and corresponded with Pierre Teilhard de Chardin, an unorthodox Jesuit priest, philosopher and palaeontologist. A Catholic version of holistic humanism (*humanisme intégral*) was influentially articulated by the philosopher Jacques Maritain, who stressed the importance of recognising the material and spiritual dimensions of the whole person.[12] Maritain helped French Catholicism to respond to Pope Pius XI's condemnation of Action Française in 1926, by proposing that Action Française's 'politics first' motto, with its emphasis on temporal power, be replaced by a new 'primacy of the spiritual'.[13] The subsequent decade became a time of Catholic intellectual and spiritual renewal, driven by new journals that followed Maritain's lead such as *Esprit* (from 1932) and *Sept* (from 1934).[14] Religious orders played a significant role in this renewal – notably the Carmelite order with its journal *Études carmélitaines*, edited from 1932 by Father Bruno de Jésus-Marie, an intellectual follower of Maritain.

This intellectual shift helped to stimulate Catholic interest in psychoanalysis. Father Bruno used Freud in his research into mysticism.[15] Another of Maritain's followers, the philosopher Roland Dalbiez, contributed significantly to disseminating psychoanalytic ideas among Catholic intellectuals with his book *La Méthode psychanalytique et la doctrine freudienne* (1936).[16] Like the psychoanalyst-medics of *L'Évolution Psychiatrique* discussed in Chapter 1, Dalbiez distinguished psychoanalytic therapeutic techniques, which he considered valuable, from Freud's theoretical standpoint which Dalbiez saw as riddled with errors.[17] From 1935, Bruno organised 'study days' in religious psychology. He encouraged psychoanalysts to attend and to publish their ideas in *Études carmélitaines*, and even to apply psychoanalytic insights to the psychology of religion itself.

These twin trends – organisational and medical holism, and Catholic humanism – were vital elements of the intellectual context in which Dolto began her career. The Dolto of *Psychanalyse et pédiatrie* was a holist in her medical orientation. She thought it essential for doctors to understand psychological as well as physiological functioning; otherwise, they would be in the situation of 'a surgeon who, faced with an abscess about to burst, tries to hide the swelling and smear it with analgesics instead of draining the abscess'.[18] Psychology was the root cause of many if not most physical symptoms, and thus should be central to medical training and treatment. Dolto emphasised general practice medicine over hospital-based specialisms. As she saw it, family doctors – who best understood their patients' personal and social circumstances because they could develop relationships with them and their families over long periods – were best placed to apply holistic and psychological insights on a day-to-day basis. In line with this holistic stance, the medical practice that Dolto opened on 1 September 1939 announced her as a 'generalist and paediatrician', not a specialist or psychoanalyst, though she clearly intended to utilise Freudian concepts. In *Psychanalyse et pédiatrie* she did not venture thoughts on religion or spirituality; the thesis was limited to outlining major concepts of Freudian theory and demonstrating how family doctors might apply them to children. She did, however, send a copy to Paul Jury, the first French priest to undergo psychoanalysis, who by 1939 was practising a kind of 'wild' psychoanalysis (often with children) in his priest's cassock.[19] Over the next fifteen years, Dolto's Christianity and her understanding of psychoanalysis became much more closely intertwined.

World War II, an inescapable part of the context for this, represented an immediate rupture in Dolto's career plans. From October 1939 until June 1940 she was requisitioned, like many female doctors, to make 'sanitary visits' to classes of refugee children in the Paris region.[20] On the German invasion in June 1940 she joined the exodus from Paris, but returned to the capital in August and remained there for the duration – one of only a handful of psychoanalysts to do so, along with John Leuba, Marc Schlumberger, Georges Parcheminey and Juliette Favez-Boutonnier.[21] In September, the Occupation authorities placed Freud's books on the 'Otto list' of banned works. The SPP disbanded, evacuated its archives and ceased producing its journal.[22] Marie Bonaparte made her way to Greece and ultimately South Africa; Rudolph Loewenstein, Raymond de Saussure and others left for the United States; Sophie Morgenstern committed suicide. Dolto took on some of their analysands.[23]

As Hanna Diamond has noted, female testimonies of the June 1940 exodus are relatively thin on the ground.[24] Dolto's experience was far from typical, since her wealth and access to a car enabled her to escape the worst of the suffering, but it may serve as evidence of attitudes among her privileged social group. She was still in Paris on 10 June 1940, when, with the German armies fast approaching, the government left for Bordeaux. That day she wrote to her friend and sometime lover Hubert Jausion expressing residual confidence in final victory – but on the eleventh she decided to leave.[25] She headed by car to Brittany, where she stayed with a friend, and visited her mother who had also left and was staying at Le Croisic, on the coast west of Nantes. On 17 June, Marshal Philippe Pétain, having been installed as Prime Minister, announced his intention to seek an armistice. That day, two of Dolto's family members were turned back from crossing the Loire by French troops. On the nineteenth, by displaying her medical card, she managed to pass through already-occupied Nantes and cross the Loire. She drove to her aunt's house in Bordeaux, where she stayed for nine days, during which time the armistice was signed. Not enjoying her aunt's company ('she gives off an aura of hostile opacity and a "morally ugly" radiance which makes me pity her'), on 28 June she moved on to friends in Puichéric, near Carcassonne, where she remained for several weeks enjoying the Mediterranean climate.[26]

Dolto therefore did not share the hardships of those who took to the roads south of Paris, often on foot, in a forlorn attempt to outrun the Nazis. She did, however, experience the general feeling of dislocation, and the widely reported sense of the *exode* as a forced extended holiday, one that enabled a reconnection with the French countryside.[27] In her letters from Puichéric in July 1940, she articulated a sense of a deep, spiritual connection to the landscape: 'I see that I like the countryside. I always believed it. But I wasn't detached. At the moment I'm completely detached from everything – context, habits – and only spiritual values abide.'[28] This renewed relationship with rural France spoke to her sense of national identity, which she now articulated using agricultural metaphors: 'A country isn't like an individual (and our leaders are at fault for not having understood this). It does not die as long as it has men on its soil, born of it and nourishing themselves from its produce. The life of a country is more like plant life than human life. It goes through periodic rebirths.'[29]

Dolto's language here resonated with that of Pétain, who three weeks earlier had contended that 'the earth does not lie. It remains your recourse, it is the Fatherland itself.'[30] Vichy would soon launch, as part of its National Revolution, policies aimed at fostering a 'return to the land'. On her return to Paris, Dolto remained convinced of the redemptive, therapeutic value of the outdoors. Her surviving case records from the Occupation period show her advising patients to spend lots of time in fresh air or to go and work with rural artisans. One patient, referred in 1942 for 'emotional backwardness, signs of mental infirmity, mutism, idleness' and diagnosed by Dolto as suffering from a 'reflected maternal neurosis and inhibitory emotional shock', became, with her encouragement, a gardener.[31] A fourteen-year-old boy, referred to her in 1941 for 'theft, masturbation, mutism', was encouraged to give up intellectual work and attend 'an open-air school'.[32]

Writing to her father from Puichéric in 1940, Dolto further stated her

> faith in France's recovery along the lines set out by Pétain. [Before the war] I loved France, but I despised her politics and those who were officially respected, and that concealed from me how much I loved France. Now I think she is very sick. Perhaps fatally wounded ... but one can try to do something and contribute to its recovery [*redressement*], and it's wonderful to be the age I am, as I may live to see that recovery.[33]

In view of such statements, Dolto critic Didier Pleux has speculated that her subsequent correspondence, which in the published volume is relatively thin for the 1941–44 period, may have been censored by the editors to hide evidence of collaborationist attitudes.[34] There is no evidence in Dolto's archives to support this. The relative lack of correspondence can be more easily explained by the fact that her family members (whose correspondence predominates in Dolto's archives for this period) rarely left Paris during the war, saw each other regularly and so had little need to write. Dolto's Pétainist sympathies are not surprising in view of her family's political and social views and her incomplete break with them, as described in Chapter

2. Pétain's explanations for France's defeat resonated with people who had been brought up to distrust the Republic. Dolto's brother Jean, who fought as an officer in 1940 and was awarded the Croix de Guerre during the French retreat, felt that 'the country was terribly contaminated, the army as well, and we're paying dearly for all the weaknesses of the recent years and for all of the lies we've had stuffed down our throats'.[35] Her mother Suzanne wrote on 28 July 1940 that 'I have absolute confidence in the patriotism and the will of the Marshal who will do everything to begin the recovery of our poor country, using quite modern ideas but safeguarding all French traditions. His task is terrible, and his self-sacrifice should bring him the gratitude and assistance of all French people.'[36]

The fact that support for Pétainism was utterly conventional for people of Dolto's background in 1940 does not mean that her views can be explained away in terms of her youth and 'naivety', as Muriel Djéribi-Valentin, the editor of her correspondence, has claimed.[37] Dolto was thirty-one in 1940, a qualified doctor and published author, and fully able to assert independence from her family's opinions where this mattered to her. Her Pétainism in 1940 was well considered. It aligned easily enough with her medical holist views. As her mother's comment about 'quite modern ideas' indicates, in sweeping away the Republic, the National Revolution offered opportunities to technicians, engineers and social reformers, many of whom were appointed to influential positions.[38] In Paris and Vichy, technocrats seized the chance to implement schemes that had become stuck in the impasses of Third Republic politics, such as the integration of Parisian public transport, carried out in 1942. The *polytechnicien* and railway engineer Jean Berthelot became Minister of Communications. Another *polytechnicien*, Jean Bichelonne, served at the Ministry of Industrial Production, alongside Pierre Pucheu from the Comité des Forges, the steel industry's co-ordinating committee. These were people to whom Dolto's father Henry Marette, himself a *polytechnicien* and steel factory director, could relate. Montbard was in the Occupied Zone, and Métal Déployé, the Marette business, appears to have rapidly adjusted to producing output for German use.[39]

It seemed likely that social policy, too, would be open to technocratic reform schemes and Pétainist regeneration. The prospect appealed to Dolto and caused her to rethink her career goals. 'I don't know if I can continue on the path I've chosen,' she wrote to her father in summer 1940. 'I would quite like to work in education, since it is finally going to be taken in a direction which seems to me to be full of promise.'[40] 'Education' did not necessarily mean 'schooling': when Pétain spoke of education he did so in terms of the transmission of morality more than of knowledge.[41] Throughout her career Dolto used the term '*éducation*' similarly broadly (or holistically) to mean something closer to 'upbringing'; her posthumous book *Les Chemins de l'éducation* (*CdE*) (*The Pathways of Education*, 1994) was concerned with parenting and medico-psychological treatment, not schools. Her desire to become involved with '*éducation*' in 1940 therefore suggests an intention to engage with how children were being raised, both by parents and by society. Pétain's statements on education suggested that Vichy would attempt an ideological reform of the school system, which it saw as a repository of republican idealism and pacifism. A measure was passed requiring primary teachers to have a classical education, with the aim of thereby changing the social and political composition of the teaching body. Teaching unions and teacher training schools were disbanded. Jews and Freemasons were banned from teaching, and Catholic religious orders returned to schools. The crucifix went up on school walls, along with Pétain's picture. There was a revival of physical education and sport. The Ministry of Education, considered a stronghold of Radical republicanism, was downgraded, with the more socially conservative Ministry of Family and Health accorded a greater role.[42] From Dolto's perspective, all of this hinted at the possibility that, since education was being withdrawn from the control of secular, universalist, positivist republicanism, it would become more open to her Freudian, Catholic, spiritual thinking. There might also be new opportunities in the broadly educational institutions being set up beyond schools, such as Vichy's new 'Mother and Baby Protection Centres' (*Centres de protection maternelle infantile*).

Dolto's September 1940 decision to take up a part-time medical role at Hôpital Trousseau, a children's hospital in the working-class twelfth arrondissement of Paris, can perhaps be understood in this context. She initially arrived at Trousseau as a doctor in the outpatient department for '*troubles fonctionnels*', meaning symptoms without a clear medical basis.[43] This replaced her job assisting

Édouard Pichon at Hôpital Bretonneau, Pichon having died in January 1940. In 1941, she began to help out unofficially in the neuropsychiatry department, taking children into psychotherapy. She saw these patients in a cloakroom four metres long and two and a quarter metres wide, which her colleagues referred to as 'a little confession booth'.[44] She gradually turned this into a semi-official, long-term but apparently unpaid role, lasting until 1978.[45] On one level, this was an opportunistic way to incorporate psychoanalysis into occupied France's public health system. This was the sense in which Dolto's daughter Catherine later spoke of the clinic taking place 'in absolute administrative secrecy, completely illegally' – thus rhetorically equating it to an act of resistance.[46] But equally, Dolto's actions may be placed in the context of her summer 1940 statements on her faith in the path to national recovery set out by Pétain. By applying her brand of holistic medicine and psychological education in a hospital setting, with working-class patients, she would have understood herself to be working to improve the physical, mental and moral health of the French race, in the spirit of the National Revolution. As she stated in a much later interview, 'doing psychoanalysis is to be at the service of people who live in the same time as me, who are from the ethnicity [*ethnie*] as me'.[47] In this way, though her ideas were not inseparably wedded to the Pétainist vision, they aligned with it smoothly enough.

This interpretation is consistent with some of Dolto's other actions in the Occupation years. In social policy, the major beneficiary of Vichy's willingness to embrace reformers and modernisers was Alexis Carrel. France's defeat and Vichy's rhetoric of renewal seemed to vindicate Carrel's 1930s prescriptions for remaking society, and the religious metaphors that became prevalent in the early 1940s chimed with his desire to see a 'spiritualisation' of politics.[48] Carrel became something of an ideological lodestar for Vichy and its institutions. Following a meeting between Carrel and Pétain, the FFEPH, headed by Carrel, became operational from summer 1942.[49] The FFEPH was to be a wide-ranging social policy unit, with a research function deliberately rivalling (or displacing) that of universities. In 1942, possibly thanks to an intervention by René Laforgue, Dolto was invited to work for the foundation's 'Mother and Child Centre' (*Centre de la mère et de l'enfant*) located on Boulevard St Germain.[50] She met

Carrel in September 1942, and began work that December on a salary of 5,000 francs per month.[51] The centre aimed to research the biological and psychological factors affecting pregnancy, birth, parenting and child development. Dolto was assigned to the 'psychobiology and mental hygiene team', housed alongside groups researching the 'development of adolescence' and 'biological lineage'.[52] The centre never really got off the ground, however, owing to management disputes and Carrel's poor health. It is not clear how much, if anything, Dolto contributed before resigning in November 1943. During her year of employment there she continued to see private patients, worked at Trousseau and gave birth to her first child. Alain Drouard's history of the FFEPH divides its 250–300 staff into a small group of Carrelite true believers, and the majority for whom participation represented a passing phase – a job and salary in uncertain times, or sometimes even cover for resistance activities – and who subsequently tended to deny or downplay their participation in this indisputably Vichyite body for reputational reasons.[53] Drouard places Dolto in the second group. Dolto wrote little about the FFEPH in her memoirs. She was not one of those engaged in resistance activities: asked about this in 1988, she replied 'but, I couldn't! I had a baby.'[54] Probably the FFEPH represented for Dolto a source of income and a potential opportunity to shape social policy in line with her holistic, Freudian orientation. But the episode also suggests that, well into 1943, she did not see that orientation as incompatible with the broader Vichy project.

Nor was the FFEPH episode the first time that Dolto had contributed to an overtly Pétainist cultural enterprise. In 1941, she published articles in *Vrai*, a forty-eight-page fortnightly describing itself as a 'social and artistic women's news magazine'. *Vrai* first appeared in October 1941, published in Paris where the Nazis strictly controlled the press. It was moderately priced, at six francs.[55] The target audience was middle-class women with a degree of leisure time. The magazine contained extracts from novels, book reviews, games and quizzes and articles on fashion, style and art. There were 'make-do-and-mend' features explaining how canny housewives could circumvent wartime shortages, such as by making jam without jars.[56] Advertisements included promotions for Linguaphone's language-learning materials, a course in advertising design at a Parisian art school and Charles Trenet's music.[57] It had a glossy style, with plenty of pictures and illustrations.

Vrai was not presented as a political publication, but was clearly Pétainist in its themes and imagery, with prominent early articles aligned with Vichy's social priorities. The first issue's cover featured a full-page photo of a smiling baby with the caption 'Birth rate, problem no. 1', trailing an interview with Vichy's Family and Health Minister Serge Huard. Every subsequent issue carried a pronatalist article and/or deplored the '600,000 little French children assassinated every year' through abortion.[58] Discussions of older children emphasised physical outdoor activity and celebrated young, Aryan, muscular, naked or semi-naked bodies.[59] The magazine promoted beauty as an important marker of the quality of children's bodies – 'Let our children be BEAUTIFUL!' was the subtitle of one pronatalist article accompanied by a picture of smiling children in swimsuits.[60] Other classic Vichy themes given conspicuous treatment included POWs – heavily featured in the run-up to Christmas 1941 – and agriculture ('farmers of Landerneau, the Marshal is pleased with you!'). Women were praised for replacing absent POWs on the land: 'What eulogy can we give to the woman left alone in the fields, battling difficulties of all kinds, during her husband's captivity?'[61] Other articles reminded women of their ultimate subservience to their husbands. A feature on famous historical couples (such as the Chateaubriands) was entitled 'The glory of a man makes his wife HAPPY'.[62]

Soon after *Vrai* first appeared, Dolto was thinking about contributing to it. She asked a friend, the Sorbonne Indologist Louis Renou, for his opinion of the publication; he replied on 3 November 1941 that 'it looks pretty good' ('*cela ne se présente pas mal*').[63] In the third issue, appearing on 15 November, an article appeared by 'F.M.', Dolto's maiden initials – the Ordre des Médecins forbade doctors to write for commercial publications under their own name. Entitled 'Get Yourselves a Family Doctor!', it appeared a few pages behind the obligatory pronatalist feature. Deploring the 'mystique of specialists', 'F.M.' encouraged her readers to trust instead in family doctors, whose holistic knowledge of patients and their family histories could place symptoms such as stomach complaints into their proper, psychological, context. She insisted on the prevalence of psychogenic aetiologies, attacking 'the custom of considering diseases or ailments ... like separate entities, accidents which have nothing to do with [the patient's] personality'.[64] Her article argued for medicine to be fully cognisant of the psychological component of physical illness:

> Intoxicated by the Pasteurian discoveries, we have lost sight of the fact that microbes are only the triggers for infections, and that in order to become activated they need to encounter hosts who are in a sufficiently vulnerable state of health ... Contrary to what many seem to believe, the psychological element plays an extremely important role in the appearance and course of development of most, if not all diseases ... There is a certain moral climate which helps disease to spawn ... Disease is not an accident.[65]

As a generalist herself at this time, 'F.M.' had a personal interest in persuading people to choose the pastoral care of a medical generalist. Doing so put her in tune with the intellectual orientation of Carrel and Coutrot, while also aligning with the nostalgic and traditionalist components of Vichy thinking. Her idealised local doctor appeared to inhabit a rural France of small-scale, ethnically homogeneous communities unsullied by industrial civilisation. She criticised Vichy's centralising, bureaucratic tendencies, as manifested in the removal of strict privacy controls on the *carnet de santé* (health record).[66] Dolto argued that the state should concentrate on renewing the patient-doctor relationship rather than on developing intrusive bureaucracy. Her anti-bureaucratic discourse and idealised vision of pre-modern rural France remained part of her thinking in much later writings.

Her November 1941 article ended by announcing a new regular feature, consisting of

> advice to parents with a view to promoting moral and physical health in their children. In everyday life, many problems arise around children which demand practical solutions. How to react in such cases ...?

This is striking for its resemblance to the concept of *Lorsque l'enfant paraît*, the radio programme which made Dolto famous some thirty-five years later. The next edition of *Vrai*, dated 1 December, began to fulfil the promise, with a column by 'M.' (Dolto once more) entitled 'Our children ... Do you know how to talk to them?' This consisted of a set of hypothetical parenting scenarios, with an outline of a 'wrong' and 'right' way to respond in each case. The thrust of the advice was that

> To win and always keep a child's confidence, all you have to do is to make sure never to use your superiority to triumph over them. You mustn't try to 'reason with' children, at least not until they are 7 or 8. Rather you have to act 'reasonably' towards them.[67]

'M.' exhorted mothers (not parents in general, as use of grammatical gender in the French made clear) not to shout, get angry or humiliate their children: 'always remain calm. Above all be compassionate':

> IF YOU ARE ANNOYED WITH YOUR CHILD
>
> NEVER SAY I'm going to buy another child! The police will come and take you.
>
> BECAUSE It's not true. You are setting them an example of lying behaviour.
>
> ACT REASONABLY
> - Never shout more loudly than the child who is acting out. Be quiet and remain indifferent. Go into another room, wait for the child to calm down ... Once they've become quiet, or have cried genuine tears, you can give them an affectionate scolding followed by a kiss if they want ...
>
> NEVER SAY Look, everybody is laughing at you. What will people think?
>
> BECAUSE
> You should never humiliate a child, especially if they're naturally proud ... Your response pushes them to focus on the effect they produce on others. You are teaching them vanity.
>
> ACT REASONABLY
> - Never scold a child in public. Don't say anything while they're acting out. Wait until it's over before you respond.[68]

The construction of this article, with its didactic headings, is more rigid than Dolto's later style, but the messaging is recognisably hers: a focus on immediate, everyday situations, and an attempt to provide direct, clear advice, drawing on Freudian concepts without explicitly naming them or employing psychoanalytic jargon. There was also a libertarian angle to her advice, following the line taken by her supervisor Édouard Pichon as described in Chapter 1 – Dolto encouraged parents to refrain from violent and impulsive punishment, and to treat children as intelligent, rational, desiring beings.

Despite being advertised as the first in a series, this article was the last that Dolto published in *Vrai*. This may be linked to the magazine's financial struggles: from December 1941 the issues shrank in size, and appeared less often, before ceasing altogether in April 1942. It reappeared from June 1943 until July 1944, without participation from Dolto or other doctors, with a heavier emphasis on prisoners' wives, war widows and cultural features. Dolto's advice column was instead eventually continued in a publication with a very different political standpoint, in the markedly different political circumstances of January 1946.

Femmes françaises ('*French Women*') was the fortnightly paper of the Union des Femmes Françaises (UFF). Though communist-dominated, the UFF attempted to bring together women from across the tripartite Resistance alliance of communists, Christian Democrats and socialists. Its paper, edited by the left-wing novelist and journalist Édith Thomas, appeared from September 1944.[69] Initially consisting of a few pages of dense type, it soon switched to a broadsheet format, with pictures and more of a 'magazine' feel. The opening pages were generally dominated by political content. The editorial line sympathised with the Soviet Union to the point of repeating its propaganda ('there are no secret camps in the USSR'), celebrated the Viet Minh and the Spanish Resistance and commemorated the anniversaries of Stalingrad and Lenin's death.[70] The back half of the paper appeared somewhat disconnected from this political activism and international focus, being devoted to lifestyle matters with columns including 'Talking Cooking by Aunt Angèle', and numerous features on fashion.

This section of *Femmes françaises* in fact had considerable overlaps with *Vrai*, especially on the subjects of children and parenting. From October 1944 there was a children's page and a column of 'advice to mothers' by Dr Ida Valentine that was not at all feminist in tone. While attacking the 'cynicism' of Vichy family policy, *Femmes françaises* remained, as Karen Adler has shown, 'reluctant to allow women to exercise functions other than the maternal'.[71] Its articles encouraged women to practise 'the elegant art of coquetry' and 'neck care', and asked 'You've put on weight, madame – WHY?'[72]

Femmes françaises also shared *Vrai*'s interest in active, muscular bodies, and like other communist publications, linked femininity to national health and hygiene, assuming that well-regulated bodies were integral to well-planned societies.[73]

Dolto had a regular column in *Femmes françaises* from January 1946 to March 1947, initially bylined 'Dr Marguerite Fradeau', but subsequently under her own name. Her first articles shared a page with a feature discussing how physical culture could be practised by women in the home (happily, it transpired, housework and physical culture could turn out to be one and the same thing).[74] As in *Vrai*, Dolto made no mention of Freud, and her first article made clear that she would not use the column to expound on theoretical matters but would strive always to give practical advice.[75] Her second column, on 25 January 1946, 'What to say to our children, how to act with them?' was a repackaging of her *Vrai* article from 1 December 1941, frequently verbatim:

> If your child is being naughty, never say 'I'm going to buy another child' or 'The police will take you away' because it's not true and therefore you're setting them an example of lying …
>
> NEVER SAY
> 'Look, everybody is laughing at you' or 'what will people think'
>
> *Because* with this response, you are teaching them vanity.[76]

Does the fact that Dolto wrote for a communist-run publication in 1946–47 mean that her politics had changed? The Marettes, like much of the French population, switched from Pétainism to Gaullism in 1942–43. When Françoise's brother Pierre (the former colonial officer in Morocco) lost his army post with the dissolution of the Armistice Army in November 1942, his father arranged a sinecure for him in a steel factory, thereby exempting him the German forced labour programme. In 1943 Pierre joined the Alliance resistance network of former army officers.[77] Her youngest brother Jacques did depart for STO in Mannheim in 1943, but took with him a transmitter destined for the German Resistance.[78]

These developments add context to Dolto's resignation from the FFEPH in November 1943. So does her marriage, in February 1942, to Boris Dolto (1899–1981), a doctor and masseur, head of the French School of Orthopaedics and Massage-Physiotherapy

(École Française d'Orthopédie et de Masso-Kinésithérapie). Boris, born into the liberal intelligentsia of the Crimea, had taken French nationality in 1929. He had arrived in France in 1922 via North Africa, where his White Army artillery unit decamped in 1920 during the Russian Civil War.[79] In the 1920s he worked as a mechanic for Peugeot and Renault, before obtaining his medical degree in 1934. He was mobilised to the French army as a doctor in 1939, and survived a serious road accident during his service.

As a doctor, physiotherapist and Orthodox Christian, Boris shared Françoise's holistic approach to medicine, and had come across *Psychanalyse et pédiatrie* while seeking out innovative works in this vein. Their common openness to esoteric forms of holistic therapy facilitated their first meeting, in 1941, at sessions of 'directed waking dream therapy' (*rêve éveillé dirigé*) organised by Robert Desoille, the technique's founder.[80] Boris was a jovial and popular figure, intellectually and spiritually curious, fond of good company and a good drink. Françoise was attracted to his generosity, maturity and ability to listen – giving her respite from her customary position both as an analyst and with her male friends such as Alain Cuny, Louis Renou and Louis Boulonnois (see below), with whom she took on a maternal role. As she wrote to Boris in August 1941:

> We spoke about nothing but me yesterday. You listened to me, and you spoke to me with the solicitude of an older brother. Normally it's me who's assigned that role, and I'm reproached for being selfish if I wish to get back a little bit of what I give to others.[81]

Their relationship progressed swiftly. Boris was invited by the Marettes for Christmas 1941, and they married on 12 February 1942 at the fifth arrondissement town hall – the administration of the Marettes' home arrondissement, the sixteenth (Passy), have declared itself unwilling to sacralise the marriage of a 'foreigner'.[82] An allocution was pronounced at the Russian Catholic Church of Paris. The couple moved to an apartment on Rue Saint-Jacques, on the Left Bank. In her memoirs Dolto claimed that they had previously declined one (in rue Chanoinesse) that had been too-obviously hastily vacated, presumably by Jews who had either been arrested for deportation or fled in advance of the roundups that took place in Paris in July 1942, when 12,884 people were arrested, most of whom were subsequently sent to Auschwitz.[83]

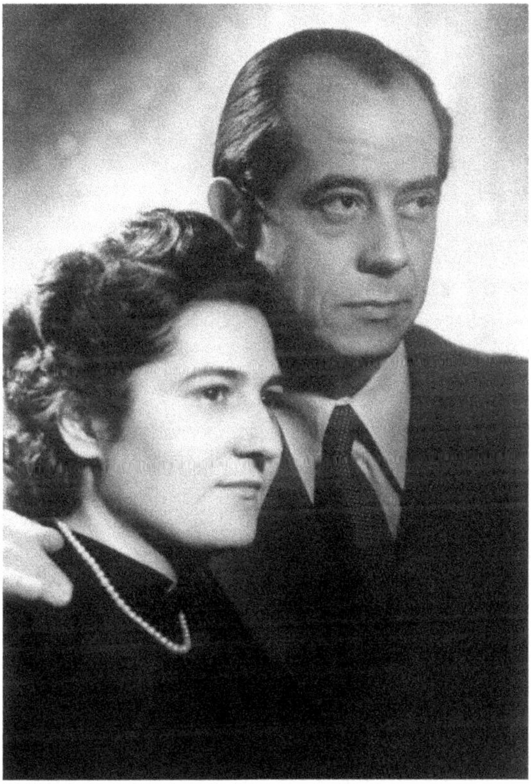

Figure 3.1 Dolto and her husband Boris, 1942

The marriage widened Dolto's social circle to include masseurs, mechanics and Orthodox Christians. Her son Carlos, born in 1943, later remembered his childhood as a chaotic whirl of comings and goings, parties, dinners and visitors of all kinds from priests and Sikh gurus to poets, actors, analysts and musicians.[84] Being of Russian (albeit anti-communist) origin, Boris came under some suspicion: Dolto later claimed that the Gestapo once forced him to strip to prove he was not Jewish.[85] In 1943–44, he offered medical services to a Resistance group, and resisters occasionally came to the Doltos' apartment for treatment or shelter.[86] However, they were reluctant to stay the night:

> Sometimes when they were coming to spend the night, they'd change their minds at the last minute: 'Listen, it's all the same to you, right?

> I've eaten well, I might be being ungrateful but I'm going.' I'd say, 'Don't you trust us?' I was humiliated because the resisters didn't feel entirely secure at our place.[87]

This passage from Dolto's autobiography is intriguing. Clearly the resisters did not see the Doltos as completely trustworthy. Was this simple prudence? Did knowledge of Françoise's earlier Vichy connections and Pétainist views play some role?

Whatever the explanation, it was not a barrier to her working closely with Vichy's opponents after the war, as a further episode from 1944–45 indicates. Henri Sellier, the Popular Front's health minister in the 1930s, was also the socialist mayor of Suresnes, a western suburb of Paris. In the interwar years, Sellier, his administrator (and town clerk) Louis Boulonnois and the medical hygienist Robert-Henri Hazemann had implemented innovative social programmes in Suresnes. These included nursery schools, crèches, vocational education schemes, a clinic-dispensary, an open-air school for children considered susceptible to tuberculosis and a 2,500-dwelling garden city. The Suresnes social care system was underpinned by *infirmières visiteuses*, health visitors/district nurses who functioned as points of contact between families and the social services, and *assistantes scolaires*, based in school infirmaries, who were in effect 'multi-purpose social workers ... the key conduits for Sellier's network of social services'.[88] In 1941 the Occupation authorities sacked Sellier as mayor, and he and Boulonnois were imprisoned for three weeks at the Royallieu-Compiègne internment camp. Sellier died in 1943. With the Liberation, Boulonnois set about re-establishing some of the interwar social services in Suresnes. In November 1944, he contacted Dolto, asking her to become involved. Boulonnois was interested in psychoanalysis, having in 1938 attempted to introduce some psychoanalytic ideas into Suresnes schools, and was aware of Dolto's thesis. Dolto agreed to take on a position with the Suresnes Public Office of Social Hygiene with responsibility for 'neuropsychiatry consultations'.[89] Boulonnois and Dolto's relationship subsequently developed to the point where Boulonnois, a year later, described her as acting 'like a mother and an analyst' towards him.[90] However, like Dolto's wartime initiatives, the project proved abortive, as Suresnes elected a communist-dominated municipal council in April 1945, displacing Boulonnois and the socialists.

For Boulonnois, Dolto was an appealing figure for her humanist-holistic ideas, and this clearly overrode previous political differences. Indeed, the Suresnes experiments may be seen as a socialist variant of the kind of holistic thinking practised by the engineers in groups like Coutrot's X-Crise in the 1930s. The Suresnes municipality tried to engineer the environments in which its residents lived, worked and were educated, in an effort to optimise their physical and mental condition. Laura Lee Downs has written that the Suresnes leaders aimed for 'ever greater technocratic control of the population' and that Sellier's reforms were 'undergirded by the neo-Lamarckian conviction that a reform of human material could be realised through systematic improvements in hygiene, housing, and education'.[91] There were overlaps between the roles of *infirmière visiteuse* and *assistante scolaire* at Suresnes, and the pastoral function of the family doctor as imagined by Dolto. The Suresnes municipality also encouraged children to form a connection with rural France, via its *colonie de vacances* (holiday camp) in the Nièvre. It is not hard to see why Dolto – once she had thrown off her family's prejudices against the republican parties, and with the defeat of Germany and of Vichy opening the way to new idealism about future reform possibilities – would be attracted to such schemes.

Like the continuities between *Vrai* and *Femmes françaises*, the Suresnes example indicates the extent to which people across the political spectrum shared interests in children, the family and 'holistic' social engineering. It also shows that there were many directions in which Dolto's career might have gone, in the fluid political context of Liberation. She did not need to change anything fundamental about her approach to medicine and parenting in order to be able to write for a communist paper in 1946. Dolto seems to have approached the Liberation years in the same spirit as she initially saw the downfall of the Third Republic: as an opportunity to renew and remake France. For Catholic reformers who were not ideologically wedded to Vichy, the 1940–41 and 1944–47 periods presented similar opportunities for national and spiritual renewal in an atmosphere tinged with a sense of guilt. However, the ideological fluidity of the Liberation years did not last: the hardening of the Cold War soon fractured the fragile Resistance unity. For Dolto, this meant a rapid end to her association with leftist figures, and a new emphasis on combining psychoanalysis with Christianity.

Postwar faith and guilt

In his Easter 1947 pastoral letter the Archbishop of Paris, Cardinal Suhard, argued that the Catholic Church needed to make radical choices, in the context of a coming global revolution brought about by scientific and technological progress.[92] Suhard argued for a new synthesis of 'tradition and Progress, transcendence and incarnation' to be achieved by Catholic scientists, sociologists, historians, psychologists and philosophers. Such intellectuals should cooperate fully with all those, believers or not, engaged in 'pure' research.[93]

At the Liberation, the Catholic Church in France was faced with a need to re-evaluate its political orientation. Having largely supported the Vichy regime in 1940–41, the Church leadership felt under pressure to demonstrate a greater openness to modernity after the war. Suhard's 1947 circular can be seen in this context. At a time when the dominant Catholic political movement was the Mouvement Républicain Populaire (MRP), a Christian democratic party born of the non-Marxist resistance, postwar Catholic theology progressed in a broadly democratic direction. Rather than emphasise the authority of the Church hierarchy, theologians undertook a 'return to the sources'. Biblical exegesis flourished, and for the first time in modern France the Bible became a bestseller.[94] Theology also moved towards 'Christocentrism', placing Jesus, rather than the Virgin Mary, at the centre of worship. This had a political dimension, as the Marian cult was stronger among the right-wing fundamentalist branches of French Catholicism. Biblical exegesis and Christocentrism thus accompanied the political shift to the centrist humanism of the MRP. These moves provoked opposition among Catholic intransigents, who often in practice overlapped with unrepentant Vichy supporters.

Increased Catholic openness to psychoanalysis can be seen as part of the same centrist trend. In the later 1940s and early 1950s, French Catholics frequently debated modernity, science and progress alongside the question of the appropriate role of sexuality in a Christian life. Should the new psychological sciences be consulted by Catholics on personal and sexual questions? Psychotherapy's relationship with religion was problematic. Its emergence represented a potential intrusion into the Church's historic territory, a challenge to the priest's primacy in the care of souls. The likes of

Roland Dalbiez had sought to fend off the issue by separating psychoanalytic technique from Freudian 'doctrine', utilising the former while preventing the latter from encroaching onto medical or religious domains. By the later 1940s, this border was no longer being effectively policed.

In 1942, Father Bruno, the Carmelite monk who had favoured a rapprochement between Catholicism and psychoanalysis in the 1930s, had published a biography of his order's founder Madame Acarie (1566–1618). The biography was partly intended to illustrate Bruno's ideas on combining psychology and religion.[95] But its main theme was marital sexuality. Bruno proposed Acarie's marriage as 'an accomplished form of conjugal perfection'.[96] He discussed the overlap between mystical union and sexual activity, arguing that (marital) sex could be a way of universalising mystical experience.[97] Bruno's valorisation of sexual ecstasy provoked opposition from conservative clerics, but enjoyed significant publishing success.[98] It seems very likely that Dolto read *La Belle Acarie*; at any rate, by the 1950s Bruno had become a close friend.[99] In 1957, Dolto and Bruno travelled to Zurich together to meet Carl Jung. Bruno's ideas fed into Dolto's re-evaluation of her Christianity, already underway in the light of her marriage to an Orthodox Christian. The first of Boris and Françoise's three children, Jean-Chrysostome (b. 1943, only later known as 'Carlos') was named after the Orthodox Church Father St John Chrysostom (*c.* 349–407). Like Bruno, John Chrysostom had advocated the enjoyment of guilt-free sexuality within marriage, arguing that sexual desire and pleasure were worthy and justified even if no children resulted.[100]

After 1945, there was considerable international interest in a potential synthesis between psychotherapy and religion. In 1946 the American rabbi Joshua Loth Liebman published a runaway bestseller (topping the *New York Times* lists for fifty-eight weeks), entitled *Peace of Mind* – a quality which, Liebman argued, could be found 'in the mighty confluence of dynamic psychology and prophetic religion'.[101] Liebman suggested that while 'religion, at its best, is the announcer of the supreme ideals by which men must live', it was 'rooted in an antiquated psychology'. In 'this psychological age', religion must not reject psychoanalysis, which was 'the newest and sharpest tool that God has given men for the examination of the human mind and its complex motives'.[102]

Liebman's work was just one example of what W. W. Meissner has called the 'more meaningful conversation between analysts and religionists' developed in this period by such works as R. S. Lee's *Freud and Christianity* (1948) and Erich Fromm's *Psychoanalysis and Religion* (1950).[103] In France, Catholic clergy and laity showed a much greater level of interest in psychoanalysis than before the war, and the theme of sexuality was central to this new interest.[104] Paul Jury's posthumously published *Journal d'un prêtre* (*Diary of a Priest*, 1956) drew attention to the secret sexual inner life of priests and the suffering caused by the insistence on celibacy.[105] The priest Marc Oraison's *Vie chrétienne et problèmes de la sexualité* (*Christian Life and Problems of Sexuality*, 1952) argued that since psychoanalysis had shown that much of human behaviour was attributable to unconscious motives, acts that the Church considered 'against nature', such as masturbation, homosexuality or fetishism, could no longer be considered mortal sins.[106] These works were the psychoanalytic end of a broader Catholic sexology literature, of which the most successful was Paul Chanson's *Art d'aimer et la continence conjugale* (*Art of Love and Conjugal Continence*, 1950).[107] The Kinsey reports, whose impact in France should not be underestimated, provided a backdrop to this, by underlining the hitherto unsuspected rarity of full sexual 'continence'.[108]

The engagement of priests and Catholic writers with psychoanalytic ideas was reciprocated by the interest shown by French psychoanalysts in Catholicism in the immediate postwar period. After the Liberation, the SPP was slow to reconstitute. Some Jewish members never returned from exile, and the *RFP* resumed publication only in 1948. In the interim, the main forum for psychoanalytic thought was *Psyché*, a journal that sought to combine psychoanalysis, Catholicism and medical holism. Largely funded by René Laforgue, *Psyché* grew out of the Centre d'Études des Sciences de l'Homme (Centre for the Study of Human Sciences), an organisation founded at Liberation and led by Maryse Choisy (1903–79). The name recalled Carrel's 'Foundation for the Study of Human Problems', and early editions of *Psyché* referred frequently to Carrel.[109] Choisy was a former investigative journalist, who had converted to Catholicism in the 1930s and been psychoanalysed by Laforgue in 1944. Over the next decade, Choisy worked assiduously for the conciliation of psychoanalysis and Catholicism.[110]

Psyché was a broad-ranging journal, with a prestigious editorial board including the psychologist Pierre Janet, the idealist philosopher and Jesuit priest Pierre Teilhard de Chardin and Prince Louis de Broglie of the Académie Française. Primarily, however, it set itself up at the interface between Catholic spirituality and psychoanalysis. Its opening editorial attacked the idea that 'we have no more need of religion, since we have psychoanalysis'.[111] The analysts who contributed to *Psyché*, including Dolto, André Berge, Georges Mauco, Angelo Hesnard, Adrien Borel and Georges Parcheminey, were almost all Catholics, and most were Laforgue's former analysands.[112] *Psyché* thus gave a platform to the Catholic section of French psychoanalysis, while encouraging Catholics in general to be open other branches of knowledge. This brought it some opposition: the fundamentalist periodical *La Pensée catholique* (*Catholic Thought*), founded in 1946, attacked Choisy and *Psyché* for engaging with evolutionary theory and psychoanalysis.[113] Dolto, Choisy, Laforgue and Parcheminey also wrote for Bruno's *Études carmélitaines*, which increasingly occupied the same crossover space. A 1951 issue of *Études carmélitaines* was devoted to asking what Catholic directors of conscience could learn from psychology and psychoanalysis.[114] A 1952 edition focused on the question of sexual continence, following a conference on religious psychology that Bruno organised in 1950.[115]

Dolto's writings on religious psychology, including those published in the 1970s and 1980s, were shaped by this context and by her experience of religion during her youth. As a Christian psychoanalyst with an interest in holistic medicine, she was well positioned to be prominent in postwar efforts to synthesise psychoanalysis and religion. Her writings in this period sought to demonstrate how Christian ideas could be rewritten in psychoanalytic vocabulary. Writing in *Études carmélitaines*, she posited a distinction between 'true' religious feelings and attitudes towards questions of sin or celibacy, from 'false' versions that she identified as neurotic. On the question of priestly celibacy, she considered that a conscious, maturely sought chastity (*une continence recherchée*) was healthy, unlike 'a chastity undertaken in masochistic fashion, through obedience to a master'.[116] For Dolto, it did not much matter whether or not priests were celibate; the important thing was that celibacy, if adopted, should be chosen from a position of psychological maturity, such that sexuality was, in Freudian terms, sublimated rather than repressed.

Behind the issue of continence, Dolto argued, lay 'the general theme of emotional guilt'. Feelings of guilt could induce priests to be celibate out of a neurotic or masochistic sense of duty, rather than as the result of a mature decision.[117] True guilt stemmed from love and confidence, whereas 'false' guilt was that provoked by the unrealistic expectations of authority figures and which became 'a source of depression and a lack of confidence in oneself'.[118] To develop a mature religious conscience, it was necessary to liberate oneself from false guilt and the 'unconscious feeling of guilt'.[119] Doctors and educators should be alert to early manifestations of guilt in young children and consider them as 'psychosomatic elements' connected to 'the embryonic stages of unconscious states of wellbeing and sickness'.[120] The concept of guilt helped Dolto to distinguish an essentially immature religious sense, imbued in children by their parents or social environment, from a mature adult spirituality free of neurotic elements. If parents invoked the name of Jesus to manage children's behaviour, they were abusing their authority, since this only instilled a false sense of religion:

> If you tell a child ... that Jesus thinks like his/her parents, then this Jesus – the supreme comforter ... appears instead like a civilised *gendarme* who keeps accounts of everyone's actions, and not a friend, a consoler ... We should never present something which is merely a custom, a matter of worldly etiquette or social conformity, as a religious rule that it would be a moral fault to transgress.[121]

For analogous reasons, in 1949 Dolto refused an invitation to write an advice column for a new Catholic magazine aimed at war widows, *Offertoire*. She refused on the grounds that the publication was built on the assumption of widowhood as a stable identity that widowed women could be pressured into adopting:

> The title itself, as well as all of the articles, implies that the whole of a widow's remaining lifespan must be dominated by the fact of having a dead husband ... I saw that it is even recommended to widows to stay faithful to their husband forever, as if he were waiting jealously for them at death's threshold.[122]

Dolto would not endorse a publication that emphasised duty to dead men over widows' right to lead full lives. The point of religion was to console and inspire, not to instil guilt. Dolto remained consistent on this point, writing in 1985 that by forcing young children to perform catechism and other rituals before they were sufficiently intellectually mature to fully understand them, 'the Catholic Church has pointlessly made every generation of our century feel guilty'.[123] When in 1958 her daughter Catherine came home with a questionnaire issued by the local parish, Dolto made extensive critical annotations. Under the question 'Do I seek to bring pleasure to those around me?', she wrote 'perversion of the sense of the sacred which is creation and not pleasure'. Under 'Do I protect the purity of my imagination and thoughts?', she wrote 'anxiety around projects for sexual encounters'. She proposed replacement questions which moved the focus from duty to spirituality, such as 'Am I continuing to deepen the meaning of my religion?'[124]

There may have been a biographical background to these attitudes, since guilt – at her failure to conform to the feminine template her family demanded, or to save her sister from cancer through prayer – was a major theme of Dolto's psychoanalysis. She subsequently identified intransigent Catholicism with the restrictive, performative aspects of her upbringing. But it is also striking to consider the wider historical context framing discussion of guilt in French Catholic circles after 1945. Guilt had been a staple of Pétainist discourse: France's culpability for its 1940 defeat was asserted as a kind of divine retribution for its alleged decadence, in an echo of previous right-wing performative expiations in 1815 and 1871. But after the full experience of occupation, collaboration, liberation and the discovery of the Holocaust, the subject became much more complex and ambiguous. How much guilt should French Catholics who had supported Vichy feel, and what exactly should they feel guilty for? How severely should collaborators be punished, and for how long should they be ostracised?

This question affected psychoanalysis, and Dolto's professional entourage, directly. In 1946 John Leuba, the new head of the SPP, argued that the society needed to 'undertake a purge before resuming our activities'.[125] Leuba's principal target was Dolto's former analyst, René Laforgue, who, following the German invasion, had attempted to work with the occupiers. In 1940, Laforgue made contact with Matthias Göring, Hermann's cousin and head of the Nazi-approved Deutsche Allgemeine Ärztliche Gesellschaft für Psychotherapie (German General Medical Society for

Psychotherapy). Laforgue offered to head up a reconstituted SPP and issue *EP* under German sponsorship. Jewish analysts would naturally be excluded; Laforgue went so far as to give Göring a list of those who could be considered 'a danger to the reconciliation of our two peoples'.[126] Laforgue probably hoped to obtain a university post and permission to publish his new book on great men and the 'psychopathology of failure'.[127] Neither hope was granted, and in 1942 Laforgue retreated to his estate at La Roquebrussanne in the Unoccupied Zone – where Dolto had joined the 'crazies' club' before the war – from where he provided some assistance to Resistance groups while also remaining in contact with Göring.[128] Not all of these details were known when Laforgue was brought before a purge tribunal in 1946. Called as a witness, Dolto delivered what Élisabeth Roudinesco describes as 'a ringing speech of homage to Laforgue'.[129] The tribunal, unaware of Laforgue's correspondence with Göring, acquitted him for lack of evidence. He retained his place in the Ordre des Médecins and the SPP, but the trial permanently tarnished his reputation. It was in the wake of this that Laforgue 'became increasingly inclined to direct his attention to spiritual concerns' and founded *Psyché*.[130] Finding himself ostracised by many former colleagues, he moved to Casablanca, Morocco, in 1956.[131]

Laforgue's former analysand Georges Mauco (discussed further in Chapter 4) also had a tarnished wartime record. So too did Dolto's friend Father Bruno, who, according to historian Agnès Desmazières, had 'fraternized with notorious collaborators' and written for the collaborationist paper *La Gerbe*.[132] French psychoanalysts were not disproportionately likely to have been collaborators or Nazi sympathisers; the SPP also contained two important resisters in Paul Schiff and Sacha Nacht. But Dolto was much closer to Laforgue, Bruno and Mauco than to Schiff and Nacht – and she, of course, had also supported the National Revolution, though not outright collaboration.

Dolto's postwar writings about guilt and religion must be understood in this light. A 1948 text on guilt that she wrote for *Psyché* positioned itself as a contribution to an approach pioneered by Laforgue in speaking 'of the solace that religions, and above all the Catholic religion, can offer to the feeling of unconscious guilt … In my capacity as a child psychoanalyst, I would like to make my modest contribution to this study.'[133] Her best-known books on religion, written with Gérard Sévérin – two volumes of *L'Évangile au risque de la psychanalyse* (published in English as *The Jesus of Psychoanalysis: A Freudian Interpretation of the Gospel*) and *La Foi au risque de la psychanalyse* (*Faith: A Psychoanalytic Perspective*) – were published between 1977 and 1981, but were based on reflections that Dolto began in the 1940s.[134] In these short, conversational books Dolto interpreted the gospels through the prism of psychoanalytic theory, arguing that 'nothing in Christ's message contradicts Freud's discoveries'.[135] Rereading the gospels as an adult, Dolto discovered in them a 'message of joy and love' which contrasted with the 'so-called Christian education' that she had received and that she now saw as 'the enemy of life and charity'.[136] The gospels now appeared to her as a 'psychodrama'. She used gospel stories as exemplars of psychoanalytic theory. For example, she interpreted the story of the boy Jesus at the Temple (Luke 2: 41–52) as a tale in which 'Jesus castrates his parents of their possessiveness ... as every child has to do'.[137]

A key part of Jesus's message, Dolto contended, was the liberation of humans from traditional sources of guilt and obligation. In her reading of the parable of the Pharisee and the tax collector (Luke 18: 9–14) she contrasted the Pharisee's loyalty to the letter of the law ('I fast twice a week and give a tenth of all I get') with the tax collector's awareness of 'God's justice and love'.[138] She compared the Pharisee to those 'militants in trade unions, parties, religions, ideologies [who] know that they are in possession of the truth, or at least know what other people must think and how they must live'. For Dolto, the message of this parable was that 'we must get beyond these emotional states and feelings of indignity and guilt'. Living according to the letter of the law, out of a sense of duty, was miserable (*malheureux*). Similarly, her reading of the parable of the prodigal son was that 'the cohesion of families is too often ordered or organised around feelings of guilt ... this is absolutely contrary to Jesus's teaching'.[139]

The keystone of the *Évangile au risque* series was Dolto's interpretation of the parable of the Good Samaritan (Luke 10: 25–37). It was after discussing this parable at a dinner with the publisher Jean-Pierre Delarge that the idea for the entire book project took shape.[140] Dolto's reading of the parable is also the most revealing of her attitudes to guilt. As a child, Dolto claimed, the parable was interpreted to her by priests as follows: 'Jesus asks us to love our neighbour, to concern ourselves with all forms of distress, to give of our time and our lives to help the unfortunate. Don't be self-centred, like the priest and the Levite who saw and walked on by.'[141] This conventional interpretation stressed that obligations of charity were not limited by social barriers; the human duty to help a neighbour in distress applied regardless of class or ethnic difference. Dolto's re-interpretation turned this on its head. In her reading, the definition of 'neighbour' is subjective and relative. The priest and Levite are not the neighbour for the injured man because, as men of God, they have nothing in common with him. Dolto emphasised that in the parable, Jesus does not blame them for not stopping. However, the Samaritan, Dolto imagined, was 'a "material" man, practical ... a merchant no doubt!' As such, he would be regularly threatened by bandits, and aware that the man lying injured could just as easily be him. Therefore, he stops to do what he can to help, without significantly inconveniencing himself – a bandage for his wounds, a lift to the nearest inn, enough money to last a couple of days. But those who did not stop need not feel guilty about this. For Dolto the moral of the parable was:

> When, like the Samaritan, you have a bit of time and means, don't turn your back on those that you see in pain ... If you aren't busy with something else and you have the energy, give what you can to those you encounter on your path who are in need. But don't do more. Don't turn away from your work. Don't turn away from your path.[142]

In the context of postwar guilt, this reads like quite a convenient theology for those with mixed wartime records. In essence, it denied that people who had resisted the Occupation, who sheltered Jews and resisters, were morally superior to those who did not – they simply happened to be in a position to act as the 'neighbour'. Those (like Dolto) who had not gone out of their way to help, who had not departed from their path, had nothing to reproach themselves for.

Shortly before her death, Dolto claimed that the Jews 'were the Christ during the war. The Jews were the Christ on the cross. The Jews incarnated Christ without even knowing it. They didn't know they were Christ-like, they incarnated it.'[143] If the purpose of Christ's suffering on the cross was to provide Christians with a model and a knowledge that redemption awaits them in heaven, then the Jews killed by Nazis seemed to Dolto to fulfil a similar function. Beyond the sheer offensiveness of Dolto's effective downplaying of the Holocaust – instrumentalising it to fit a Christian theological narrative – this idea appears to fulfil a function in respect of Dolto and her friends' own feelings of guilt and humiliation about their wartime actions: if the Jews' suffering served a spiritual purpose, then perhaps there was less reason to feel guilty about not having acted to prevent it.

Politics of the 1953 split

In 1949, the French Communist Party condemned psychoanalysis as a reactionary ideology. Attacking psychoanalysis as essentially conservative, American and capitalist – 'a technique of adaptation to bourgeois society' – the party accused analysts of attempting to neutralise political radicalism by medicalising it.[144] For the communists, Freudian techniques could only offer a partial liberation from psychological afflictions, since they could not reveal the socio-economic relations that underpinned them.[145] This attack came in the context of escalating Cold War tensions, which included an element of Soviet antisemitism – New York had become the leading global centre of postwar psychoanalysis, thanks to the wave of Jewish analysts fleeing Hitler. The refugees included Rudolph Loewenstein, who in the 1930s had analysed three men who became leading figures of postwar French psychoanalysts: Jacques Lacan, Daniel Lagache and Sacha Nacht. They also included Heinz Hartmann, Nacht's second analyst and president of the IPA between 1953 and 1957. By that time, Hartmann and Loewenstein were known in France as founders of 'ego psychology', which was vigorously attacked by Lacan as a technique that encouraged conformist adjustment to the social realities of capitalism.

From 1949, just as the *rapprochement* between Catholicism and psychoanalysis was in full swing, French communists sympathetic to psychoanalysis were required to renounce that sympathy, or at least affirm the primacy of their communism. The hardening of the Cold War prompted some Catholic intransigents to soften their hostility to psychoanalysis, realising that the *Psyché* group, whatever its theological faults, was at least decidedly anti-communist.[146] In 1951, Dolto even got a favourable review in the Vatican journal *L'Osservatore Romano*, which described her presentation to an international congress of Catholic doctors, on 'the training of children's moral conscience', as 'brilliant and deep'.[147]

From 1948, the re-formed SPP was led by Nacht, a Romanian-born Jewish doctor and former Resistance fighter. Arrested by the Gestapo in 1943, he escaped from a concentration camp and became a medical officer in the Free French army.[148] Nacht's vision for the SPP was very different from the spiritual-holistic direction of *Psyché*. Nacht saw psychoanalysis as first and foremost a branch of medicine. He wanted to restrict its practice to qualified physicians and integrate French psychoanalysis more closely with state medical structures and the IPA. *Psyché*, by contrast, sought to open up psychoanalysis to non-medical ('lay') practitioners and forge links with the Catholic Church and holistic therapies.

These differences contributed to the SPP's split in 1953. In December 1951, the Ordre des Médecins brought a case for illegal practice of medicine against a non-medical American child psychoanalyst. Margaret Clark-Williams had worked since 1946 at the Claude Bernard 'psycho-pedagogic centre' (see Chapter 4), and joined the SPP in 1950. Clark-Williams testified that she practised 're-education therapy' and was thus a pedagogue, not a psychoanalyst: therefore, she was not appropriating a medical role. The problem with this defence was that it implicitly recognised that psychoanalysis did indeed require medical supervision. Clark-Williams's supporters, including Marie Bonaparte and Maryse Choisy, nonetheless wanted to use the trial to defend the principle of lay analysis and the notion that undergoing one's own personal analysis was the only necessary qualification. In 1953, an appeal court imposed a symbolic fine on Clark-Williams and threw the affair back to the internal regulation of the SPP, citing its recommendation that trainee analysts should be medically qualified.[149]

By that time, the SPP was dividing into those who wanted to uphold the medical restriction, such as Nacht and Georges Heuyer, and those, including Dolto, Lagache and Lacan, who supported lay analysis. This division overlapped with a battle for control of the SPP's training institute, now being re-established following its dissolution in 1940 – an important fight since it determined how psychoanalysis would be taught to postwar students and analysands. Here, the divide was between supporters of the 'orthodox' training advocated by the IPA, notably the principle that sessions should always last around fifty minutes, and those who felt that analysts should be freer to innovate. Particularly contentious were the methods employed by Lacan, already an idiosyncratic theorist and rising star of the movement. A training programme run by Lacan, whose sessions were of unpredictable but often very short lengths, would be very different to one run by the 'orthodox' Nacht.

Dolto was prominent among the 'dissidents', as those who supported both Lacan and lay analysis were called. The *Psyché* group were united against Nacht. Advocates of the rapprochement between Catholicism and psychoanalysis lined up behind lay analysis, not least because most priests did not have medical degrees and thus risked being completely shut out from psychoanalytic training. For similar reasons, most of the SPP's women also opposed Nacht, since women with medical degrees were still rare; restricting psychoanalysis to doctors would thus instantly render it a much more male profession. It felt deliberate that the conservative, corporatist Ordre des Médecins had targeted a non-medical, foreign, and *female* analyst in Clark-Williams.[150] Lagache and Juliette Favez-Boutonnier, as academic professors of psychology, likewise did not wish to see psychoanalysis restricted to a medical sub-discipline. Fifty-one out of the eighty-five analysts in training also supported Lacan over Nacht.

Nacht's authoritarian management style contributed to the opposition to him. Writing to the trainee analysts in May 1953, Dolto denounced Nacht's 'coercive paternalist management' and argued that he and his supporters appeared 'more like religious traditionalists than scientists, more concerned with protecting their professional privileges … than putting themselves at the service of real-live people'.[151] But this was not the only objection, at least not on the part of the analysts referred to approvingly by Laforgue as 'those who have reacted against Nacht's policy with French instincts'.[152] In private letters, Dolto attacked Nacht as a 'gorilla gangster' and 'a fearful comrade with animal cunning' – and, in a section excised from her published correspondence, denounced 'the gang of Jewish communists' running the SPP.[153]

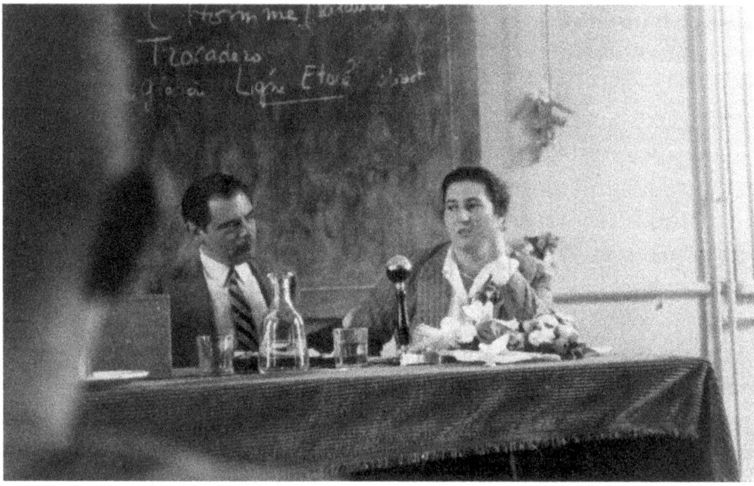

Figure 3.2 Dolto and Sacha Nacht, early 1950s

Any flirtation Dolto had once had with the radical Left was very much over. Her holistic visions of health now aligned, once again, with the right-wing, antisemitic views that were prevalent in her family and in her professional circle in the interwar years. Dolto argued for lay analysis for the same reasons that she had promoted the idea of the family doctor in 1941. She valued human connection and authentic desire to help others over formal medical qualifications, believing that this was the way to solve 'human problems', as Alexis Carrel had termed them. For Dolto in the 1940s and 1950s, just as for Carrel in the 1930s, this approach was linked to ensuring the flourishing of the French race (or *ethnie*) in a modernising world. If psychoanalysis succumbed to high entry barriers enforced by the state, especially if this was combined with bringing it under the control of a left-wing, foreign-born, Jewish leadership, then from Dolto's perspective it could not contribute to the spiritual and moral *redressement* of the French populace that Pétainism had promised, and which Dolto still hoped to see emerge after 1945. Dolto's promotion of a liberal and psychologised version of Catholicism was connected to this outlook. She developed a theology of guilt that felt progressive, since it rejected the intransigence of the interwar church and incorporated much of the new psychological thinking – but which also, conveniently, served to justify her and her colleagues' failure to do more to resist the Nazi Occupation. Dolto had integrated psychoanalysis with Christianity in a way that could help defuse lingering antisemitic prejudice against analysis as a 'Jewish science', but that also denied any Jewish specificity to Freudian ideas. In *L'Évangile au risque de la psychanalyse*, Dolto treated Freud as a second Jesus, an inspirational teacher whose message resonated beyond Judaism into human universality. Implicit in that equivalence was that French psychoanalysis did not need to be limited by Freudian orthodoxy (as represented by Nacht or the IPA), any more than Christianity needed to be constrained by Jewish theology. Conversely, Jesus also belonged in a Freudian tradition – as Dolto presented him, Jesus mainly performed acts of individual psychological healing with few societal implications. He did not demand that Christians go out of their way to help others, or that they should feel guilty for failing to do so – a comforting idea not just for those with undistinguished wartime records, but also for people of means who did not support the kind of radical wealth redistribution that some scriptural readings seemed to require.

Dolto was comfortable, politically, to end up in a position where she was opposing both the forces of bureaucracy (as represented by the Ordre des Médecins or the IPA) and Jewish analysts led by Nacht. Nacht's vision of a medicalised, standardised psychoanalysis was anathema to Dolto because it seemed to risk reverting to the interwar situation where psychoanalysis existed on the margins of an exclusive, secular, male, empiricist medical establishment. Faced with this threat, Dolto became a 'dissident', meaning that she reverted to the pluralistic, humanist, anti-bureaucratic Catholic holism that had developed in right-wing circles in the 1930s and subsequently proved adaptable to various political situations. When a different form of dissidence developed in the 1960s, associated in Dolto's orbit with the rise of radical (anti-)psychiatry and Lacanian psychoanalysis, Dolto embraced that too (Chapter 5). From that point onwards, the deep roots of her ideas in the earlier period of 1930s right-wing holism became obscured in the French public mind.

Not everyone, however, was prepared to forget her past stances. In 1960, the Société Française de Psychanalyse (SFP), the organisation created by the 'dissident' psychoanalysts after the 1953 split, sought to join the IPA. The IPA made the SFP's accession conditional on Lacan and Dolto leaving the organisation, or at least on preventing them from taking part in the training of new analysts.[154] It was predictable that Lacan would be singled out, since his short sessions, theoretical innovations and charismatic cultivation of a personal following had by that stage become notorious. Dolto's exclusion, however, was a surprise. Roudinesco speculatively attributed it to British analyst Donald Winnicott's judgement that Dolto 'had too much intuition and not enough method to be a training analyst'.[155] However, documents unearthed by the SPP's in-house historian Alain de Mijolla strongly suggest an alternative explanation. The rump SPP, led by Nacht, had sent a dossier to the IPA in reference to the new group's application for admittance, material which was particularly hostile towards Dolto, accusing her of 'thaumaturgical practices' and of maintaining improper contact with patients.[156] The dossier also attacked Laforgue, noting his wartime collaboration, and Angelo Hesnard, the most senior surviving member of the pre-war SPP's right-wing nationalist tendency. Both, along with Dolto and Lacan, were ultimately excluded from the IPA: political scalps, perhaps, obtained by Nacht in exchange for his acquiescence in the SFP's admission.

If this was Nacht's revenge for Dolto's words and actions in 1953, it hit home: Dolto's exclusion from the international movement left her deeply disconcerted for a time. In the longer run, however, it did her no harm. Lacan cleverly redefined the exclusion as an 'excommunication', thus implicitly recognising the religious dimension of the split while casting himself as a latter-day Spinoza.[157] The episode fed the narrative of Lacan and Dolto as radical, pioneering outsiders – thereby helping them subsequently to create new orthodoxies of their own.

Notes

1 See Fishman, *Vichy to the Sexual Revolution*, introduction.
2 René Spitz to Dolto, 13 September 1946, in Djéribi-Valentin, *Une vie de correspondances*, p. 157.
3 Clarke, *Age of Organization*, introduction; Philip Nord, *France's New Deal: From the Thirties to the Postwar Era* (Princeton, NJ: Princeton

University Press, 2010), Ch. 1; Marjorie Beale, *The Modernist Enterprise: French Elites and the Threat of Modernity, 1900–1940* (Stanford, CA: Stanford University Press, 2000).

4 Alexis Carrel, *Man, The Unknown* (New York: Harper & Brothers, 1939 (first published 1935)), p. 7.

5 Jean Coutrot, *De quoi vivre* (Paris: Grasset, 1935); Clarke, *Age of Organization*, pp. 14ff.

6 Carrel, *Man, The Unknown*, p. 16.

7 Clarke, *Age of Organization*, pp. 70ff.

8 Fette, *Exclusions*, pp. 80–1.

9 Clarke, *Age of Organization*, p. 10.

10 Tumblety, *Remaking the Male Body*, pp. 6–7.

11 Cited in Clarke, *Age of Organization*, pp. 107–8.

12 Jacques Maritain, *Humanisme intégral: problèmes temporels et spirituels d'une nouvelle chrétienté* (Paris: Le Cerf, 1936).

13 Jacques Maritain, *Primauté du spirituel* (Paris: Plon, 1927). Simone de Beauvoir echoed its title in her book *Quand prime le spirituel* (Paris: Gallimard, 1979), written between 1935 and 1937 and originally titled *Primauté du spirituel.*

14 Étienne Fouilloux, *Une église en quête de liberté: La pensée catholique française entre modernisme et Vatican II 1914–1962* (Paris: Desclée de Brouwer, 1998), p. 85.

15 See Desmazières, *L'Inconscient au paradis*, pp. 63ff.

16 Roland Dalbiez, *La Méthode psychanalytique et la doctrine freudienne* (Paris: Desclée de Brouwer, 1936). On the reception of this, see Mijolla, *Freud et La France, 1885–1945*, p. 682.

17 Desmazières, *L'Inconscient au paradis*, pp. 70–1.

18 Dolto, *Psychoanalysis and Paediatrics*, p. xxiii.

19 Dolto to Paul Jury, 11 July 1939, *Une vie de correspondances*, p. 16. On Jury, see Desmazières, *L'Inconscient au paradis*, pp. 93–5.

20 Mijolla, *Freud et la France, 1885–1945*, p. 783.

21 On French psychoanalysis under the Occupation, see Ohayon, *L'Impossible Rencontre*, pp. 229–71; Mijolla, *Freud et la France, 1885–1945*; also Alain de Mijolla, 'La Psychanalyse en France (1893–1965)', in Roland Jaccard (ed.), *Histoire de la psychanalyse*, 1 (Paris: Hachette, 1982), pp. 9–105; Roudinesco, *Jacques Lacan*, pp. 152–70.

22 Ohayon, *L'Impossible Rencontre*, p. 242.

23 Dolto, *Autoportrait*, p. 156.

24 Hanna Diamond, *Fleeing Hitler: France 1940* (Oxford: Oxford University Press, 2007), p. 6.

25 Dolto to Hubert Jausion, 10 June 1940, *Une vie de correspondances*, p. 39.

26 Françoise to Henry Marette, 21 July 1940, *Une vie de correspondances*, p. 54.
27 For Richard Cobb, 'the *exode* was for many a voyage of discovery of a wealth and freshness that no travel agent could achieve'. *Promenades: A Historian's Appreciation of Modern French Literature* (Oxford: Oxford University Press, 1980), p. 53. See also Diamond, *Fleeing Hitler*, p. 160.
28 Françoise to Henry Marette, 21 July 1940, *Une vie de correspondances*, pp. 54–5.
29 *Ibid.*
30 Philippe Pétain, 'Appel du 25 juin 1940', in Jean-Claude Barbas (ed.), *Philippe Pétain: Discours aux Français: 17 juin 1940–20 août 1944* (Paris: Albin Michel, 1989), pp. 63–6.
31 AFD, box labelled 'Cas 2', case of 'Serge F.', treated 1942–44. Typed summary by Dolto.
32 AFD, Cas 2, case of 'Roland F.', treated from 1941. Typed summary by Dolto.
33 Françoise to Henry Marette, 21 July 1940, *Une vie de correspondances*, p. 54.
34 Didier Pleux, *Françoise Dolto, la déraison pure* (Paris: Autrement, 2013), pp. 109ff.
35 Jean Marette to Françoise, 15 July 1940, *Une vie de correspondances*, p. 48.
36 Suzanne Marette to Françoise, 28 July 1940, *Une vie de correspondances*, pp. 59–60.
37 Muriel Djéribi-Valentin, preface to *Une vie de correspondances*, p. xiii.
38 See Clarke, *Age of Organization*, pp. 128ff.
39 This is suggested by Henry's letter of 22 July 1940, *Une vie de correspondances*, p. 56. By this date, Henry had returned to Paris from Montbard, 'where everything is being put back in order'.
40 Françoise to Henry Marette, 21 July 1940, *Une vie de correspondances*, p. 54.
41 See Robert O. Paxton, *Vichy France; Old Guard and New Order, 1940–1944* (New York: Knopf, 1972), p. 37.
42 Fishman, *Battle for Children*, p. 8.
43 Patrice Josset, *Hôpital d'enfants Armand-Trousseau* (Paris: Assistance Publique, 1999), pp. 32–3.
44 Cited by Catherine Dolto, 'Intervention au Colloque pour les 100 ans de l'Hôpital Trousseau' (2001), www.dolto.fr/archives/siteWeb/english/docs_a_garder/trouscat.htm, accessed 29 January 2021.
45 Hivernel, '"The Parental Couple"', 506.
46 Catherine Dolto, 'Intervention au Colloque'.

47 Françoise Dolto, 'Françoise Dolto: Ma vie et la psychanalyse', in Antoine Hess, *Les Analystes parlent* (Paris: Belfond, 1981), p. 100.
48 See Andrés Horacio Reggiani, *God's Eugenicist: Alexis Carrel and the Sociobiology of Decline* (Oxford: Berghahn, 2006).
49 Alain Drouard, *Alexis Carrel (1873–1944): De la mémoire à l'histoire* (Paris: L'Harmattan, 1995), p. 206. See also Drouard, *Une inconnue des sciences sociales: la Fondation Alexis Carrel, 1941–1945* (Paris: Editions de la Maison des sciences de l'homme, 1992); Schneider, *Quality and Quantity*, pp. 272ff; Ohayon, *L'Impossible Rencontre*, pp. 256–62.
50 On Laforgue's intervention, see Annick Ohayon, 'Psychoanalysis under the Vichy Regime', in Joy Damousi and Mariano Ben Plotkin (eds), *Psychoanalysis and Politics: Histories of Psychoanalysis Under Conditions of Restricted Political Freedom* (New York: Oxford University Press, 2012), pp. 35–56, 50.
51 Suzanne and Henry Marette to Dolto, 6 October 1942, *Une vie de correspondances*, pp. 99–100, and n. 21; Ohayon, *L'Impossible Rencontre*, p. 261. A compte-rendu from the FFEPH's Comité de direction, dated 24 November 1942 (reproduced in Drouard, *Une inconnue*, p. 429), records Dolto's employment. Her salary was roughly average for doctors hired by the foundation.
52 Drouard, *Alexis Carrel*, pp. 211–14; *Une inconnue*, pp. 262–9, 429.
53 Drouard, *Alexis Carrel*, p. 210.
54 Dolto, *Autoportrait*, 182.
55 For comparison, the official price of a litre of milk was 4F60. See Fabrice Grenard, *La France du marché noir (1940–1949)* (Paris: Payot, 2008).
56 'Des conserves sans boîtes', *Vrai*, 3, 15 November 1941, 34–5.
57 *Vrai*, 3, 15 November 1941, 2; *Vrai*, 2, 1 November 1941, 37.
58 *Vrai*, 1, 15 October 1941, 20–3.
59 *Vrai*, 2, 1 November 1941, 6–7.
60 *Vrai*, 3, 15 November 1941, 21–3.
61 *Vrai*, 2, 1 November 1941.
62 *Ibid.*, 24–5.
63 Louis Renou to Françoise Marette, 3 November 1941, *Une vie de correspondances*, p. 83.
64 'F. M.', 'Ayez votre médecin de famille', *Vrai*, 3, 15 November 1941, 28–9.
65 *Ibid.*
66 The *carnet*, introduced in 1939 and which parents were required to maintain for their children, was a compulsory record of vaccinations, growth milestones and illnesses. See Schneider, *Quality and Quantity*, pp. 268–70, 287–91.

67 'M.', 'Nos enfants ... Savez-vous leur parler?', *Vrai*, 4, 1 December 1941, 23.
68 *Ibid.*
69 On Thomas, see Claire Gorrara, 'Crises of Witnessing: Édith Thomas and the War Years', *Modern & Contemporary France*, 4:3 (1996), 361–3; Dorothy Kaufmann, 'Uncovering a Woman's Life: Édith Thomas (Novelist, Historian, *Résistante*)', *The French Review*, 67:1 (1993), 61–72.
70 *Femmes françaises*, 25 January 1946, 10.
71 Adler, *Jews and Gender*, p. 52.
72 *Femmes françaises*, 19 January 1946; 2 December 1945; 16 March 1946.
73 See Joy Damousi, 'Representations of the Body and Sexuality in Communist Iconography, 1920–1955', *Australian Feminist Studies*, 12 (1997), 59–75; Vassil Girginov, 'Totalitarian Sport: Towards an Understanding of its Logic, Practice and Legacy', *Totalitarian Movements and Political Religions*, 5 (2004), 25–58.
74 'Culture physique avec matériel "maison"', *Femmes françaises*, 15 February 1946.
75 'Dr Marguerite Fradeau', 'Introduction à une page d'éducation', *Femmes françaises*, 18 January 1946, 14. Dolto's 1946 *Femmes françaises* columns are reprinted in Dolto, *Les Chemins de l'éducation* (Paris: Gallimard, 1994), pp. 137–202.
76 'Dr Marguerite Fradeau', 'Que dire à nos enfants, comment agir avec eux?', *Femmes françaises*, 25 January 1946.
77 Dolto to Nicole Marette, 8 June 1943, *Une vie de correspondances*, p. 110, and n. 12. Steelworkers were exempt from STO under an agreement between Jean Bichelonne and Albert Speer classing steel as a protected industry. Resisters could thus be sheltered by sympathetic factory managers. Luc-André Brunet details creative measures taken by steel bosses to protect underemployed workers in *Forging Europe: Industrial Organisation in France, 1940–1952* (London: Palgrave, 2017).
78 Suzanne Marette to Dolto, 12 August 1943, *Une vie de correspondances*, pp. 113–14, and n. 22.
79 Françoise Dolto's 1988 preface to Boris Dolto, *Le Corps entre les mains* (1976) (Paris: Vuibert, 2006).
80 The technique interested psychoanalysts because it promised access to the unconscious thoughts of patients unable to recount their dreams. See Robert Desoille and Georges Mauco, 'La Technique du rêve éveillé et ses applications', *Psyché*, 4 (1947), 150–8.
81 Françoise Marette to Boris Dolto, 3 August 1941 (draft), reproduced in Potin (ed.), *Archives de l'intime*, p. 156.

82 Suzanne Marette to Boris Dolto, 22 December 1941, *Une vie de correspondances*, p. 85.
83 Dolto, *Autoportrait*, p. 179.
84 Jean-Chrysostome Dolto, *Je m'appelle Carlos* (Paris: Ramsay, 1996), p. 26.
85 Dolto, *Autoportrait*, pp. 182–3.
86 *Ibid.*
87 *Ibid.*, p. 181.
88 Laura Lee Downs, *Childhood in the Promised Land: Working-Class Movements and the Colonies de Vacances in France, 1880–1960* (Durham, NC: Duke University Press, 2002), pp. 125–6; Reynolds, *France between the Wars*, pp. 142–4.
89 Louis Boulonnois to Dolto, 21 November 1944, *Une vie de correspondances*, p. 137.
90 Boulonnois to Dolto, 24 October 1945, *Une vie de correspondances*, p. 143. Boulonnois had undergone an (apparently unproductive) analysis with Jacques Lacan in 1937.
91 Downs, *Childhood*, pp. 128, 131.
92 See Colin W. Nettelbeck, 'The Eldest Daughter and the Trente glorieuses: Catholicism and National Identity in Postwar France', *Modern & Contemporary France*, 6:4 (1998), 445–62, 451.
93 Emmanuel Célestin (Cardinal Suhard), *Essor ou déclin de l'Église: Lettre pastorale, Carême de l'an de grâce 1947* (Paris: A. Lahure, 1962), pp. 151–2.
94 Fouilloux, *Église*, pp. 220ff.
95 Bruno de Jésus-Marie, *La Belle Acarie, bienheureuse Marie de l'Incarnation* (Paris: Desclée de Brouwer, 1942), p. ix.
96 *Ibid.*, pp. vi, 191.
97 *Ibid.*, pp. 487.
98 Desmazières, *L'Inconscient au paradis*, p. 68.
99 See e.g. Bruno to Dolto, 1 January 1953, *Une vie de correspondances*, p. 224.
100 St John Chrysostom, 'Homily 12', in *On Marriage and Family Life*, trans. Catherine P. Roth and David Anderson (Crestwood, NY: St Vladimir's Seminary Press, 2003), p. 76. (Thanks to Maroula Perisanidi for this reference.) The Doltos' two further children were Grégoire (b. 1944) and Catherine (b. 1946).
101 Joshua Loth Liebman, *Peace of Mind* (New York: Bantam, 1946), p. 27. See Herzog, *Cold War Freud*, p. 37.
102 Liebman, *Peace of Mind*, pp. 21–3.
103 R. S. Lee, *Freud and Christianity* (London: James Clark, 1948); Erich Fromm, *Psychoanalysis and Religion* (New Haven, CT: Yale University

Press, 1950). See W. W. Meissner, 'Psychoanalysis and Catholicism – Dialogues in Transformation', *Psychoanalytic Inquiry*, 28:5 (2008), 580–9.

104 Desmazières, *L'Inconscient au paradis*, p. 92.

105 Paul Jury, *Journal d'un prêtre* (Paris: Gallimard, 1956).

106 Marc Oraison, *Vie chrétienne et problèmes de la sexualité* (Paris: Lethielleux, 1952).

107 Paul Chanson, *Art d'aimer et la continence conjugale* (Paris: Editions familiales de France, 1950). See Desmazières, *L'Inconscient au paradis*, pp. 145–6.

108 See Fishman, *Vichy to the Sexual Revolution*, pp. 52–4; Coffin, *Sex, Love, and Letters*, Ch. 2; Judith Coffin, 'Beauvoir, Kinsey, and Mid-Century Sex', *French Politics, Culture and Society*, 28:2 (2010), 18–37.

109 See Alain de Mijolla, *La France et Freud Tome 1 1946–1953: Une pénible renaissance* (Paris: Presses universitaires de France, 2012), pp. 11–14; Ohayon, *L'Impossible Rencontre*, pp. 323–35; Roudinesco, *Jacques Lacan*, pp. 192–205.

110 See Ohayon, *L'Impossible Rencontre*, pp. 324ff.

111 'Où en sommes-nous', *Psyché*, 1 (1946), 2–6.

112 Dolto's articles were 'Hypothèse nouvelle concernant les réactions dites de jalousie à la naissance d'un puîné', *Psyché*, 7, 9 and 10 (1947); 'Les Sensations coenesthésiques d'aise ou de malaise, origine des sentiments de culpabilité', *Psyché*, 18 and 19 (1948); 'Rapport sur l'interprétation psychanalytique des dessins au cours des traitements psychothérapiques', *Psyché*, 17 (1948).

113 See Desmazières, *L'Inconscient au paradis*, pp. 141ff.

114 *Direction spirituelle et psychologie: Études carmélitaines* (1951).

115 *Mystique et continence. Travaux scientifiques du VIIe congrès international d'Avon: Études Carmélitaines* (1952/1).

116 Françoise Dolto, 'Continence et développement de la personnalité', *Études carmélitaines* (1952/1), 209–19, reprinted in Françoise Dolto, *La Difficulté de vivre* (Paris: Vertiges-Carrère, 1986), pp. 251–66, 265.

117 Dolto, 'Continence et développement', *La Difficulté de vivre*, p. 266.

118 Françoise Dolto, 'Comment on crée chez l'enfant une fausse culpabilité', *Etudes carmélitaines* (1949/2), 43–56, reprinted in *La Difficulté de vivre*, pp. 267–84, 267.

119 Françoise Dolto, 'La Psychanalyse chez les enfants atteints des troubles du comportement', in *Ve Congrès international des Médecins Catholiques, Paris 6–9 juillet 1951* (Paris: l'Expansion scientifique française, 1952), 71–89. Copy in AFD, box 5: Psychanalyse et pédagogie, fiche A7. See Desmazières, *L'Inconscient au paradis*, pp. 122–5.

120 Françoise Dolto, 'Les Sensations coenesthésiques d'aise ou de malaise', *Psyché* (1948), reprinted in Françoise Dolto, *Au jeu du désir: Essais cliniques* (Paris: Seuil, 1981), pp. 18–59, 21.
121 Françoise Dolto, 'Comment on crée chez l'enfant une fausse culpabilité', *La Difficulté de vivre*, p. 280.
122 Dolto to Mme François Jacquemin, 20 December 1949, *Une vie de correspondances*, pp. 182–3.
123 Dolto, *Cause des enfants*, p. 41.
124 AFD, box 47 ('Religion – La Foi'), fiche 4.
125 Quoted in Ohayon, *L'Impossible Rencontre*, p. 247.
126 Alain de Mijolla and Elisabeth Roudinesco, who exposed Laforgue's collaboration in the 1980s, absolved him of antisemitism. Annick Ohayon, having found Laforgue's diary, disagrees. See Ohayon, *L'Impossible Rencontre*, pp. 243–9; Roudinesco, 'René Laforgue et la collaboration manquée Paris/Berlin, 1939–1942. Documents concernant l'histoire de la psychanalyse en France durant l'Occupation', *Cahiers Confrontation*, 16 (1986), 243–78.
127 René Laforgue, *Psychopathologie de l'échec (Napoleon, Robespierre, Rousseau)* (Paris: Payot, 1944).
128 Roudinesco, *Jacques Lacan*, p. 159; Ohayon, *L'Impossible Rencontre*, p. 245.
129 Roudinesco, *Jacques Lacan*, p. 161.
130 *Ibid.*, p. 162.
131 Ohayon, 'Psychoanalysis under the Vichy Regime', pp. 51–2.
132 Desmazières, *L'Inconscient au paradis*, p. 91. On *La Gerbe*, see Richard Golsan, 'Ideology, Cultural Politics and Literary Collaboration at *La Gerbe*', *Journal of European Studies*, 23:89–90 (1993), 27–47.
133 Dolto, 'Les Sensations coenesthésiques', 18.
134 Her correspondence shows that she had been working on a reinterpretation of St John's gospel from as early as 1943. Louis Renou to Dolto, 22 October 1943, *Une vie de correspondances*, p. 20.
135 Françoise Dolto and Gérard Sévérin, *L'Évangile au risque de la psychanalyse, tome 1* (Paris: Delarge, 1977), p. 13.
136 *Ibid.*, p. 10.
137 *Ibid.*, p. 35.
138 Dolto and Sévérin, *L'Évangile au risque de la psychanalyse, tome 2* (Paris: Delarge, 1977), pp. 103–17.
139 Dolto and Sévérin, *La Foi au risque de la psychanalyse* (Paris: Seuil, 1981), p. 40.
140 Dolto and Sévérin, *L'Évangile au risque 1*, pp. 10–11; 145ff. for Dolto's reading of the parable.
141 *Ibid.*, p. 146.

142 *Ibid.*, p. 155.
143 Dolto, *Autoportrait*, p. 186.
144 Lucien Bonnafé et al., 'La Psychanalyse, idéologie réactionnaire', *La Nouvelle Critique*, 7 (1949), 57–72, 57. See also Roudinesco, *Jacques Lacan*, pp. 178–89.
145 Bonnafé et al., 'La Psychanalyse', 63.
146 Desmazières, *L'Inconscient au paradis*, p. 144.
147 *Ibid.*, pp. 122–3.
148 Ohayon, *L'Impossible Rencontre*, pp. 248–9.
149 On the Clark-Williams trial, see Roudinesco, *Jacques Lacan*, pp. 209–12; Mijolla, *La France et Freud 1946–1953*, entries for 1950, 1952, 1953.
150 See Roudinesco, *Jacques Lacan*, p. 208.
151 Dolto 'au docteur Jenny Roudinesco et aux analystes en formation', 27 May 1953, *Une vie de correspondances*, pp. 227–8.
152 Cited in Ohayon, 'Psychoanalysis under the Vichy Regime', p. 52.
153 Dolto to Lacan, 16 May 1953; Dolto to Arturo Prat, 30 May 1953, *Une vie de correspondances*, pp. 224, 229.
154 See Pierre Turquet (head of the IPA's enquiry commission into the SFP), 'Report on a visit to the Société Française de Psychanalyse, 21 June 1960 with some statistical material', in Alain de Mijolla, *La France et Freud Tome 2: D'une scission à l'autre 1954–1964* (Paris: Presses universitaires de France, 2012), pp. 275–9.
155 Roudinesco, *Jacques Lacan*, p. 319.
156 Mijolla, *La France et Freud 1954–1964*, pp. 319ff.
157 Jacques Lacan, *Le Séminaire de Jacques Lacan, livre XI – Les quatre concepts fondamentaux de la psychanalyse, 1964*, ed. Jacques-Alain Miller (Paris: Seuil, 1973).

4

Family politics: popularising psychoanalysis, 1945–68

If the interwar years were when psychoanalysis began to occupy a central place in western intellectual and popular culture, it was in the postwar decades that this centrality translated into significant impacts on ordinary lives and public policy.

Historians of psychological thinking argue that the postwar period crystallised the shift away from the 'Victorian culture of character' in Western Europe and North America, towards the 'permissiveness' of the later twentieth century.[1] After 1945, there was an increased sense that people needed new sources of advice and information on how to handle the problems of daily life. Questions of child-rearing, in particular, were seen as being of societal importance if future generations were to avoid succumbing to totalitarian politics. An array of doctors, clinics, authors and media figures sought to respond, and often drew on psychoanalysis in doing so. A notable example in the United States was Benjamin Spock's *Baby and Child Care* (1946), which used psychoanalytic ideas to encourage liberal, democratic parenting practices and displace the discipline-, obedience- and hygiene-driven approach of earlier behaviourist writers such as Truby King or John B. Watson. In Britain, psychoanalytic ideas transformed judicial policy and social expectations around selfhood, citizenship, mental health and democracy, as Michal Shapira has shown.[2] British psychoanalysts such as Donald Winnicott and John Bowlby intimately connected parenting practices to the survival of democratic societies. In France, magazines and other aspects of popular culture regularly foregrounded psychological thinking, helping to create a form of 'psychologised society' in which, as Sarah Fishman writes, 'the habit of seeing others, children, spouses, and the self, in psychological terms spread'.[3] As the last chapter showed, this tendency reached institutions such as the Catholic Church that had previously been relatively resistant to the new psychological disciplines. Another institution being won over was academia. The Sorbonne created an undergraduate degree programme in psychology, run by the psychoanalyst Daniel Lagache; one of its first graduates, in 1949, was the future philosopher Michel Foucault.[4]

This was a promising situation for Dolto, who from the beginning of her career had consistently sought to popularise psychoanalytic thinking and promote its use in parenting, medicine, education, religion and wider public culture. Her public engagement took numerous forms: magazine articles, press interviews, public lectures, books, radio and television broadcasts. More concretely, she shaped French society by creating or participating in institutions that gave psychoanalysts and psychoanalytically informed educators access to large numbers of young children. This reached its height with the Maison Verte children's centres (Chapter 6), which leveraged the fame of Dolto's 1970s radio broadcasts to obtain public funding and spread across the country. This chapter focuses on an earlier set of institutions, the École des Parents (EdP – The School for Parents) and the Centres Médico-Psycho-Pédagogiques (CMPPs), in which Dolto participated from the 1940s. The section on the EdP argues that it became a vehicle for Dolto and other Laforguian psychoanalysts to disseminate psychoanalytic thinking, and especially their ideas about family structures and gender roles. The CMPPs are shown to have been successful in terms of providing analysts with a state-funded opportunity to engage with families from far lower down the income spectrum than they would have encountered in their private practice. However, their location within the medical bureaucracy made them less effective in spreading enthusiasm for psychoanalysis among ordinary French people. The chapter goes on to examine Dolto's interventions on French radio in 1950 on the subject of sex education, showing how she used this platform both to promote the acceptance of psychoanalysts as experts on such questions, and to disseminate her views on the importance of bringing up children according to a strongly binary conception of gender roles.

Schooling the parents

As the influence of behaviourism weakened and that of psychoanalysis grew, the idea that babies are fully human subjects with delicate psyches, requiring attentive nurturing and significant freedom to develop in accordance with their internal rhythms and desires, became commonplace. The interwar pioneers of this approach, such as Susan Isaacs in Britain or Édouard Pichon in France, frequently combined this notion with a liberal approach to education drawn from the child-centred pedagogies advocated by John Dewey, Maria Montessori, Célestin Freinet and Friedrich Froebel. Pichon's views, as set out in his 1936 textbook on education, were considered in Chapter 1. Isaacs (1885–1948) was a teacher and writer who worked to convert psychoanalysis into common-sense recommendations for popular consumption, and who to that extent can be seen as a precursor or comparator for Dolto.[5] Having studied philosophy at Manchester University and then undergone psychoanalysis in the early 1920s, Isaacs ran the Malting House School from 1924 to 1929, where she developed a child-centred, discovery-based pedagogy.[6] In 1929 she published *The Nursery Years* (1929), a seventy-five-page manual on child psychology which sold 100,000 copies.[7] From 1929 to 1936 Isaacs wrote a column on 'Childhood problems' under the pseudonym 'Ursula Wise' in *Nursery World*, a magazine aimed at nannies, and from 1933 she ran courses in child development at the University of London targeted at early-years educators. Her example demonstrates that a psychoanalytic approach to education could lead to a diverse career, informing interventions in areas ranging from medicine to schools, higher education and the popular press – a similar range of fields to that in which Dolto would also intervene several decades later.

Whereas Isaacs was a socialist, the dominant political orientation of the liberal-psychoanalytic approach to education in France was that of the holistic-technocratic-Catholic Right described in the previous chapter. The example of the EdP, to which Dolto contributed in the early 1950s, illustrates how that approach could be deployed alongside the gender-normative conception of the family advocated by interwar conservatives and, after 1940, promoters of the National Revolution.

A Parisian institute offering parenting training and marriage counselling, the EdP was set up in 1929 by the bourgeois Catholic Marguerite Lebrun, better known as Madame Vérine, and run by Catholic intellectuals and pro-family campaigners.[8] Created in the context of interwar pronatalist and familialist efforts to improve the quantity and quality of France's population, it can also be interpreted as an attempt to reclaim educational space from the secular republican state. Supported by interwar family lobbying groups such as the Alliance Nationale pour l'Accroissement de la Population Française (National Alliance for the Growth of the French Population) with a board comprising social Catholics, educators, parents and priests, the EdP aimed to teach parents how to inculcate moral and social values in their children.[9] In doing so, as Annick Ohayon has shown, it became a pioneer of psychosociology and an early site for the popularisation of psychoanalysis.[10] Pichon gave talks at the École in the 1930s, as did other psychoanalysts including notably André Berge, Dolto's friend and fellow analysand of René Laforgue. Berge, later also president of the French Montessori society, took on a leadership role in the EdP, as Vérine's deputy.

Madame Vérine blended Catholic familialism with a libertarian educational approach, emphasising the importance of according children space for inquisitiveness, play and expression. Her book *La Mère initiatrice* (*The Initiating Mother*, 1928) argued that, rather than focus on control, repression and punishment, mothers should encourage children's curiosity, and answer their questions (including sexual ones) frankly.[11] At the same time, Vérine believed that the French family had become debased – and that this helped explain France's geopolitical woes. In 1940, Vérine and other EdP leaders enthusiastically signed up to the National Revolution. Vérine was the only woman to write a section of the Vichy manifesto *France 1941: La Révolution nationale constructive* (*France 1941: Building The National Revolution*). Vérine's text exalted the patriarchal family and deplored young women who resisted it: 'Woman – wife and mother – is made for Man, for the home, for children. Until all of France's young wives understand this, and live out this natural truth, nothing of civic value will be built.'[12]

After Vérine's death in 1946, the EdP reorganised, losing its confessional character and political links. It tried to widen its popular audience by launching an in-house magazine with a print run of 10,000 copies.[13] Under the patronage from 1949 of Georges Heuyer, the psychiatrist of juvenile delinquency who supported psychoanalysis in interwar France (Chapter 1), its emphasis became less moralist, and more medical and technical. Psychiatrists, psychologists and psychoanalysts of different theoretical persuasions became involved. Psychoanalysis, in particular, seemed a promising addition to the toolkit of the parenting school since it claimed the ability to explain how the parenting practices and childhood experiences of individuals were connected to macro-scale political and social developments. Depending on political persuasion, it thus offered the hope of either preventing moral degeneration and/or forestalling the development of proto-totalitarian thought patterns.[14]

These changes did not, however, mean that the École's attitude to women and gender had changed – just as the postwar period as a whole saw a reassertion, rather than an undermining, of patriarchal power.[15] Within the EdP, these attitudes were now recast in the psychoanalytic terminology associated with Laforgue and his understanding of family neuroses and penis envy. In 1946 André Berge, the EdP's vice-president, argued in *Psyché* that the roles women had recently assumed in the workplace, politics and warfare had unbalanced their families. Drawing on penis envy theory, Berge claimed that 'blinded by the discovery of their new possibilities, women are sometimes tempted to reject the old ones … [thereby] compromising the balance of life'.[16] Berge thus continued to romanticise women's exclusively maternal role after the war, and justified this using psychoanalytic concepts. Unlike Dolto, however, Berge subsequently became a supporter of the family planning movement, which sought to give women greater control over their fertility.[17]

Dolto spoke at the EdP at least six times between 1950 and 1954. Her talks covered topics such as parental separation, the only child, the appropriate role of grandparents and children's sleep.[18] In them, Dolto seized on everyday parenting questions as opportunities to disseminate psychoanalytic ideas, by explaining concepts like 'neurosis', 'complex' and 'castration' in ordinary language and emphasising their relevance to everyday life. Thus in one text she defined a neurosis as 'the fact of feeling impotent, of feeling completely stuck in an impossible situation'.[19] This definition left out some central elements of Freud's concept, such as the conflict between different psychical entities, or the return of the repressed. Rather than broach these more technical ideas, Dolto applied the word to the commonplace feeling of being blocked or trapped, effectively inviting her audience to incorporate the psychoanalytic term into their everyday language. She also promoted childhood determinism, the idea that children's psychological problems could be 'heavily consequential' for their future psychological constitution and that psychological education on the part of parents could help prevent this.[20] She suggested that many apparently minor aspects of a child's life, such as their relationship to animals and plants, could be very psychologically significant. The clear implication was that parents should be very attentive to, and seek to optimise, their children's psychological states: something that necessitated close, emotionally sophisticated parent-child relationships rather than austere, disciplinarian ones.

Dolto also used her EdP talks to stress the importance of large families, presenting this as a nugget of wisdom gleaned from her psychoanalytic clinic, and not discussing the political component of the concept or its importance in her own upbringing. At the beginning of her talk on one-child families, Dolto hastened to affirm that 'being an only child doesn't make you ill' – but the rest of her text contained several more or less severe warnings about the psychological dangers.[21] As products of 'a household which has refused to generate other lives', such children – Dolto contended – struggled to develop both physically and emotionally, and were unable to see their parents in their proper capacity as 'progenitors'.[22] Having difficulty in developing manual dexterity, they took refuge in intellectual pursuits and thus succeeded at school, but not necessarily socially or, later, romantically. Used to being on their own, they could not cope with competition and lacked team spirit: 'the great obsessives are often from one-child families, people whose muscular impotence has led to an excessive flight into the mental realm'.[23] Growing up surrounded by other children was, for Dolto, vital for a child's 'cohesion'; parents who really cared about their child's psychological well-being would therefore ensure that siblings were provided. Maud Mannoni, who met Dolto in 1947, testified to the pressure that Dolto put on her to marry and procreate: 'Her conservative opinions about families implied that one got married in order to have children: I managed to provide … one child, but I couldn't resolve myself to give her three.'[24]

On the question of parental separation, Dolto did not speak out against divorce directly, finding it to be less generative of psychological conflicts than situations where parents maintained a false appearance of unity: 'There are fewer neuroses, including serious neuroses, in children who are presented with a clear, defined situation – where people aren't spending their lives "pretending."'[25] Nonetheless, she also argued that divorce risked causing juvenile delinquency, since adolescents could operate an unconscious linguistic slippage from the 'delinquency' of their parents' act in getting divorced, to carrying out 'delinquent' petty crime themselves.[26] For Dolto, what mattered was that, regardless of the family structure, the parents or people *in loco parentis* provided appropriate psychological role models that children could (spontaneously, unconsciously) internalise. This required men and women to embody clearly distinguished masculine and feminine roles: 'as living examples, the father and mother, through their way of being, structure the child's concepts of "masculine" and "feminine"'.[27] Parents therefore needed to model the idea of a 'complementary fecundity' in order to foster the 'cohesion' and 'vitality' of their children's psyches.[28] Indeed, as Dolto saw it, this was one of the key tasks of parenting.

As Camille Robcis has pointed out, there are resemblances between Dolto's argument here and the 'structuralist social contract' suggested by the work of Claude Lévi-Strauss in *The Elementary Structures of Kinship* (1949), especially after Lévi-Strauss's conclusions had been taken up by Jacques Lacan. As Robcis sees it, what Dolto was doing in her EdP texts was effectively to transform Lévi-Strauss's descriptive language about the functioning of human societies into a prescriptive or imperative mode.[29] However, though Dolto had begun to use the language of 'structure' and 'cohesion' by the 1950s, it is not obvious that there is a direct link: there is no evidence that Dolto had read Lévi-Strauss, and Lacan only took up structuralism in earnest in his 'Rome discourse' of 1953. At most, it would seem that, at a time when structuralist ideas were beginning to be widely discussed in intellectual culture, people like Dolto saw the potential to adopt structuralist language to give existing familialist concepts a further degree of scientific justification. The structuralist connection was not clearly fundamental to the success of the psychoanalytic-familialist ideas of Dolto and her fellow

Laforguians, since their implementation into public culture and medical institutions was already well underway.

The Centre Claude Bernard and the Centres Médico-Psycho-Pédagogiques

Dolto's talks at the EdP show her seeking to popularise psychoanalytic thinking, and promote the importance of close, attentive parenting relationships – alongside a gendered conception of the ideal family, as characterised by a strong and vigorous male presence at the head of a plentiful crop of physically robust, non-intellectual offspring. At the Centre Claude Bernard (CCB), formed in 1946, she sought to translate these ideas into clinical practice with patients from poor or averagely off backgrounds, to whom she would have been unlikely to have had access through her private practice. The CCB was a new, psychoanalytically oriented children's clinic whose ideology and personnel overlapped with those of the EdP. Describing itself as a 'centre psycho-pédagogique' (later amended to 'centre médico-psycho-pédagogique' or CMPP), the centre aimed to make psychoanalytic therapy available to families of modest means.[30] It was created by Georges Mauco, a psychoanalyst and demographer, along with his fellow medically qualified analysts Berge, Dolto and Juliette (Favez-)Boutonnier. Marc Schlumberger, who had studied medicine alongside Dolto and worked at Summerhill, A. S. Neill's experimental school in Suffolk, was also involved. By restricting itself to medically qualified analysts, the centre avoided the kind of controversy that affected the SPP with the Clark-Williams affair. Perhaps more significantly, it was able to access new public funding available following an extension of state-supported health insurance in 1945 that permitted families unable to afford private treatment to recoup the cost of specialist consultations. Parents could thus book an effectively free or low-cost appointment with a medically qualified analyst to discuss problems with their children's character or behaviour. As Mauco explained in an article for *Psyché*, these might include 'shyness, emotionalism, enuresis, anxiety, tics, nervousness, petty delinquency, anomalous sexual behaviour, etc'.[31] The centre offered children, adolescents and their parents the benefits of psychoanalytic, medical and psychological expertise, communicated in a friendly setting designed not to feel like a hospital.

The CCB's creation was assisted by Mauco's political connections. Mauco had gained a degree of recognition in the 1930s for his doctoral thesis on immigration, which was informed by a racist, Lamarcko-Jungian understanding of the collective unconscious and acquired group characteristics. His thesis ranked different races and nationalities according to their perceived assimilability to French society, and was welcomed across the political spectrum as a scientific contribution to the question of how the French state should approach immigration.[32] Mauco joined the fascist Parti Populaire Français in the 1930s, and during the Occupation wrote a piece for the anthropology journal *L'Ethnie française*, edited by extreme antisemite Georges Montagnon. Mauco's article combined psychoanalysis with racism by postulating the existence of a 'Jewish neurosis'.[33] At the Liberation, De Gaulle nonetheless appointed Mauco as secretary to the Haut Comité Consultatif de la Population et de la Famille (High Committee on Population and the Family), thus giving him the opportunity to advise on how many, and which, displaced persons and immigrants France should accept.[34] Thereafter Mauco, who had trained as a teacher in the 1920s, reinvented himself as an expert on child psychology and education, apparently successfully concealing his wartime activities and antisemitism from colleagues and the young psychologists and analysts he trained and directed. He remained head of the CCB until 1971. In 1982, Dolto wrote a preface to Mauco's autobiography, *Vécu*, which highlighted his moral qualities and claimed that Mauco 'had known how to resist Nazi barbarism'.[35]

The analysts who worked at the CCB in its early years were all former analysands of Laforgue, trained in his ideas of family neuroses and focused on the immediate nuclear family as the site of aetiology. Most were from Catholic, bourgeois backgrounds. This contrasted with the patients, who judging by the surviving records in Dolto's archive were generally from lower-middle-class families: artisans or small businessmen with 'mediocre' living standards.[36] Dolto appears to have ceased working formally with the centre after 1949, but her case records are sufficient to indicate the kinds of problems treated and the orientation of her responses. In effect, situations that the CCB categorised as 'médico-psychologique' were those in which a child's behaviour presented cause for concern to a parent, a doctor or, most frequently, a teacher. Patients sent to Dolto at the CCB were variously described in their referral documents as 'obsessional and anxious', 'antagonistic to everyone' or suffering from 'character disorders', 'poor academic performance' or 'personality disturbances confirmed by all the tests'.[37]

Dolto's diagnostic comments on these patients show her working to (re)construct the unconscious intra-familial conflicts and psychosexual tensions that she was convinced lay at the heart of almost every case. For one boy – referred on the grounds that he was 'distracted, headstrong. Lacks concentration in class. Fearful, shy, hypersensitive' – Dolto diagnosed 'a castration complex lived out in the anal mode. Schizophrenic behaviour. Severe maternal and paternal neurosis.'[38] The themes of her talks at the EdP, such as the importance of the models of virility and femininity transmitted by parents to children, recur in her case notes. The importance of a strong paternal figure is particularly prominent: of one boy, she wrote that 'his father is far too soft for him ... a weak man with a "victim" mentality'.[39] Her diagnostic conclusion for a nine-year-old daughter of a *lycée* teacher, treated for lack of motivation and 'temperamental attitude', was 'Obsessive parents. Affective inversion of the couple & older mother. Psychoanalytic psychotherapy urgent ++.'[40] While Dolto did not ignore the wider social context surrounding her child patients – such as their participation in religious or scout groups, or in one case the 'nationality difficulties' encountered by a parent of Italian origin – she always looked to the family dynamic as the ultimate source of the problem. She frequently described that dynamic in terms that disapproved of, indeed pathologised, any deviation from her ideal of a fecund family with a virile fatherly presence.

This is visible even in the case of her most famous CCB patient, the future novelist Georges Perec, whom she treated in 1949. Perec, then thirteen, was living with an aunt and uncle following the deaths of his father (in fighting in 1940) and mother (in Auschwitz). Dolto told Perec's aunt that while Georges's difficulties were mainly down to the war, they were also partly caused by being part of a family of strong women and weak men, and the relative professional success of his aunt in comparison to his father.[41] It was not that Dolto was oblivious to wider contexts beyond the family or completely insensitive to the psychological impact of what Perec, playing on a

French homonym, would later call '*l'Histoire avec sa grande hache*' ('History with a capital H'/'History with its big axe').[42] But in her final analyses and public statements, such factors tended to fade into the background, while family dynamics came to the fore. Dolto very rarely publicly mentioned the impact of World War II in causing childhood trauma, for example, even though her case records indicate that she saw numerous examples of this occurring. When she did discuss it, she did so only to highlight its effects on family dynamics – such as the supposed link between POW fathers and juvenile delinquency – rather than as a traumatising factor in its own right. By contrast, she repeatedly wrote and spoke publicly about the harmful effects of growing up in a family in which patriarchal gender norms were not respected, for which the formula of 'strong mother, weak father' could stand as a kind of shorthand. (Chapter 5 will return to this theme in the context of autistic children.)

The CCB proved a success, at least from the point of view of the analysts involved and from that of the medical structures that funded it. The model that it established subsequently became widely replicated. From the 1960s, some 400 CMPPs spread throughout France, becoming a significant vector for the diffusion of psychoanalytic concepts in wider French society. As well as the CCB, Dolto worked at (and received a salary from) the Étienne Marcel CMPP in central Paris after its creation in 1961 (this was also the setting for the 'Dominique' case discussed in Chapter 5). The CMPPs indirectly gave rise to a later set of institutions, the Lieux d'Accueil Enfants-Parents (LAEPs), which will be discussed further in Chapter 6.

The CCB initially wore its psychoanalytic orientation somewhat lightly, partly for fear of triggering the wrath of the Ordre des Médecins, but by the 1960s many CMPPs were openly psychoanalytic in orientation.[43] Some were set up with the explicit aim of improving awareness of psychoanalysis among psychiatrists and the general public. Researching in the mid-1970s, Sherry Turkle found that CMPPs had been the principal site in which her working-class interviewees had encountered psychoanalysis. This, Turkle suggested, might partly explain the relatively negative impression of psychoanalysis provided by working-class interviewees in comparison to middle-class or intellectual respondents. Poor families often found that, via the CMPP system, they would be assigned (not choose) an analyst only after passing through a series of offices and

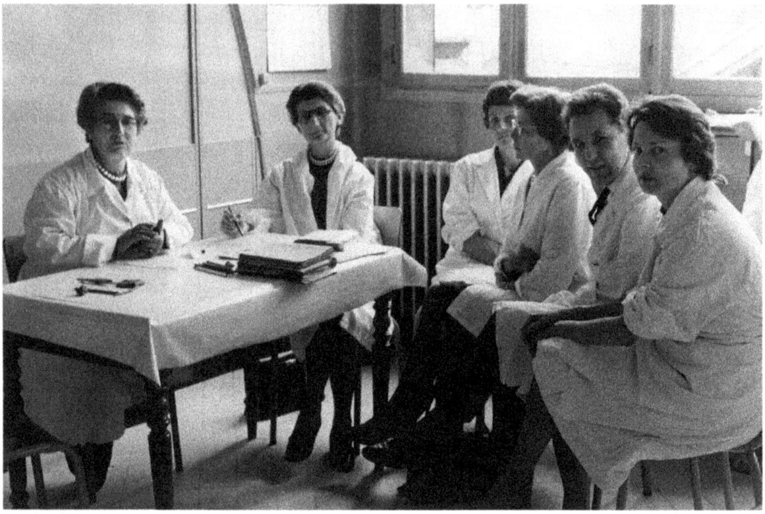

Figure 4.1 Dolto with junior colleagues, probably at the Centre Médico-Psycho-Pédagogique Étienne Marcel, Paris, 1963. L–r: Dolto, Antoinette Huot, Christiane Guillemet, Ursula Huber, Bernard This, Françoise Ledoux

a battery of tests. For them, 'the sense of personal humiliation associated with public health facilities interfered with any sense of psychoanalysis as liberating'.[44] Turkle's research, conducted just before Dolto's breakthrough into popular consciousness with *Lorsque l'enfant paraît*, suggests why use of the mass media was important to the continued advance of psychoanalysis into French culture. Medico-psychological institutes and clinics operating on top-down lines and within bureaucratic constraints were limited in their ability to implant psychoanalytic thinking into popular child-rearing practices. Achieving that would require charismatic advocates able to connect with a broad section of the French public.

Sex(ed) education

Dolto's inclination from the very beginning of her career had been to look beyond the small circles of the psychoanalytic movement and to spread her core ideas by engaging with the mass media and popular audiences. As early as autumn 1939, she wrote to the Service de la radiodiffusion at the Ministère des Postes with a (now lost) proposal for some kind of radio broadcast, probably aimed at parents and children in response to the psychological difficulties caused by the outbreak of war.[45] It was after this idea had proved unviable that Dolto sought to engage with a popular audience via the magazine *Vrai*, as described in the previous chapter.

It is not clear when Dolto first spoke on radio. The earliest evidence is a letter from her husband in February 1947 praising her contribution to an unspecified broadcast.[46] More definitively, on 6 February 1948 Dolto appeared on *La Tribune de Paris*, a national radio programme, as a participant in a debate on 'the resurgence of juvenile delinquency'. Dolto was introduced simply as a doctor, appearing alongside the children's author Paul Faucher (famous for the popular book series *Albums du père Castor*) and a scout leader. She spoke on *La Tribune de Paris* again in December 1949, advising parents on which toys would make the most psychologically beneficial Christmas presents for children. Dolto recommended Guignol puppets, which, she said, allowed children to verbalise otherwise forbidden words and ideas. She also suggested toys that children could be allowed to break and smash, since aggressive actions were part of the discovery process of play.[47]

In 1950 *La Tribune de Paris* invited Dolto to take part in a series of five debates on sex education, broadcast on five successive Tuesday evenings at 11.00 p.m., a slot selected so that children would be in bed, or 'if they're not, perhaps there'll be nothing to teach them'.[48] Joining the moderator Raymond Thévenin and Dolto, presented as a '*doctoresse*' and psychoanalyst, were three men: Joseph Logre, a psychiatrist; Père Charles Larère, a Catholic spokesman; and Louis François, Inspecteur Général de l'Instruction Publique (Inspector General of State Education), who had represented France at UNESCO and chaired a government committee on sex education in schools. These broadcasts, or rather the reaction to them, can be seen as a marker of the progress of 'psychologisation' in France in 1950. They were seen as being of sufficient public interest for *Marie France* to publish extracts over a series of editions, and for *Elle* magazine (which by 1955 was read by one in six French women) to publish the entire transcript over five issues.[49] *Elle* presented the broadcast as of interest to young parents seeking enlightenment on child psychology and sexuality, helping them to answer questions such as

> How can you make your child into the harmonious, balanced man or woman that you want them to be? How can you, in short, teach them things that you, their parents, doubtless were never taught but which you feel are an awkward but urgent necessity for them?[50]

The transcripts thus show how the subject of sex education encapsulated a cultural move towards more permissive parenting attitudes, and an attentiveness towards young people's thought and experiences that was presumed to have been absent for earlier generations. Much of the dramatic tension in the broadcasts came from the fundamental opposition between the stances of Dolto and Louis François. Dolto advised parents to be direct and clear when discussing sexuality, so as to disarm it of its shameful or dirty connotations; François preferred 'a more evocative, even poetic language'. He maintained that the sexual instinct was 'fearsome … left unconstrained, [it] risks leading to all kinds of perversions and ruining an individual's mental balance'.[51] He argued that children under the age of seven or eight were largely ignorant of sex; there was no need to disturb their imaginative world with such discussions. Dolto countered that children should be told the truth, frankly and honestly, to help them avoid developing anxieties around sexuality. She subsequently received letters from listeners praising her 'frank and clear' stance in contrast to the unworldly 'innocence' of François.[52] Yet this contrast should not mask the broader agreement between all four participants on the importance of consulting psychological experts on such issues. At one point, Pére Larère cited a 1929 papal encyclical on education, which, he claimed, 'expressly asked Christian parents to undertake [sexual] education in good time … I turn to Doctor Dolto-Marette so that she can tell us at what age we can begin that education.'[53] This was a creative reading of Pius XI's text, which in fact condemned 'the error of those who with dangerous assurance and under an ugly term propagate a so-called sex-education, falsely imagining they can forearm youths against the dangers of sensuality'.[54] Larère's theological flexibility here, and deference to Dolto's medico-psychological authority, illustrates the willingness of parts of the postwar church to incorporate psychological expertise, and to set aside the more reactionary interwar attitudes of the high church.

Taking advantage of such deference, Dolto continually turned the focus of discussion away from adolescence and onto early childhood, bringing the debate into her domain of expertise and accentuating the contrast between her, as a woman and mother, and the male participants. 'You are a man, therefore a father ... it's therefore natural that you don't know how to respond', Dolto told François at one point. 'I'm particularly speaking to mums.'[55] Dolto thus both exploited and reinforced the assumption that it was natural for mothers to be better acquainted with children than were fathers. Focusing the discussion on early childhood also allowed Dolto subtly to change the key question from 'how to talk about sex' with older children to 'how to be sexed' for young children – that is, how to teach children the gendered roles they would perform later in life:

> Education begins in the cradle – not, of course, sex education in the sense of learning about reproduction, but sexed education, that which teaches children how to become like Daddy, for a boy, like Mummy, for a girl ... the goal of education is to preserve among little ones the intuitive sense of the *big boy* or *big girl* that they should become.[56]

Dolto thus switched the focus from sex acts to sex roles, conflating the question of telling children the facts of life with that of preparing them for the expected gendered norms of adulthood. This move discouraged wider conversations about schools, or the place of sex in society, and directed the audience's attention towards the family as the primary educational site. Correspondence she received following the broadcasts indicates that this message was well received by at least some parents. For example, 'Rolande B.' wrote to thank Dolto for her on-air advice, informing her that 'my little girl aged six-and-a-half has been brought up to speed thanks to your words, and it all seemed natural to her ... At the same time, she has become aware of her role as a future wife and mother, and little by little will be able to prepare herself for her duties.'[57] Dolto thus clearly had at least some success in conflating a permissive approach to sex education with a message about reinforcing conventional gender roles and family structures.

Claire Duchen, in her history of French women's postwar lives and rights, showed that the dominant atmosphere regarding 'women's place' and 'women's role' in these years was a 'generally hostile context' towards women who sought to resist being confined to a deferential role of housewife and mother. After 1945, new anxieties arose regarding the 'modern woman' – more self-assertive and inclined to pursue professional work – and her potential to 'dominate' her husband and children.[58] The so-called liberal professions of medicine, law and banking remained 'bastions of reaction, hostile to women's participation'.[59] Nonetheless, Sarah Fishman argues that the misogyny of much 1950s discursive output should not obscure the differences with Occupation-era views.[60] Whereas Vichy celebrated the sacrifices and self-abnegation of motherhood, 1950s and 1960s mothers, 'while still primarily viewed as focused on their families and homes, were advised to strive for equilibrium in their lives, to save a part of themselves'.[61] Fathers, though still clearly seen as the heads of families, could now be censured for excessive authoritarianism, indifference or not playing enough of a collaborative role in everyday family life – issues that would not have been considered a problem in 1940.[62] Fishman thus suggests that historians need to look past the conventional surface-level misogyny of 1950s discourse on the family and instead ask what was new or changing. In particular, the interest shown in the works of Simone de Beauvoir, Alfred Kinsey and Sigmund Freud in the early 1950s suggests a population beginning to think about the psychology of gender and sexuality in ways that were not possible a decade earlier.[63] *Elle*'s framing of the 1950 sex education debate, with its focus on the importance of children growing up to be 'harmonious' and 'balanced', is suggestive of a society in which the premise of the crucial importance of childhood experience in shaping future adult minds was becoming widely accepted – something that can be contrasted with the late and marginal development of psychoanalysis in the interwar years.

Dolto's texts from this period can be considered as both a part of and response to this discursive shift. As the example of the *La Tribune de Paris* broadcasts illustrates, her attempts to influence parenting and education along liberal lines were inseparable from her views on family structures and gender roles, but Dolto often seemed keen to emphasise that the one should not be promoted without the other. Alongside her liberalism or libertarianism on parenting methods, Dolto upheld a vision of the family centred on paternal authority and mothers' subservience to fathers' desires and children's needs. She claimed that families in which the father's authority was too weak, and the dominance of the mother too strong, were liable to provoke mental disturbance in children, especially boys. In doing this, she was to some extent echoing a conventional wisdom of the time: concerns about dominant and domineering mothers were widespread in 1950s juvenile court reports, for example.[64] But Dolto also encouraged 1950s social attitudes to move away from Vichy-era hierarchies and authoritarianism, towards more attentive parenting, more respect and indulgence for children, more child-centred pedagogies and more freedom for women to consider their own sexuality and needs and be less self-sacrificing. Dolto thus contributed to the establishment of new cultural visions of the family and new ideas about the self, oriented more towards individual fulfilment than self-sacrifice. As someone who clearly was not seeking to threaten the normative, patriarchal vision of gender roles – rather the contrary – she could be relied on to not create too much controversy, or offend the largely Catholic audiences of the EdP or *La Tribune de Paris*. In the context of the early 1950s, Dolto's conventional conservatism on gender questions may have bolstered her credibility in arguing for more liberal attitudes to parenting and education. However, as time went on, and social mores moved towards more liberal parenting while Dolto's views on gender remained unchanged from her early-1950s positions, her stance began to appear more noticeably conservative.

Some perspective can be gained by comparing Dolto's views with those of groups that fought for women's rights in the 1950s and 1960s, such as the Mouvement Démocratique Féminin (MDF – Women's Democratic Movement), and the Mouvement Français pour le Planning Familial (MFPF – French Family Planning Movement). The doctors and journalists who led the MFPF were frequently ex-resisters, many from Protestant or Jewish backgrounds, which gave them a very different perspective from the Catholic Vichy-sympathisers in Dolto's circle. Some of them indeed saw the battle to defeat medical moralists and the Catholic Church as a continuation of the wartime struggle, since the Ordre des Médecins, which opposed family planning, remained dominated by conservative, xenophobic, anti-feminist currents. The MDF and MFPF contributed to the wider change in social attitudes between 1945 and 1968. By the time that reforms – improving women's legal position within marriage in 1965, increasing the length of paid maternity leave in 1966 and implementing access to contraception in 1967 – were finally passed, they were seen as belatedly sanctioning long-widespread attitudes and common practices.[65] Nonetheless, the family as an institution remained sufficiently central to political discourse that the campaigns for these reforms had to be framed in terms of strengthening and improving family life. As Lisa Greenwald has argued, only after conservative senators were reassured that the institution of the family would be protected 'could the government begin providing for wives' equality in law as it was being increasingly lived out in fact'.[66] The contraception campaigners' key gambit was to move the emphasis from large families to happy ones, by deploying the term 'happy motherhood' (*maternité heureuse*): rather than trying to maximise family sizes, the state should ensure that every birth was truly desired.

Some psychoanalysts joined this cause, arguing that avoiding unwanted pregnancies would result in fewer unhappy children and avoid the trauma of clandestine abortions.[67] Dolto was not among them. Although the marriage law reform that was ultimately passed in 1965 disappointed women's rights advocates – granting married women control over their solely owned financial assets but leaving the husband's legal position as the head of the family intact, along with his ability to control shared assets and veto his wife's employment choices – Dolto still felt that it had gone too far.[68] In a text written for (but not finally included in) Ménie Grégoire's book, *Le Métier de femme* (*Women's Work*, 1965), which appeared as the reform was being debated, Dolto deployed the authority of psychoanalysis to reinforce the biological essentialism that lay at the heart of opposition to the measure:

> Psychoanalysis has brought to light in irrefutable fashion that, just as in biology not one cell of a female body resembles a cell of the male body, *not one of the emotional states, acts or thoughts of a woman is neutral*. All of her psychology and all of her behaviour develop in a feminine key, according to highly-gendered impulses ... Man and woman are to humanity as the right and hands are to a functioning human body ... [woman is] by her genital form passively open to the

> future of time, whose rhythms resound in her womb [*qu'elle scande en ses entrailles*].[69]

If the laws of states accorded civic rights disproportionately to men, this was, Dolto wrote, an unconscious compensation for the excessive strength of the 'real' power of women within the home:

> If over such a long period, in our civilisation of detribalized Christian couples which has conquered the world, written laws appear to deny freedom to individual women and accord civic rights only to men, it's because the *real everyday power of women, at home, has been unconsciously recognized as too strong*. That's without doubt the reason for the fact that, at all times in human societies, authority has been the province of men.[70]

Dolto here stuck to the widespread 1950s claim that it was women, not men, who possessed the power to dominate their children, with potentially severe consequences for their psychological well-being. She was also echoing the Gaullist speaker of the National Assembly, Henri Collette, who claimed that the law was unnecessary since France had informally established 'a rather strong matriarchy in which the husband does not act before consulting his wife'.[71] Such claims were not sufficient to clinch the argument; opponents of women's liberation were defeated in 1965, 1967 and above all in 1975 with the legalisation of abortion. But, as Sandrine Garcia argues, the emphasis on women's supposedly excessive (if informal) power in the family, rather than on the fact of their legal inferiority, suggested a possible new strategy for social conservatives in the wake of these defeats.[72] If women were powerful to the point of being 'too strong' on an everyday level within their homes, then children needed protection from them – protection that could only come from a strong and legally empowered father figure.

In the decade following the abortion reform, Dolto developed a new emphasis on children and children's rights as a crusading cause. In her 1985 book *La Cause des enfants*, she deployed language which presented all children, collectively, as a neglected or persecuted minority. 'Parents educate children like princes govern peoples', she wrote. 'To an adult, the idea that a human being in its child form could be considered their equal is scandalous.'[73] In the context of post-1968 anti-authoritarianism, she claimed that parental authority was one more 'hierarchy between those who command and those who obey' in need of challenge.

But Dolto's mission to create 'a society at the service of childhood' – the title of one of the sections of *La Cause des enfants* – had another aspect. As will be shown in Chapter 6, Dolto's vision for a society built around the needs and desires of children, and her advice to individual parents, often assumed a level of parenting commitment that would in practice make it impossible for women to work outside the home. Dolto, whose own childhood and parenting experience had featured assistance from numerous nannies and various other paid workers, rarely displayed much understanding of the difficulties faced by working mothers of limited means. Asked by a current affairs television programme in 1963 whether it was preferable for schools to open on Thursdays or Saturdays – the French state school system being in the process of adjusting its timetables so as better to align with the standard working week – Dolto answered 'neither', since 'it's necessary [for children] to have at least one day a week with nothing to do – really nothing! That's to say lose track of time, look at things, think, tinker, sew.'[74] The implications for working parents should not, she implied, be a consideration. As social attitudes changed, and feminism became an important force in French social politics in the 1970s, Dolto saw no reason to change her views on women's equality. 'It doesn't surprise me that I give the impression of being retro', she said in 1977. 'But it's neither retro nor not-retro, it's eternal ... It's something that is unconsciously written into everyone's biology ... It can't go out of fashion, because you can't change your biology.'[75]

Statements like this give the lie to Dolto's claim to association with post-1968 radicalism, which will be discussed further in the next chapter. To some extent they may have had a strategic element: her inflexible views on sex difference, gender roles and women's rights offered her rhetorical protection from ultra-conservatives, cover from which she could advocate for more liberal educational methods, or for more attentive, empathetic parenting from fathers as well as mothers, without it being possible to dismiss her as a neurotic feminist seeking to destroy the institution of the family. But there is no indication that her views were not sincerely held; indeed, they aligned closely with her psychoanalytic version of childhood determinism. Sex differences and gender roles must, Dolto felt, be a red line at which progressive change had to halt, or else both individual psyches and societal structures would be put at risk. Her insistence on these matters was to have wide-reaching consequences in subsequent decades.

Notes

1 Mathew Thomson, *Psychological Subjects: Identity, Culture, and Health in Twentieth-Century Britain* (Oxford: Oxford University Press, 2006), p. 10. Thomson developed this argument in *Lost Freedom: The Landscape of the Child and the British Post-War Settlement* (Oxford: Oxford University Press, 2013).
2 Shapira, *War Inside*; also her article 'Psychoanalytic Criminology, Childhood and the Democratic Self', in Matt Ffytche and Daniel Pick (eds), *Psychoanalysis in the Age of Totalitarianism* (Abingdon: Routledge, 2016), pp. 73–86.
3 Fishman, *Vichy to the Sexual Revolution*, p. xxiv.
4 See Ohayon, *L'Impossible Rencontre*, pp. 277–90.
5 Thomson, *Psychological Subjects*, pp. 135–6.
6 Philip J. Graham, *Susan Isaacs: A Life Freeing the Minds of Children* (London: Karnac, 2009), p. 98. On Malting House, see Graham's article 'Susan Isaacs and the Malting House School', *Journal of Child Psychotherapy*, 34:1 (2008), 5–22.
7 Susan Isaacs, *The Nursery Years: The Mind of the Child from Birth to Six Years* (London: Routledge, 1929). Graham, *Susan Isaacs*, p. 202, for the sales figure.
8 Annick Ohayon, 'L'École des Parents ou l'éducation des enfants éclairée par la psychologie (1929–1946)', *Bulletin de psychologie*, 449 (2000), 635–42; Muel-Dreyfus, *Vichy et l'éternel féminin*, pp. 181–4.
9 Robcis, *Law of Kinship*, p. 119.
10 Ohayon, 'L'École des Parents'; also *L'Impossible Rencontre*, pp. 184–9.
11 Madame Vérine (Marguerite Lebrun), *La Mère initiatrice* (Paris: Spes, 1929).
12 Madame Vérine, 'La Famille', in André Bellessort and Raymond Postal (eds), *France 1941: La Révolution nationale constructive, un bilan et un programme* (Paris: Alsatia, 1941), p. 197. See Muel-Dreyfus, *Vichy et l'éternel féminin*, pp. 181–4.
13 Ohayon, *L'Impossible Rencontre*, p. 189.
14 I explore this further in my article 'Democratic Babies? Françoise Dolto, Benjamin Spock and the Ideology of Postwar Parenting Advice', *Journal of Political Ideologies*, 24:2 (2019), 201–19.

15 Greenwald, *Daughters of 1968*, pp. 31–4.
16 André Berge, 'La Crise de la condition féminine et ses répercussions sur la Famille et la Société', *Psyché*, 1 (1946), 51–60.
17 Greenwald, *Daughters of 1968*, p. 78.
18 Françoise Dolto, 'Les Parents séparés', *L'École des Parents* (March 1950), reprinted in Dolto, *Les Chemins de l'éducation* (hereafter *CdE*), pp. 281–303; 'L'Enfant unique', *L'École des Parents* (April 1950), *CdE*, pp. 103–17; 'Les Grands-parents', *L'École des Parents* (December 1950), *CdE*, pp. 233–50; 'Les troubles du sommeil', *L'École des Parents* (April 1952), reprinted in Dolto, *Les Étapes majeures de l'enfance* (Paris: Gallimard, 1994, hereafter *EME*), pp. 138–61; 'L'Influence des animaux et des plantes', *L'École des Parents* (1953), *EME*, pp. 349–73; 'L'Âge des parents', *L'École des Parents* (February 1954), *CdE*, pp. 211–32.
19 Dolto, 'Les Parents séparés', *CdE*, p. 289.
20 *Ibid.*, p. 282.
21 Dolto, 'L'Enfant unique', *CdE*, p. 103.
22 *Ibid.*, p. 114.
23 *Ibid.*, pp. 113, 115.
24 Maud Mannoni, *Ce qui manque à la vérité pour être dite* (Paris: Denoël, 1988), p. 28.
25 Dolto, 'Les Parents séparés', p. 283.
26 *Ibid.*, pp. 292–3.
27 *Ibid.*, p. 283.
28 *Ibid.*
29 Robcis, *Law of Kinship*, p. 139.
30 On the CCB, see Robcis, *Law of Kinship*, pp. 114–27; Geissman and Geissmann, *A History of Child Psychoanalysis*, pp. 298–301; Ohayon, *L'Impossible Rencontre*, pp. 290–2; Mijolla, *La France et Freud 1946–1953*, pp. 14–16.
31 Georges Mauco, 'Consultations psycho-pédagogiques', *Psyché*, 3 (1947) 47–53.
32 Georges Mauco, *Les Étrangers en France: leur rôle dans l'activité économique* (Paris: A. Colin, 1932).
33 See Élisabeth Roudinesco, 'Georges Mauco (1899–1988): Un psychanalyste au service de Vichy. De l'antisémitisme à la psychopédagogie', *L'Infini*, 51 (1995), 69–84; Patrick Weil, 'Georges Mauco, expert en immigration: Ethnoracisme pratique et antisémitisme fielleux', in Pierre-André Taguieff (ed.), *L'Antisémitisme de plume, 1940–1944: Études et documents* (Paris: Berg, 1999), pp. 267–76.
34 See Tara Zahra, *The Lost Children: Reconstructing Europe's Families After World War II* (Cambridge, MA: Harvard University Press, 2011), Ch. 5; Adler, *Jews and Gender*, Ch. 5; Greg Burgess, 'The Demographers'

Moment: Georges Mauco, Immigration and Racial Selection in Liberation France, 1945–46', *French History and Civilization*, 4 (2011), 167–77.

35 Dolto, preface to Georges Mauco, *Vécu 1899–1982: Histoire de l'apparition de la psychanalyse en France* (Paris: Émile Paul, 1982).

36 See e.g. AFD, box labelled 'Cas 5'. Résumé of case of 'Muriel', treated 1955.

37 AFD, Cas 5. Cases of 'Jeannette', treated 1949, 'Résumé de Séances: 1, 2, 3 juin'; 'Rémi', treated 1953, 'Feuille de renseignements scolaires'; 'Muriel', treated 1955.

38 AFD, Cas 4. Case of 'Claude', treated 1951. Typed summary document, undated.

39 AFD, Cas 1. Case of 'Serge', treated 1942–44. From a fourteen-page typed summary dated 1946.

40 AFD, Cas 1. Case of 'Avrille', treated 1948. 'Feuille de synthèse', dated 17 November 1948.

41 David Bellos, *Georges Perec: A Life in Words* (London: Harvill, 1995), p. 370. The notes from this case are not preserved in Dolto's archive, and Perec did not discuss his analysis with Dolto in his published writings. According to Bellos (p. 96), Dolto was recommended to Perec's family by André Berge as an expert interpreter of children's drawings, after Perec's cousin showed him some of Georges's drawings. Perec had drawn an imaginary island, 'W', which became the basis for *W ou le souvenir de l'enfance* (Paris: Denoël, 1975), written during his subsequent analysis with J.-B. Pontalis.

42 Perec, *W ou le souvenir de l'enfance*, p. 17.

43 See Geissmann and Geissman, *A History of Child Psychoanalysis*, p. 300.

44 Turkle, *Psychoanalytic Politics*, p. 321, n. 15.

45 J. Duhamel of the 'Service de la radiodiffusion', to Dolto, 25 October 1939, *Une vie de correspondances*, p. 25. Dolto's original proposal is lost. The reply was encouraging, but warned that Dolto would need the approval of the Ministère de l'Hygiène Publique to proceed.

46 Boris to Françoise, 11 February 1947, AFD, box labelled 'correspondance Françoise-Boris'.

47 *Une vie de correspondances*, p. 190, n. 5.

48 Suzanne Catelain, secrétaire générale de *La Tribune de Paris*, cited in Mijolla, *La France et Freud 1946–1953*, pp. 159–60.

49 *Elle*, 253–7, October–November 1950. 'One in six', Ross, *Fast Cars, Clean Bodies*, p. 209, n. 14.

50 'Comment instruire les enfants de la question sexuelle', *Elle*, 253, 2 October 1950, 14–16, 14.

51 'Ce qu'il faut dire à vos jeunes enfants', *Elle*, 254, 9 October 1950, 38–40.
52 'Françoise E.' to Dolto, 31 May 1950, *Une vie de correspondances*, p. 195.
53 *Elle*, 253, 2 October 1950, 15.
54 Pope Pius XI, *Divini Illius Magistri*, 31 December 1929.
55 *Elle*, 254, 9 October 1950, 40.
56 *Elle*, 253, 2 October 1950, 14–15. Original emphasis.
57 Rolande B. to Dolto, 29 November 1950, *Une vie de correspondances*, p. 199.
58 Duchen, *Women's Rights*, pp. 165–6.
59 *Ibid.*, p. 143.
60 Fishman, *Vichy to the Sexual Revolution*, introduction.
61 *Ibid.*, p. xxiv.
62 *Ibid.*, p. 20.
63 *Ibid.*, p. 31.
64 *Ibid.*, pp. 82–3.
65 Duchen, *Women's Rights*, p. 175.
66 Greenwald, *Daughters of 1968*, p. 70.
67 Garcia, *Mères sous influence*, pp. 91ff.
68 Duchen, *Women's Rights*, p. 178.
69 Dolto, 'Texte pour le livre de chez Plon sur la femme demandé par Ménie Grégoire en 1967', AFD, box 20 – 'La condition féminine' – fiche A1, p. 12. Dolto's emphasis. The 1967 date is presumably an archiving error, since Grégoire's book appeared in 1965 and given the relevance of these extracts to the marriage law debate.
70 Dolto, 'Texte pour le livre de Ménie Grégoire', p. 12. Dolto's emphasis.
71 Cited in Greenwald, *Daughters of 1968*, p. 69.
72 Garcia, *Mères sous influence*, p. 9.
73 Dolto, *Cause des enfants*, p. 13.
74 Jean-Pierre Chartier, *L'Avenir est à vous*, RTF, 16 September 1963.
75 'Le Métier des parents', *Questionnaire*, TF1, 4 December 1977, interview by Jean-Louis Servan-Schreiber. Transcript published in *CdE*, pp. 7–44; here pp. 34–7.

5

Autism, antipsychiatry and the pathogenic family: Dolto and the psychoanalytic approach to autism in France

In 2004, the European Committee of Social Rights, part of the Council of Europe, ruled that France's provisions for autistic people were inadequate. The committee upheld a complaint brought by an autism rights association, Autism Europe, concluding that France had failed to uphold the rights of disabled children to adequate levels of care, assistance, education and training, as enshrined in the European Social Charter.[1] Provisions for autistic children in France had such a bad reputation that thousands of parents were sending their children to specialist schools in Belgium instead.[2] The Council of Europe made further similar findings in several subsequent cases.[3] In 2016, the UN Committee on the Rights of the Child also worried that autistic people in France continued 'to be subjected to widespread violations of their rights' to education and support.[4]

From the mid-1980s, a variety of associations of autists and parents of autistic children campaigned to change the way autism was treated in France. They argued that autistic children were less likely to be diagnosed (or were diagnosed much later) in France than their counterparts in the United States and United Kingdom; that under 30 per cent of autistic children attended mainstream schools, compared to around 80 per cent in the United Kingdom (instead attending psychiatric hospitals or day hospitals); and that treatment methods based on cognitive behavioural psychology, such as Treatment and Education of Autistic and Related Communication Handicapped Children (TEACHH), Picture Exchange Communication System (PECS) and Applied Behaviour Analysis, were not widely available in France.[5] Instead, autistic children were approached through the prism of psychoanalytic concepts, to the detriment, the campaigners argued, of their life outcomes.

The concept of autism is a relatively recent one in the history of medicine, and in its twenty-first-century definition encompasses far larger numbers of people than was thought to be the case fifty or one hundred years ago. Contemporary thinking, considerably shaped by autistic people themselves, has moved towards conceiving of autists as a 'neurotribe' who experience the world in a distinct way that is no less valid than 'neurotypical' experience.[6] In 2019, the Swedish climate campaigner Greta Thunberg's reference to her Asperger's syndrome as a 'superpower' was widely reported.[7] For most of the twentieth century, however, the condition was considered a severe form of mental illness. The term was coined in 1911 by a Swiss psychiatrist, Eugen Bleuler, who also created the diagnosis of schizophrenia. Bleuler conceived of autism as the process by which a child, wishing to avoid unsatisfying realities, replaces them with fantasies and hallucinations. Bleuler's definition was close to, and indeed influenced by, Sigmund Freud's terminology of 'autoerotism' (and later, 'primary narcissism').[8] Autism in this framework was understood to be an exaggeration of a trait that was present in all humans, but one that was pathological and connected to adult schizophrenia. The concept was taken up in the 1920s by Jean Piaget, who saw autistic thinking as characteristic of early infancy, and later by psychoanalytic thinkers in Britain in the 1930s such as Susan Isaacs and Melanie Klein. Isaacs preferred the term 'childhood schizophrenia', but wrote of it as characterised by a 'flight to phantasy' caused by early childhood anxiety over aggressive impulses that caused the child to 'withdraw from contact with real people and real situations'.[9]

As Bonnie Evans has argued, this background means that the two psychiatrists often considered as the fathers of the autism diagnosis for their work in the 1930s and 1940s – Hans Asperger and especially Leo Kanner – were not in fact striking out in a particularly new theoretical direction.[10] Asperger (1906–80), based at the Heilpädogigik Station Kinderklinik at the University of Vienna from 1932 onwards, saw autism as a 'psychopathology' that probably had a genetic cause and applied to a range of people – not only the so-called high-achieving autists with whom he is often associated.[11] As Edith Sheffer has shown, his work had some deeply problematic aspects, and bore the imprint of its development in the context of a Nazi psychology which served as the justification for the wartime child euthanasia programme in which Asperger was complicit.[12] These aspects were not recognised, however, when his work was taken up and popularised by the English psychiatrist Lorna Wing in the 1980s, prior to which it was largely unknown. Meanwhile Kanner (1894–1981), a Ukrainian Jewish émigré based at Johns Hopkins University in Baltimore, produced a 1943–44 definition of 'early infantile autism' as a rare, monolithic condition characterised by 'a will to self-isolation' and an 'anxiously obsessive desire for the maintenance of sameness'.[13] He highlighted the 'affective' and emotional aspects of autism, rather than seeing it as primarily an intellectual defect, but his main contribution was probably the set of clear case studies that he published, and his work was not accepted as definitive at the time.[14]

Kanner, already prominent as the author of a widely used textbook, *Child Psychiatry* (1935), initially suggested that autism was inborn, but later argued for a psychogenic aetiology.[15] His ambiguity here may well have been strategic, in view of the increasing prevalence of psychoanalysis in American psychiatry and in American culture more generally between approximately 1945 and 1963.[16] In this period psychoanalysts were extending their insights to areas of medicine and psychiatry such as asthma and schizophrenia. Their explanations frequently led back to the family, and specifically to pathogenic mothers. The Hungarian-American psychoanalyst Franz Alexander wrote that asthmatics, for example, suffered from 'excessive, unresolved dependence' upon 'asthmatogenic' mothers.[17] Other US-based analysts such as Harry Stack Sullivan, Frieda Fromm-Reichmann and Theodore Lidz similarly described 'schizophrenogenic mothers'.[18] The idea that mothers were generally to blame for their children's psychiatric symptoms was a powerful concept. It had the attraction of offering simple narrative explanations for conditions that remained poorly understood, while also speaking to anxieties about the changing postwar status and role of women.[19] Influenced by these writers, some of whom were his colleagues at Johns Hopkins, Kanner applied the same line of thinking to autism.[20] It was Kanner, not Bruno Bettelheim, who coined the phrase 'refrigerator mothers' to describe what he saw as the coldness and distance of mothers towards autistic children.[21] Bettelheim popularised the idea with his 1967 book *The Empty Fortress*, which synthesised Kanner's work with that of other theorists of toxic parenting.[22] Bettelheim added a striking image by drawing an analogy between autistic children and concentration camp victims, implicitly placing parents in the role of camp guards who caused their children to 'withdraw from the world before their humanity ever really develops', just as victims of Nazi camps 'had lost their humanity in response to extreme situations'.[23] This implied that the best place for autistic children was in an institution, well away from their toxic parents.

Reversing this notion in the United States took years of action by activist groups, legislative change such as the 1975 Education for All Handicapped Children Act and the development of new educative techniques. It also required a reduction in the influence of psychoanalysis in American psychiatry, as crystallised in the removal of psychoanalytic terminology from the third edition of the American Psychiatric Association's Diagnostic and Statistical Manual (DSM) in 1980. By the 1990s, thanks to the achievements of the women's movement and to changing cultural perceptions of autism, accelerated by the film *Rain Man* (1988), the 'refrigerator mother' theory was waning. Changes in diagnostic criteria meant that many more children were diagnosed with autism or related conditions. This change was in part driven by the activism of parents' associations, such as the National Society for Autistic Children led by Bernard Rimland, who also conducted his own research into the condition (published in *Infantile Autism*, 1964).[24] This pattern was also in evidence in the United Kingdom, where the Society for Autistic Children, in alliance with the researchers John and Lorna Wing (who were also parents of an autistic child), helped to propel a new research agenda in the 1960s that transformed conceptions of autism by the 1970s – dismantling the psychoanalytic concept of childhood schizophrenia and developing the modern understanding of a sensory and communicative disorder affecting the ability to form social relationships.[25]

In France, a similar pattern played out, but at later dates than in the United Kingdom or United States, a delay which corresponds to the relatively late rise (and later fall) of psychoanalysis as a dominant force within psychiatry. Parents' associations only became a significant factor in the 1980s in France, where the peak of psychoanalytic influence on psychiatry occurred not in the 1950s as in the United States, but after 1968, with the rise of Lacan and the arrival of many of his former trainees and analysands in important psychiatric positions. French psychoanalytic psychiatrists protested the removal of Freudian concepts from the DSM, and in response developed their own Classification française des troubles mentaux de l'enfant et de l'adolescent (CFTMEA – French Classification of Child and Adolescent Mental Disorders) which retained psychoanalytic vocabulary. As late as the 1990s, many French psychiatrists continued to define autism in broadly psychoanalytic terms – that is, as a severe psychosis. French psychoanalysts continued to propose causal links between the family environment – especially the mother – and the development of autistic disorders. Women who presented an autistic child for psychiatric assessment risked being told that they, or at least troubles in the mother-child relationship, were responsible for their child's condition. One recalled being told that her son was autistic 'because he suffered separation issues from breast-feeding. This the analyst gleaned from watching him spin round objects (which reminded him of his mother's breasts) and chase after one that he had "lost" when it fell and rolled under a piece of furniture.'[26] Another woman received a psychiatric report explaining her son's autism in terms of 'sexual phobias being liquefied … It was all texts by Lacan, and she was trying to put Guillaume in them. It didn't sound like Guillaume.'[27] The mother of a son born in 1988, asking what had caused his condition, was told 'maybe you didn't cuddle him enough'.[28] Only 7 per cent of parents of autistic children born in France between 1960 and 1990 reported being happy with the treatment their children received.[29]

Parents' associations formed in the 1980s and 1990s pressed the French state to redefine autism as a medical disability and a genetic condition, rather than one caused by family dynamics. They invited geneticists and neuroscientists to their meetings and called for further medical research into the condition.[30] The French state initially responded with limited reforms. A 1996 law recognised autism as a disability, rather than part of the domain of psychiatry and mental health, and from 1999 regional resource centres (Centres Ressources Autisme) were set up to improve early diagnosis and provide services.[31] Following the 2004 Council of Europe judgement, the government produced a series of 'Plans Autisme' designed to direct investment towards increasing early detection and diagnosis, improving educational provision and supporting families. The first three plans (spanning 2005–7, 2008–12 and 2013–17, respectively) led to various improvements, such as an increase in the number of autistic children attending mainstream school from 12,500 in 2008 to 30,000 in 2015. Nonetheless, in 2017 the Cour des comptes noted that out of an estimated total of 700,000 autistic people in France, still only 75,000 had a diagnosis.[32] Recognising that it still needed to go further, the government inaugurated a fourth Plan Autisme in 2018 with a budget of 400 million euros.[33]

Dolto played a significant role in developing and popularising the psychoanalytic approach to autism in France. She did so in two ways. First, her collaboration on the subject with Maud Mannoni in the 1960s. Second, when she was at the height of her career, her case study of an (arguably) autistic boy published as a popular book in 1971, *Le Cas Dominique* (*The Dominique Case*). Dolto helped popularise the idea that autism, psychosis and so-called backwardness were the results of childhood trauma, and ultimately caused by poor parenting. This approach followed from Dolto's general theoretical positions concerning childhood determinism, family neuroses and gender roles. Just as René Laforgue had suggested in the interwar period that 'family neuroses' were caused when mothers became overly dominant in the family or sought professional advancement, so Dolto and Mannoni presented the type of pathogenic family that gave rise to autism as one in which the mother was overly strong, and the father weak or absent. They provided accessible case studies to illustrate this idea, which helped convince French public opinion of the existence of such families. As will be shown below, there were clear continuities between these ideas as promoted by Dolto and Mannoni in the 1960s and the attitudes of some French psychoanalysts towards autism in the twenty-first century. To understand how their thinking developed, it is necessary first to examine their relationship to the radical psychiatry or antipsychiatry movement.

Antipsychiatry/radical psychiatry

The 1960s saw a shift from the incarceration of the mentally ill in asylums and other institutions to community-based treatment. In the United States, the asylum population peaked between 1955 and 1961 (at 560,000) and declined sharply thereafter.[34] In France, the rate of psychiatric incarceration peaked in 1961 at 244 per 100,000 people, declining to 193 per 100,000 by 1976.[35] These declines were the result of a combination of clinical and cultural changes. The clinical change was the availability, from the mid-1950s onwards, of demonstrably effective pharmacological remedies for some severe mental illnesses. New drugs such as chlorpromazine, imipramine and lithium enabled many asylum patients to return to the community and live relatively normal lives, reducing psychiatrists' reliance on crude and often inhumane older methods like straitjackets, cold packs, lobotomies, fever induction and insulin shock.[36]

The cultural shift was antipsychiatry, or – as it was also termed to be inclusive of psychiatrists who wanted to practice in very different ways without abandoning the discipline altogether – 'radical psychiatry'.[37] From the 1950s onwards, radical psychiatrists in a number of western countries attacked the carceral practices of asylums and mental hospitals, seeing the use of violent restraints and shock treatments as inhumane. These critics contended that madness could not be seen outside its social context, and that psychiatrists needed to move, in R. D. Laing's words, 'from a clinical to a social phenomenological perspective'.[38] Asylum inmates were not ill, but rather victims of social circumstance in need of liberation and political empowerment – much like other marginalised or oppressed groups. Three foundational texts of this approach appeared in 1961, two in the United States and one in France. Thomas Szasz's *The Myth of Mental Illness* argued that the entire concept of mental illness was a category error, since it ascribed a medical condition to people who were in fact simply 'disabled by living'.[39] Erving Goffman's *Asylums* deplored the conditions in what he called 'total institutions' for the mentally ill, drawing attention to patterns of interaction that dehumanised patients.[40] In France, Michel Foucault's *Madness and Civilisation* argued that the beginnings of confinement in the sixteenth and seventeenth centuries represented a decision to silence madness on the part of a polity that found unreason scandalous.[41] Such publications were accompanied by a range of institutional experiments. In 1961, Franco Basaglia was appointed to run the asylum in Gorizia, Italy. Refusing to restrain his patients, Basaglia set about democratising the institution and creating a 'therapeutic community'.[42] His work eventually inspired the 1978 Basaglia Law, which closed Italian asylums altogether. In Britain, R. D. Laing and

David Cooper ran institutional experiments such as the so-called anti-hospitals of Villa 21 and Kingsley Hall. At Elliott Barker's Oak Ridge asylum in Ontario, Canada, the experience of undergoing mental distress was compared to a shamanic journey into the psyche, one that could provide valuable insights analogous to the experience provided by perception-altering drugs.[43] Some radical psychiatrists, including Laing and Barker, supplied psychoactive substances to some of their patients.

The relationship of psychoanalysis to the burgeoning radical psychiatry movement differed according to the local intellectual context, as can most obviously be seen by comparing the situation in the United States to that in France. In the United States, psychoanalysis had achieved widespread cultural ascendancy and a degree of hegemony within psychiatry by the 1950s, such that the American Psychiatric Association and most major university psychiatry departments were run by psychoanalysts. This domination was never total, and American psychoanalysis was far from monolithic, but as Nathan Hale has written, to a significant extent it 'became identified with the "establishment" in psychiatry and society, reconciled with conventional moral and religious values and sexual conventions'.[44] In France, however, psychoanalysis – especially its Lacanian or, in the terminology used in Chapter 3, 'dissident' variant – was only beginning its cultural ascendancy in the 1960s, and was not yet predominant within psychiatry. In 1955, despite the 'psychologisation' of French society by that date (as explored in the previous chapter), *Femme* magazine could write that 'psychoanalysis is still seen as an obscure discipline'.[45] It followed that French psychoanalysis could be an ally, rather than a target, of radical psychiatry, since psychoanalysis had not presided over the system of mental health institutions that was coming under attack.

In addition, many French radical psychiatrists were either psychoanalysts themselves or had a strong interest in Freud. As Sherry Turkle has written, the distinctiveness of French antipsychiatry was that it was 'both "psychoanalytic" and deeply embedded in a Marxist tradition of political action'.[46] In the 1950s and 1960s the influence of Lacan, in particular, had gone a long way to repositioning psychoanalysis as a left-wing and avant-garde system of thought.[47] Lacan presented the École Freudienne de Paris, founded following his and Dolto's exclusion from the International Psychoanalytic

Association in 1964, as an anti-authoritarian, anti-hierarchical, anti-capitalist body.[48] In the later 1960s members of Lacan's circle, including his daughter and son-in-law, became affiliated with Maoist politics.[49] Lacan allied himself with the Marxist philosopher Louis Althusser, who provided a room at the École normale supérieure for Lacan's seminars. This deepened a trend, already in evidence from the 1950s, of interest in Lacan from young thinkers and psychiatrists on the radical far left – 'radical' here in the sense of advocating egalitarian transformations in social organisation without being affiliated to the Communist Party or other long-standing socialist political structures. Several of the leading names of French anti- or radical psychiatry, especially Jean Oury, Félix Guattari and Maud Mannoni, had a personal connection with Lacan. The Lacan connection helps explain how Dolto, too, came into contact with thinkers whose political orientation was very different from the Catholic, holistic, anti-communist direction of *Psyché* and *Études carmélitaines* that she had followed in the initial postwar years.

Jean Oury (1924–2014) was a psychiatrist who had begun his career at the Saint Alban asylum in Lozère.[50] Saint Alban's history as a pioneering site of psychiatric reform dated back to the 1930s. During the Occupation, it became a centre for the Resistance as well as innovative psychiatry. Under the direction of the Catalan/Spanish republican psychiatrist François Tosquelles, Saint Alban removed its outer walls and prison-like bars and opened its front doors. After the war, Frantz Fanon worked there as an intern, while the communist psychiatrist Lucien Bonnafé, who later campaigned for recognition of the 40,000 French mental health patients who died (mostly of starvation) during the Occupation, also passed through.[51] When Oury arrived in 1947, Saint Alban was known as a centre of psychiatric reform with politically (far-)left-wing inflections. Institutional psychotherapy, the reform movement that originated there, had a similar political flavour. Tosquelles and his colleagues were also among the first doctors to make use of Lacan's structural understanding of human personality.[52]

In 1953, Oury left Saint Alban and founded a private clinic at La Borde, near Cour-Cheverny in the Loire. He was joined as co-director by Félix Guattari (1930–92). Guattari's early career, before he achieved national fame as the co-author with Gilles Deleuze of *Anti-Oedipus* (1972), illustrates how the worlds of left-wing politics, radical psychiatry and Lacanian psychoanalysis overlapped. Guattari was from a right-wing family – his father was a former member of the interwar extreme nationalist Croix de Feu – but he became active in the anti-Stalinist Left, organising protests against French colonialism in Vietnam and Algeria, and visiting China in 1954.[53] He came into contact with Oury through the Youth Hostel movement. In addition, Oury's younger brother Fernand, an innovative pedagogue and educational reformer, had taught Guattari at *lycée*. (On Fernand, and his connection to Dolto, see Chapter 6).

Oury and Guattari turned La Borde into a humane, egalitarian community, in deliberate contrast to the repressive, carceral atmosphere of most asylums. La Borde's nurses did not wear white smocks, but dressed indistinguishably from the patients. Spaces were permeable and patients free to move around. Patients ran group therapy sessions and creative projects themselves, and were brought into the centre's decision-making processes. Guattari, in charge of work schedules, constantly assigned staff to work outside their specialist areas as a way of furthering the egalitarian spirit. All responsibilities were shared equally, every employee alternated between manual and intellectual labour and all received the same salary. Oury, responsible for psychiatric treatment, looked for what he called the 'truth' in patients' discourse, seeking out creative or transcendental dimensions to their speech and actions. While not denying the somatic basis of his patients' conditions, he was moving the focus onto social, environmental and linguistic elements.

Both Oury and Guattari were strongly influenced by Lacan. Oury was inspired by a 1947 text by Lacan on psychic causality, and in 1951 recommended Lacan's work on the mirror stage, aggression and the family to Guattari.[54] Guattari soon began attending Lacan's seminars – later claiming to be the first non-physician to do so – and generally, as he put it, 'bugging everyone about Lacan'.[55] Oury commenced an analysis with Lacan in 1953 that continued for the next twenty-seven years, and made Lacan's work central to his understanding of psychosis.[56] Guattari and indeed most of La Borde's staff soon followed him into Lacan's consulting room. On Wednesday afternoons the clinic emptied out as the staff decamped to Paris for Lacan's seminar.[57] For his part, Lacan valued Oury and Guattari for their connection with an avant-garde psychiatric clinic, and for conversations that helped him think about psychosis. For a time, Lacan even considered giving Guattari a special position as his 'preferred interlocutor' – i.e. chosen heir – an idea that definitively ended with the publication of *Anti-Oedipus*.[58]

Via Lacan, the ideas behind institutional psychotherapy spread into the psychoanalytic movement. This is particularly evident in the writings of Maud Mannoni (1923–98). A product of the Belgian Psychoanalytic Society, Mannoni moved to Paris after World War II and quickly came under Dolto's wing. 'Françoise Dolto welcomed me like a member of the family', Mannoni later recalled.[59] It was Dolto who introduced Maud to her future husband, Octave Mannoni, a philosophy professor turned Lacanian analyst.[60] (Maud) Mannoni observed Dolto's child psychotherapy consultations at Hôpital Trousseau and decided to specialise in work with (so-called) psychotic children. Mannoni's Belgian analyst Maurice Dugautiez wrote to Dolto in 1949, praising her training of Mannoni and her methodology for child psychoanalysis.[61] Subsequently, Mannoni visited Donald Winnicott in London and did a control analysis with him – as well as undertaking a further personal analysis with Lacan, who was keen to draw Mannoni into his circle and hear about her clinical work.[62] But Mannoni also looked beyond psychoanalysis and made connections with radical psychiatrists. While in England, she visited Kingsley Hall and befriended R. D. Laing.[63] In 1969 she founded an experimental school in Bonneuil-sur-Marne, an outer Parisian suburb, aimed at children diagnosed as autistic, psychotic or '*arriéré*' ('backward' or, in the now even more offensive term used by her English translator, 'retarded').

Mannoni became an important figure in the synthesis between radical psychiatry and psychoanalysis. Her writings explored how psychoanalysis could harness the insights of the radical psychiatrists – most fully in her 1970 book *Le Psychiatre, son 'fou' et la psychanalyse* (*The Psychiatrist, His 'Fool' and Psychoanalysis*), but the direction of her thinking had already been clear in *L'Enfant arriéré et sa mère* (*The Retarded Child and the Mother*, 1964).[64] This appeared as the first book in Lacan's new '*Champ freudien*' (Freudian field) collection at Éditions du Seuil – Lacan's own *Écrits* (*Writings*, 1966) was the second – and Lacan recommended it to his seminar audience.[65] *The Retarded Child and the Mother* appeared in the same year as an important work in British radical psychiatry, R. D. Laing and Aaron Esterson's *Sanity, Madness and the Family*.

Laing and Esterson had spent many hours with the families of schizophrenic young women, trying to understand how family dynamics could give rise to schizophrenia. Their thesis was that schizophrenic behaviour was an existential response to a certain kind of family environment (which was not quite the same thing as saying that parents made their children schizophrenic – not least because Laing and Esterson doubted that schizophrenia existed at all as a physiological condition). Mannoni attempted to do something similar for the problem of children with learning difficulties – including, in practice, many children who would likely today be diagnosed as autistic. In *The Retarded Child and the Mother*, she argued that a child's 'backwardness' (*arriération*) occurred in the context of the family dynamic. This was a nuanced version of psychogenesis theory: Mannoni did not claim that all *arriération* had a psychological origin, but rather that the family and societal environment could aggravate or perpetuate it. In her words,

> An illness, however organic it may be, may assume in the Other (parent or doctor) a function and a status that result in an additional alienation on the part of the 'handicapped' child … it is not a question of denying the existence of mental retardation or psychosis, but rather of examining the way in which … we confront it in our society, aggravate it, and transform it into alienation.[66]

For Mannoni, so-called objective measurements of children, such as low IQ scores or poor school reports, should not suffice as a basis for diagnosis. Rather, these were probably symptoms of something else, such as a disturbance in the mother-child relationship – something with a history, a meaning that could be uncovered by a perceptive observer: a mystery to be solved.

Whereas Laing and Esterson made multiple visits to their subjects' family homes, Mannoni's case studies were based only on in-clinic observations. Mannoni nevertheless played detective, seeking the meaning of a child's illness in the parents' – especially the mother's – neuroses:

> The climate favouring the development of a psychosis exists even before the birth of the child. From conception, the child plays a very definite role for the mother on the fantasy plane; his destiny is already marked out; he will be an object without desires of his own, whose sole purpose will be to fill the maternal void.[67]

Despite her occasional hints in the direction of a social model of disability (holding large-scale social and economic structures responsible for the alienation of disabled people from mainstream society), the majority of Mannoni's examples pointed to 'pathogenic parents' and psychogenic causes. Most of the mothers that she mentioned in the case studies in *The Retarded Child and the Mother* came in for criticism. Simply to be a mother was to be in error: 'From the outset, the mother will be mistaken about her child.'[68] Each of the following quotes refers to a different family:

> The child reacted to the mother's anxiety by passive opposition … [He] showed … signs of disturbance.
>
> The mother appeared rigid, totally lacking in affection … The most striking thing about her was her refusal to have children, while in fact she had had three …
>
> This unwanted child is the object of maternal hypersolicitude, to which he reacts by vomiting, behaviour disorders, and refusal to learn.[69]

The most likely key to the mystery of *arriération* was that it resulted in some way from parental, almost certainly maternal, behaviour. 'The child does not know that he is being called upon to play a role in order to satisfy his mother's unconscious wishes', Mannoni wrote. 'Unknown to him, he is in a sense being "ravished" in the desire of the mother.'[70]

Mannoni clearly acknowledged Dolto's influence on this thinking: 'I am indebted to Françoise Dolto for the benefit of her enormous experience; the accuracy of her clinical sense in psychoanalysis proved decisive in the direction that my work took.'[71] They did not agree in every particular, and Mannoni had a greater tendency to refer explicitly to Lacan's theories. But they approached children's mental disturbances in very similar ways. Following Dolto's methodology – drawn in turn from Laforgue and the idea of the family neurosis – Mannoni considered that the family history and dynamics were the key elements in explaining children's problems. She doubted 'whether we are dealing with the case of the accidental arrival of an abnormal child in a family that is no way responsible', suspecting that instead, usually 'it was the family destiny that drove [the child] to abnormality'.[72] Her focus was on 'behaviour whose origin is not so much organic as the result of a reaction to a pathogenic family situation'.[73] Like

Dolto, Mannoni argued that the analyst should look beyond the parents to the preceding generation, since 'the nexus of the drama already exists at the level of the grandparents'.[74] Dolto's inquiries into her patients' family histories were unusually thorough, encompassing grandparents, great-grandparents, aunts and cousins. In *Le Cas Dominique* (of which more shortly) she expressed her belief in the fundamental importance of this background in provoking psychoses, in a formulation which became somewhat famous: '*It takes three generations for a psychosis to appear*: two generations of neurotic parents and grandparents in the subject's genetic make-up [are required] for the subject to be psychotic.'[75] Dolto wanted to know about any historic traumatic events experienced by close relatives, believing that their impacts could be unconsciously transmitted to the family's children.

By probing family histories in this way, Dolto elicited a wealth of material that could be incorporated into her interpretations and case explanations. Dolto, like many psychoanalytic writers, enjoyed storytelling, and her case studies are generally engaging to read. However, their literary quality also gives rise to a suspicion that she approached them as a kind of creative writing challenge. Her patients supplied the ingredients of a narrative; her task was to unravel the mystery and bring the whole story together in a narratively and psychoanalytically satisfying way. The more details about the family history that Dolto obtained, the more chance she had of constructing a plausible story explaining the psychological disturbance in terms of that history. Steve Silberman has written of Leo Kanner, who also had a flair for dramatic narrative, that in his 'refrigerator mother' phase he 'turned the detailed notes that parents had provided to him … into a weapon'.[76] Much as Pierre Bourdieu noted with the concept of the 'biographical illusion' (see the Introduction of this book), immersion in particular cultures of storytelling could make doctors prone to write case histories which satisfied the conventions of those cultures. Dolto, as will be seen in the *Dominique* case, had a tendency to write case histories as if they were works of detective fiction. The danger, of course, was that such writers might fall prone to the narrative fallacy – falsely assuming a connection between the events recorded in the case history and the psychiatric outcome, and ignoring or obscuring other possible causes or explanations. Another danger was confirmation bias: looking only for those facts or events that would support a pre-formed narrative or conviction about the causes of a psychiatric condition.

The story that Dolto and Mannoni seemed keenest to tell in the 1960s was one in which deviation from normative patriarchal family dynamics led to children's mental disturbances. This is especially evident in Mannoni's second book, *Le Premier Rendez-vous avec le psychanalyste* (*The First Meeting With the Psychoanalyst*, 1965), to which Dolto contributed a substantial forty-five-page preface. Dolto and Mannoni concurred as to the importance of the father-mother-child family triangle and the critical position of the paternal signifier within that triptych. For both, the archetypal pathogenic family could be summarised by the labels applied by Mannoni to the book's first case study: 'depressed mother'; 'resigned/absent man'; 'child-toy'/'child-object'.[77] Depressed mothers and unimposing fathers created passive, disturbed children. A toxic environment was one in which the father was psychologically (not necessarily physically) absent from the child's upbringing, whether out of negligence or – more commonly in Dolto and Mannoni's case studies – an inability to withstand the mother's excessive desire for control. Bad fathers were ones who abandoned their child to a 'couple-like situation with the mother' from which the 'Paternal Law' (*Loi du Père*) was lacking.[78] 'Any substitution of the role of the father by the mother is pathogenic', wrote Dolto.[79] The child risked becoming subjugated, a support or adjunct to the mother's emotional needs, lacking the ability to become truly autonomous or independent. 'Any situation where the child serves as a prosthetic to one of their parents … is pathogenic, especially if it isn't made clear to the child that such a situation is wrong.'[80]

Mannoni provided numerous examples of such situations. Her patient 'Nicolas' was 'trapped in the maternal world [and] living as the mother's echo'.[81] The absence of her father left another patient, 'Bernadette', 'in danger of being *devoured*' by her mother.[82] 'Roger' was 'trapped in his mother's fantasy. His illness gave his mother all the rights, and caused his father enough guilt to justify his withdrawal.'[83] The (often depressed) mothers of these patients were presented as destructive figures, with dangerous desires that their children were powerless to resist. Only a father's resolute intervention could prevent disaster. Mannoni represented mothers' desires as pathogenic, and fathers' ability to intercede and frustrate these as bringing autonomy and psychological health to the child.

This simplistic, recurrent pattern of family relations and causality of disturbance was largely absent from the work of Laing and Esterson, who presented their cases at greater length and with more complex discussion of wider socio-economic considerations. Laing and Esterson deliberately pared their interpretative commentaries on individual cases down to a minimum, underlining instead the relatively basic general point 'that the experience and behaviour of schizophrenics is much more socially intelligible than has come to be supposed'.[84] Dolto and Mannoni went much further, proposing that psychotic behaviour in children was explicable in terms of psychoanalytic theory and especially the Lacanian paternal signifier. They were channelling the antipsychiatric impulse in a specifically psychoanalytic, but also anti-feminist direction.

Dolto and Mannoni's interpretation of autism – or, in their terminology, autistic behaviour as part of child schizophrenia – had clear resemblances to that of Kanner and Bettelheim. Bettelheim's *The Empty Fortress* appeared in French translation in 1969, and his reputation spread considerably in 1974 when, during a TV strike, all three national channels broadcast a four-part documentary, *Portrait de Bruno Bettelheim*, on the same evening.[85] Dolto and Mannoni's version of the psychogenetic mother – devouring, incestuous – diverged from Bettelheim's cold, distant, inhuman figure. But the implications were similar. If the family environment provoked the child's disturbance, then isolating children from their families must be the logical response. In one case, Bettelheim only admitted a child to the Orthopedic School in Chicago after receiving written assurances from her mother 'that they would leave her with us until such time as we had either affected her rehabilitation or felt unable to help her any further'.[86] Mannoni, given her commitment to opposing incarceration, did not go to these lengths. Her institution at Bonneuil-sur-Marne was somewhere between a specialist school and a day hospital (*hôpital de jour*), though it also had facilities for children to stay overnight. At Bonneuil – presented to the French public via a documentary, *Vivre à Bonneuil* (*Life at Bonneuil*), on TF1 in 1975 – Mannoni worked with the pedagogue Fernand Deligny to develop a new type of educational programme, designed to reach children with learning disabilities through psychoanalysis.

Bonneuil had a model of communal organisation modelled to some extent on La Borde, where Deligny had also worked.[87] It became seen as a model institution of its type. After 1975, as asylums closed and French mental health provision became more localised, day hospitals became a major feature of the system.[88] Very often, French children with autism or learning disabilities were assigned to day hospitals rather than mainstream schools, frequently as the result of a referral by a psychoanalytically trained psychiatrist.

Dominique

The case studies presented in Mannoni's work were no more than fragmentary sketches: nineteen cases in twenty-five pages in *The Retarded Child and the Mother*, thirty in sixty pages in *The First Meeting with the Psychoanalyst*. In 1967, Dolto decided to present something much longer, giving a more representative impression of the reality of psychotherapeutic practice. She chose the case of 'Dominique Bel' (not his real name), a fourteen-year-old boy from the outer Parisian suburbs. Dominique had been referred to Dolto in 1962 in her capacity as a consultant at the Étienne Marcel CMPP in central Paris, for advice on a school placement. She presented the case at a two-day workshop on child psychosis (*l'enfance aliénée*) at the EFP in October 1967. Organised by Mannoni with a number of participants from the world of antipsychiatry/radical psychiatry – including Guattari, Jean and Fernand Oury, Tosquelles, Laing and Cooper – the event was intended as a dialogue between the structuralist approach of the Lacanian group and the 'existential' framework of the English attendees.[89] The proceedings were edited by Guattari and published in *Recherches*, a journal he had created in 1965 to present the work of a federation of groups bringing radical left-wing perspectives to healthcare, education and social work.[90]

Dolto's text on Dominique followed the structure of her clinical sessions with him, with a chapter dedicated to each of the twelve consultations.[91] Most chapters were built around a verbatim transcript of part of the clinical session, accompanied by Dolto's (often much longer) interpretative glosses. Such transcripts were available because Dolto, who since 1955 had been running seminars on child psychoanalysis, had also opened up her Étienne Marcel consulting room to trainee psychoanalysts.[92] The trainees could observe her work, and in return assisted her by taking detailed notes of the sessions. When Dolto revised the text for publication as a book in 1971, she added two further chapters of interpretative commentary, plus an appendix on 'the Freudian theory of instances of the psyche during the evolution of sexuality, in relation to the Oedipus complex'.

The preliminary facts of the case ran as follows. Dominique attended a special needs school, having repeatedly failed to pass the grades in mainstream schools. He was innumerate, forgetful and distracted, living somewhat in his own world. His father described him as being 'from another planet. He's not like the rest of us.'[93] His mother reported that he made the family's home life impossible, but without being able to say exactly how. Dominique had phobias, tics and some strange and obsessive behaviours. He was 'completely disoriented in time and space', and 'so distracted that he'd go out in his pyjamas ... if you didn't remind him'.[94] He liked drawing planes and cars – always the same ones – making models and inventing stories that his family thought made little sense.

Until the age of two and a half, Dominique's development had been normal. He was toilet trained early, and at age two began attending a Montessori nursery school with his elder brother Paul-Marie. At this time his mother was pregnant with his sister, Sylvie. After she was born, Dominique had violent jealous reactions. He began to soil his clothes, resulting in his expulsion from nursery. At six, he started school, where he was 'extremely unstable and without contact with others'.[95] He was sent to a psychiatrist, who prescribed medication which seemed only to over-excite Dominique. He also spent six months in psychoanalysis, which focused on his jealousy and sibling rivalry, to no discernible benefit. After two years in school he had not learned to read, nor made any friends. Thereafter, he spent around a year living with his grandparents in a rural area near Perpignan, where he had apparently been happy and learned to read – only to regress after returning to Paris.

The doctor who referred the adolescent Dominique to Dolto described him as 'simply an imbecile' (*un débile simple*), and feared that 'since he hit puberty, a progression towards schizophrenia' was occurring.[96] But Dominique was not aggressive, and no one had seriously suggested confining him to an institution. 'He was a child who expressed himself well. He just wasn't sociable.'[97] In short, no one knew quite what to do with him. Dominique's father thought that his son's condition was inborn and that, unless corrective brain surgery became possible, there was nothing to be done. His mother was unsure, but reluctantly agreed to Dolto's suggestion of further psychoanalytic psychotherapy.

Before seeing Dominique, Dolto spent some time talking to his mother alone, in which she ran through the wider family history. Madame Bel (Dolto did not provide a first name) had spent an unhappy childhood in Africa. Her father had been a colonial officer in French Equatorial Africa and the Congo, and she was educated by missionary nuns in a boarding school. The family returned to France during the Occupation, where Madame Bel took a degree in German and became a German teacher. Dominique's father, Georges, was an engineer. The son of an army officer, he too had had an unhappy childhood. He had been in the army in 1940 and taken prisoner, but had escaped. He now (i.e. in 1962) worked for a small industrial export company, with a business partner who was in a failing marriage – the two men spent a lot of time away together on business trips. Probing further, Dolto discovered that Georges had had two younger brothers with tragic histories. One had died aged eighteen months after swallowing a piece of a toy train – Georges therefore forbade his children to play with train sets – while the other disappeared on a mountain trip aged seventeen and never returned. These events were potentially prime material for a Laforguian family neurosis-style interpretation of Dominique's case. But Dolto had already hit upon her own interpretation, one that did not require these elements.

Almost as soon as he entered the room, Dolto provided Dominique with her pre-formed conclusion. Based on her conversation with Madame Bel, Dolto was already certain that Dominique's condition was not innate or inborn, but a result of how he had reacted to his family environment, a mask that he had assumed. 'You've disguised yourself as a loon so as not to get told off', she told him. 'You've disguised yourself as a fool or an idiot and you're not that.' Their first recorded interaction in the book ran as follows:

Dominique: Well, I'm not like everybody else, sometimes when I wake up, I think that I've lived through a true story.

Dolto: That's made you false.
Dominique: That's it![98]

Primed by the theories that she and Mannoni had developed, Dolto was sure that the explanation for Dominique's condition would lie in family circumstances and, more specifically, in a 'depressive/devouring mother'; 'resigned/absent man'; 'child-toy/child-object' pattern. Dolto's lack of doubt about this, from the outset and throughout, is striking. Other possibilities are not considered. At the end of the first session (which Dominique's father did not attend), Dolto added an interpretation on Dominique's innumeracy: 'I repeated to Dominic in front of his mother that it's not because his father wasn't often there that he didn't count (sic).'[99] The '(sic)' indicates the deliberate double meaning: Dolto was suggesting that Dominique could not count numbers because of a sense that he 'did not count' for his father (or that his father 'did not count' for his mother), because of his frequent absences.

In the following sessions, occurring at intervals of a month or more, Dolto proceeded according to her standard methodology. She had Dominique draw pictures and make clay models, which she then discussed with him, searching his language for clues about his psychic structures and anxieties. She ran IQ-style tests that put Dominique's mental age at around five. In the fourth session, she began to make sexualised interpretations of Dominique's play in terms of the family dynamic. For example, here is Dominique playing with a Plasticine dog and mouse:

> *Hey, let's teach him to walk! But where's the mouse? Ah, it's true, he's eaten it, there's nothing left.* He stood the dog up again and at that moment, removed its head and stretched the tail down to the floor. Pause ... *Ah and then, we started off with a dog and, well, we're going to end up with a cow.*[100]

For her readers, Dolto glossed this as follows:

> He has projected onto the dog the fantasy of losing your head just at the moment you start to walk. Well, isn't that what's happened in Dominique's life? Walking means straightening up, putting the body in a phallic posture ... After, there's the transformation of the dog into a cow by its 'tail'.[101]

To Dominique himself, Dolto suggested that there was transference at work, i.e. that Dominique had a bit of a crush (*béguin*) on her.

Dominique's response – 'I don't want that! That's not good! I want to love only my parents!' – gave Dolto the opportunity to tell him what she termed 'the law', i.e. the incest taboo: 'It's good to have crushes, that doesn't remove the love for the parents, it's not the same; and later, after lots of crushes like this, a bigger crush arrives and that one's for getting married and having children.'[102]

Dolto suspected that Dominique had never been clearly told this 'law', and that his condition was in some way the result of this ignorance. In the text, this episode serves the purpose of preparing the reader for later interpretations according to which Dominique's woes were attributable to his family's deviance from patriarchal, heterosexual norms. The account of this session is followed by a ten-page 'summary of the clinical situation' in which Dolto introduced two further important elements of interpretation, based on her suppositions about Dominique's early childhood. First, she noted his tendency to lower his voice when admitting to something he considered secretive or shameful, labelling this a 'phobia of being heard and hearing'. This she attributed to 'the primal scene both glimpsed and experienced', i.e. the fact that since Dominique slept in his parents' bedroom until his sister's birth, he presumably witnessed their lovemaking.[103] Dolto's confidence in this interpretation is remarkable. Dominique's sense of shame seems, on the face of it, fairly commonplace. Furthermore, Dolto ignored another possible source of shame around sexuality in Dominique's family, one that Dominique himself spontaneously mentioned: his mother's possible relations with German soldiers during the Occupation: 'When she met Germans, you know, my mum. And well, she would speak to them. … What had she done? I think she'd been hanging about in the streets in the evenings.'[104] Dolto's failure to pursue this aspect of the family history is noteworthy in view both of her commitment to exploring such background aspects as a fundamental part of her methodology, and of her indulgent attitude towards colleagues with records of collaborating with the Germans.

The second new interpretation Dolto introduced at this stage was to seize on Madame Bel's comment that Dominique, as a baby, had sometimes banged his head violently against the side of his cot. Dolto interpreted this as a manipulative act on the part of the young Dominique: 'His mother, he dominated (living up to his name). Through force of will and masochistic behaviour, he mastered her, making her into his attentive slave, and thereby separating her from his father.'[105] This was a key interpretation for Dolto, permitting her to bring the case into her 'devouring mother'/'absent man'/'child-object' template. The failure of Georges Bel to prevent an over-close relationship between his wife and child had turned Dominique into 'mummy's phallus'. Having initially dominated his mother, Dominique now became dominated by her, fearing the 'devouring contact from a devouring other with an eroticised and devouring outcome'.[106] Dolto reinforced her hypothesis in the following session, when she learned (from Dominique's older brother Paul-Marie) that Madame Bel was in the habit of taking her children into her bed at night, during her husband's absences, to keep her company. She now asserted that 'it's the temptation of incest which is the principal cause of the regression', and, invoking racist stereotypes to help her, provided Dominique with what she believed to be the central interpretation of the case:

> In the law of all humans, everywhere on Earth, even for those Blacks who live completely naked, it's prohibited for boys to sleep with their mother ...
>
> The human law is that the sex of the son can never encounter the sex of the mother.[107]

From this point in the text, Dolto's language towards Madame Bel becomes increasingly severe. She accuses her of reducing her children to the status of 'space-heater fetishes, partial objects, warm-blooded animal dolls', and of behaving 'like a perverse passive homosexual, masochistic and paedophiliac towards her own children, all while babbling virtuously, like a sort of innocent Snow White surrounded by her dwarves, who are dependent on her and sworn to celibacy'.[108] This last comment was part of the sections added for the 1971 Seuil publication, in which Dolto made various textual revisions which further underlined the role of the pathogenic mother. During the consultations themselves, she held back from clearly stating this interpretation, beyond a gentle question to Madame Bel ('do you know that it may disturb [*gêner*] the children, the boys especially [to go to bed with you]?').[109]

Completing the picture of the pathogenic family, Dolto increasingly portrayed Georges as absent and insufficiently manly: it was the 'absence of the spouse's penis' that had caused Dominique to be 'fetishised by his mother'.[110] She hinted that both Georges and in particular his eldest child Paul-Marie might be homosexual, suggesting that the latter had chosen 'the homosexual ethic' or a 'passive homosexual structure' as his solution to the same family dynamic afflicting Dominique.[111] Dolto described Georges as being 'mothering' (*maternant*) towards his wife, and insufficiently 'castrating' or imposing of his will within the family – thus failing to prevent Madame Bel from perverting their children. 'If we wanted to find an allegorical equivalent, we'd need to consider the male roundworm, unobtrusive ... camouflaged and protected by the giant female, a male only in the sense of his reproductive function.'[112] Again, this fitted Dolto's standard template of the weak father in a toxic family: as she commented in an interview with *Les Temps modernes* in 1963, 'in refusing to be a castrator, he becomes perverting, and delivers his wife over to the child's abusive prerogatives'.[113]

After Dominique's twelve sessions with Dolto, it was Georges who decided to discontinue the treatment – on the grounds that the therapy was not working, and that psychotherapy in general was in any case '*baratin*', hot air. Dominique's parents had been divided on the value of the sessions. Madame Bel reported that Dominique had made significant progress at school, become more sociable and less distracted and used more complex language. She praised Dolto – 'you've made him sociable like the others' – while noting that 'arithmetic remains the weak point', thus indicating that Dolto's interpretations of 'counting for somebody' had not proved effective.[114] Georges thought that Dominique's improvements were marginal, and probably due to him getting older rather than any fundamental change. If they were to keep spending money on him, it would be better directed to specialised education and arithmetic lessons.

Dolto welcomed Georges's decision to end the therapy. This action placed him in the role of '*père castrateur*', imposing his will on the family, the very thing Dolto had been worried about him failing to do. In another striking comment, she also suggested that stopping the treatment was no bad thing since there was a risk that, in her desire to find a way to help Dominique, Madame Bel might end up destabilising her family structure. Madame Bel had talked to Dolto about going back into teaching, and specifically into special needs teaching – likely hoping to learn more about how she might help her son and other children like him. Dolto feared that this would destroy the family's equilibrium, which depended on the mother being restricted to the home: 'All this leads me to think that it's not such a bad thing if the father shows himself to be somewhat opposed to a treatment which risks modifying too quickly the total dependence of his wife on the family and home, and restoring her to the circuit of social relations.'[115] Dolto was thus happy to stop the sessions, despite seeing the case as just a partial success that had only cured Dominique's 'psychotic regression'. Only attaining financial independence, she argued, would ultimately free Dominique from 'the prohibitions on his development'.[116] There was always the option of a further psychoanalysis later in life.

***

It is obviously not possible to provide a definitive retrospective diagnosis for Dominique. Nonetheless, from a twenty-first-century perspective, Georges Bel's belief that his son's condition was inborn seems more convincing than Dolto's attempts to force the case into her pathogenic family template. Much of Dominique's behaviour is consistent with twenty-first-century definitions of autism spectrum disorder. The onset of his symptoms at age two and a half, when his sister was born, is consistent with regressive autism, in which children initially develop normally but begin to lose speech and motor skills between the age of fifteen and thirty months.[117] Dolto's own commentary referred to Dominique's 'autistic reclusion' and stated that at the time of his sister's birth 'he entered into autism' as a way of coping with the new family dynamic.[118] But 'autistic' was not generally used as a diagnostic category in 1960s France. Children broadly fitting the modern diagnosis would be labelled as schizophrenic, psychotic, retarded or, like Dominique, fall into gaps between these conceptual labels. Many such children were confined to institutions, but doctors had little to offer those less severely affected. Dolto, after all, was far from the first doctor to see Dominique, and no previous consultant had offered a satisfactory diagnosis or successful treatment. Psychoanalysis at least had the attraction of holding out hope: that the source of the distress could be identified, ameliorated, even cured, without the need to take the drastic step of institutionalisation. Dolto had a track record of trying to keep similar children out of carceral institutions, and argued in 1985 that 'society would benefit from a better integration of [autistic] children into everyday life'.[119] As her biographer Jean-François de Sauverzac argued, Dolto set herself 'against a psychiatric vision which labels autistic people incurable'.[120]

But parents of children like Dominique who consulted psychoanalysts also ran a risk that they would find themselves being blamed for their children's condition. Where Dolto is most open to criticism regarding this case is in her efforts to make it fit the preconceived archetypal explanation that she and Mannoni applied to so-called 'retarded' children. With flimsy evidence, she turned Dominique into an illustration of the dangers posed by pathogenic mothers and the need for strong patriarchal authority within conventional bourgeois family structures. She did this at a time when those structures were being called into question more than ever before, and when the rise of French psychoanalysis and her own growing profile were beginning to confer on her a significant degree of cultural authority. By the 1990s, the *Dominique* case had become a reference point in the training of child psychoanalysts. Jacques Hochmann has written that the Dolto-Mannoni vision of 'the mother in the guise of a murderous Medea ... was imposed onto numerous professionals, who passed it on and transmitted it to their teams, without supporting evidence, in a way that pretty much terrorised the affected families'.[121]

On its publication by Seuil in 1971, *Le Cas Dominique* was a surprise hit with the book-buying public. It was favourably reviewed by many of France's leading national, regional and specialist literary newspapers and magazines. Most reviewers understood the book as carrying a hopeful message. *Sociologie politique*'s review argued that Dolto 'makes us understand how psychosomatics, psychotics, and neurotics can all be psychoanalysed, and thereby regain their lost libido and use it for communication and creativity'.[122] For Jean-François Cornier in *Témoignage chrétien*, the book had a universal message applicable well beyond the world of psychoanalytic specialists: 'there is something deeply moving – on a human level – in the way a young boy, for whom the psychotic universe had been hell, is awakened to life, to self-identity, to the recognition of others'.[123] Cornier's review, which argued that 'this book will certainly become a work of reference', was not the only one to frame what

Dolto had done in Christian terms. Jacques Brosse in *Nouvelles littéraires* described Dolto as having carried out 'the resurrection of a soul' by bringing Dominique back into the realms of human communication.[124] This is a useful reminder that Dolto was writing for and in a culturally Christian context, and that many of her readers approached the text from a Christian perspective.

Several reviewers commented on the literary quality of Dolto's text. Raymond Bellour in *Magazine littéraire* praised Dolto's 'great sharpness in writing and gift for scene-setting' and suggested that she be considered for a literary prize.[125] Philippe Nemo in *Le Nouvel Observateur* noted that '*Dominique* begins like a crime novel and is gripping in the same way. We are given, one by one, the elements of the investigation. And at the end the culprits are revealed. For there is indeed a crime here.'[126] Nemo's reaction illustrates that many readers, carried along by Dolto's literary skill, were entirely persuaded by the narrative of the pathogenic family that she constructed and her gradual unmasking of Madame Bel as the guilty party. The review in the liberal-Catholic *Chronique sociale de France* emphasised that a crucial lesson of the book was that '*any substitution of family roles is pathogenic* … The absence of the father or mother … must not lead to the concentration of the paternal and maternal functions in the *same* person.'[127] Readers of the review could be forgiven for concluding that Dolto had effectively provided a scientific case against single parenting: 'The masculine and feminine [functions] can't be represented and taken on by a sole representative, whether masculine or feminine. The negation of this principle leads to troubles and disorders in the child.' Such conclusions took Dolto's thinking out of the domain of psychiatry and into that of sexual politics, providing ammunition to opponents of any deviation from nuclear, patriarchal families.

Some reviewers did raise objections. The Protestant paper *Réforme* was concerned that the book risked provoking unhelpful feelings of guilt among parents: 'It's not by being made to feel guilty that we will become better parents, nor that we will learn how to avoid our children becoming neurotic adults … Is it really desirable to put into the hands of all parents, material that is difficult to understand and thoroughly guilt-inducing?'[128] The review in the Catholic paper *La Croix* suggested that Dolto's focus on the immediate family as the cause, and psychotherapy as the solution to psychosis, neglected the wider social context of mental illness. By blaming parents, Dolto 'releases our society from the guilt that it feels when faced with mental illness'.[129] However, these objections were relatively rare. As most reviewers saw it, Dolto had given ordinary parents a new tool for understanding and preventing mental illness in their children, and celebrated it accordingly.

Le Mur: autism and the mother revisited

The psychoanalytic view of autism and learning disabilities that Dolto promoted in *Le Cas Dominique*, seeing them as products of nurture rather than nature and specifically of the psychological dynamics within families, became widely accepted in French society. Although it was challenged by parents' associations, resulting in the court judgements and policy changes described at the start of this chapter, it was arguably only in the 2010s that attitudes in wider French society turned decisively away from the psychoanalytic approach. A particular flashpoint was a 2011 documentary film, *Le Mur: La psychanalyse à l'épreuve de l'autisme* (The Wall: Psychoanalysis Put to the Test By Autism), made by Sophie Robert in conjunction with the parents' association Autistes Sans Frontières and resulting in a lengthy legal battle.[130]

The film's standpoint was not only that the psychoanalytic approach to autism was ineffective, but that its imposition by psychiatrists was actively harmful, causing children to be denied access to therapies with a better track record. The film presented and contrasted two autistic children. Julien, fourteen, had spent his early childhood in a day hospital. He was mute, and completely dependent on others. Guillaume, eleven, had been diagnosed as autistic at age four. His parents, rejecting psychoanalytic explanations of his condition, had arranged for Guillaume to be treated according to cognitive behavioural methods such as PECS and TEACHH. By eleven, Guillaume was well socialised, successfully integrated into a mainstream school and performing well academically. Robert interspersed footage of these children and their families with that of interviews she had conducted with eleven psychoanalysts. Her interview questions pushed the analysts to make explicit the logical conclusions of their approach to autism, and to reveal what Robert clearly regarded as the absurdity or offensiveness of those positions. Several of the analysts interviewed articulated ideas closely resembling those of Mannoni and Dolto from the 1960s, as the following exchanges make clear:

Yann Bogopolsky:	The father is there to make it clear what is forbidden and at the same time to protect the child ... from the mother's incestuous desires.
Robert:	All mothers have incestuous desires?
Bogopolsky:	Yes, whether they're aware of them or not.
Genevive Loison:	When the mother takes on board the father's words, the child discovers speech.
Robert:	If the child doesn't speak, it's because the mother disregards the father's words?
Loison:	Well, we don't have many of those here, they're mostly in psychiatric hospitals ... the profoundly autistic ones.
Aldo Naouri:	Most of the time, the child's symptom is no more or less than the symptom that's been imparted to it, chiefly by the maternal unconscious.[131]

As these extracts indicate, some of Robert's questions seemed designed to elicit sweeping dogmatic statements from the analysts in order to subject them to ridicule. The film was a polemic as much as a documentary, and did not, for example, explore internal debates within French psychoanalysis as to the nature of autism. Controversy erupted when, before the film had been screened in cinemas or on television, three of the analysts sued Robert for libel. Alexandre Stevens, Éric Laurent and Esthela Solano-Suarez, all from the École de la Cause Freudienne (the Lacanian successor organisation to the EFP), alleged that Robert had edited the footage in such a way as to misrepresent their position. In January 2012, a Lille court accepted their case and banned the film, ordering Robert to pay thousands of euros in damages.

The reaction to this development, however, illustrated the change in attitudes since the 1970s. Reporting of the judgement in France and internationally was largely sympathetic to Robert, interpreting it as an attack on freedom of expression and an attempt by the psychoanalytic lobby to censor criticism and avoid ridicule.[132] The international journalist association Reporters Without Borders spoke out in Robert's defence.[133] Politically, too, the mood was turning against the analysts. The same month, Prime Minister François Fillon declared autism a 'Grande cause nationale' for 2012, and a parliamentarian from the centre-right UMP party suggested a law forbidding psychoanalysts from treating autism. In 2014, an appeal court overturned the ban on *Le Mur*.[134] By April 2016, Ségolène Neuville, the socialist secretary of state for disabilities, was declaring that 'psychoanalysis is not among the [treatment] methods recommended for autistic children … It's no longer acceptable to blame mothers.'[135] In a question to Neuville in the National Assembly, socialist deputy Gwendal Rouillard won applause for denouncing 'the psychoanalytic approach [to autism], an approach which I consider a moral sham, an intellectual sham, a medical sham and an ethical sham'.[136]

Le Mur did not mention Dolto or Mannoni, instead attributing the psychoanalytic view of autism to Lacan, Bettelheim and, to a lesser degree, Donald Winnicott. But as this chapter has shown, any account of the French psychoanalytic view of autism that leaves out the role of Dolto and Mannoni is incomplete. Lacan, as mentioned above, praised and encouraged Mannoni's work in his 1964 seminar. In his seminar of 1969–70 (thus not long after Dolto's presentation of the Dominique case at the 1967 '*enfance aliénée*' workshop and its 1968 publication in *Recherches*), he gave his own version of the devouring mother idea:

> The mother's desire is not something that is bearable just like that, that you are indifferent to. It will always wreak havoc. A huge crocodile in whose jaws you are – that's the mother. One never knows what might suddenly come over her and make her shut her trap. That's what the mother's desire is.[137]

With *Le Cas Dominique*, Dolto had seemed to show that such mothers were found not just in theoretical statements but in real families and clinical situations. Her novelistic depiction showed the French public what a toxic family might look like, and offered a clear and reassuringly familiar prescription – paternal authority – for ameliorating situations of great suffering and life-altering distress. The enthusiasm with which the book was received indicates the strength of the underlying desire to obtain insight and solutions into such issues in the early 1970s. This was how, in the words of Dolto's biographer Jean-François de Sauverzac, the Dominique case became 'a kind of paradigm' that shaped the way many French people and professionals thought about autism and mental illness in children.[138]

Meanwhile, the real Bel family continued to lead their lives. By 1970, Dominique had finished school and become a potter, sporting hippy clothes and long hair. Madame Bel, by now separated from Georges, had contacted Dolto again, concerned that Dominique was being sexually exploited by some co-workers. Dolto responded by helping to arrange a placement with a specialist social worker in the south of France. Later, Dominique worked for a time in Belgium, but rather than settle there was eventually persuaded to return home by his mother, who – according to Dolto – thereupon turned him into a 'native laundry houseboy' (*boy à faire la lessive*).[139] This label referenced Madame Bel's colonial upbringing – with a pejorative racial stereotype – while also appearing to vindicate Dolto's original interpretation of the case: i.e. that Dominique was being prevented from developing his independence by a tyrannical mother. Madame Bel would presumably tell a different story. When *Le Cas Dominique* was published, she threatened to sue Dolto for defamation, but was talked out of it by her son's social worker. Dolto subsequently – out of guilt, her biographer suggests – donated part of the book's royalties towards funding Dominique's professional training.[140] Having thus been spared a possible scandal, Dolto was free to continue her rise to national celebrity.

Notes

1 Decision taken at a Ministers' Deputies' meeting, 14 January 2004.

2 Caroline Piquet, 'Ces enfants handicapés obligés de s'exiler de France pour aller à l'école', *Le Figaro*, 7 November 2014.

3 See e.g. the 'Report to the Committee of Ministers', dated 11 September 2013, in *European Action of the Disabled (AEH) v. France*, Complaint No. 81/2012. https://search.coe.int/cm/Pages/result_details.aspx?ObjectID=09000016805c8e97, accessed 29 January 2021.

4 UN Committee on the Rights of the Child (CRC), *Concluding Observations on the Fifth Periodic Report of France*, 29/12016, CRC/C/FRA/CO/5, www.refworld.org/docid/56c17fb64.html, accessed 29 January 2021.

5 Brigitte Chamak, 'Autism as Viewed by French Parents', in V. B. Patel, V. R. Preedy and C. R. Martin (eds), *Comprehensive Guide to Autism*

(New York: Springer, 2014), pp. 2533–43; Brigitte Chamak and Béatrice Bonniau, 'Changes in the Diagnosis of Autism: How Parents and Professionals Act and React in France', *Culture, Medicine, and Psychiatry*, 37:3 (2013), 405–26.

6 Steve Silberman, *Neurotribes: The Legacy of Autism and How to Think Smarter About People Who Think Differently* (London: Allen & Unwin, 2015).

7 'Greta Thunberg responds to Asperger's critics: "It's a superpower"', *Guardian*, 2 September 2019.

8 Bonnie Evans, *The Metamorphosis of Autism: A History of Child Development in Britain* (Manchester: Manchester University Press, 2017).

9 Cited in *ibid.*, p. 56.

10 *Ibid.*, p. 41.

11 Hans Asperger, 'Die "Autistischen Psychopathen" im Kindesalter', *Archiv für Psychiatrie und Nervenkrankheiten*, 117:1 (1944), 132–5.

12 Edith Sheffer, *Asperger's Children: The Origins of Autism in Nazi Vienna* (New York: W. W. Norton, 2018).

13 Silberman, *Neurotribes*, p. 182. Leo Kanner, 'Autistic Disturbances of Affective Contact', *Nervous Child*, 2 (1943), 217–50; 'Early Infantile Autism', *Journal of Pediatrics*, 25:3 (1944), 211–17.

14 Evans, *Metamorphosis of Autism*, pp. 113–14.

15 Leo Kanner, *Child Psychiatry* (Springfield, IL: C. C. Thomas, 1935 – several subsequent editions).

16 Silberman, *Neurotribes*, p. 192; Nathan G. Hale, *The Rise and Crisis of Psychoanalysis in America: Freud and the Americans 1917–1985* (New York: Oxford University Press, 1995), p. 258.

17 Franz Alexander, *Psychosomatic Medicine* (1950), cited in Hale, *Rise and Crisis*, p. 260.

18 Hale, *Rise and Crisis*, pp. 266ff.

19 See e.g. Jonathan M. Metzl, '"Mother's Little Helper": The Crisis of Psychoanalysis and the Miltown Resolution', *Gender & History*, 15:2 (2003), 228–55; Ilina Singh, 'Bad Boys, Good Mothers, and the "Miracle" of Ritalin', *Science in Context*, 15:4 (2002), 577–603.

20 Hale, *Rise and Crisis*, p. 253; Silberman, *Neurotribes*, p. 192.

21 Leo Kanner, 'Emotional Interference with Intellectual Functioning', *American Journal of Mental Deficiency*, 56:4 (1952), 701–7.

22 Bruno Bettelheim, *The Empty Fortress: Infantile Autism and the Birth of Self* (New York: Free Press, 1967). Bettelheim consulted such papers as Louise Despert, 'Some Considerations Relating to the Genesis of Autistic Behavior in Children', *American Journal of Orthopsychiatry*, 21 (1951), 335–50; C. E. Goshen, 'Mental Retardation and Neurotic

Maternal Attitudes', *Archives of General Psychiatry*, 9 (1963), 168–75; Leon Eisenberg, 'The Fathers of Autistic Children', *American Journal of Orthopsychiatry*, 27 (1957), 715–24.

23 Bettelheim, *Empty Fortress*, p. 7. On Bettelheim and his legacy in France, see Jonathyne Briggs, 'The Enduring Fortress: The Influence of Bruno Bettelheim in the Politics of Autism in France', *Modern Intellectual History* 17:4 (2020), 1163–91.

24 Bernard Rimland, *Infantile Autism: The Syndrome and its Implications for a Neural Theory of Behavior* (London: Methuen, 1964). On parents' associations and their influence in the United States, see Chloe Silverman, *Understanding Autism: Parents, Doctors, and the History of a Disorder* (Princeton, NJ: Princeton University Press, 2011).

25 See Evans, *Metamorphosis of Autism*, Ch. 4.

26 Chantal Sicile-Kira, 'Autism and Education in France', *Huffington Post*, 14 June 2010.

27 From the documentary *Le Mur* (dir. Sophie Robert, France, 2011).

28 From an interview conducted in 2005–6 by Chamak and Bonniau. 'Changes in the Diagnosis of Autism', 411ff.

29 *Ibid.*, 419.

30 Chamak, 'Autism as Viewed by French Parents', pp. 2533–4.

31 The text of the law ('Loi no. 96–1076 du 11 décembre 1996 modifiant la loi no. 75–535 du 30 juin 1975 rélative aux institutions sociales et médicosociales et tendant à assurer une prise en charge adaptée de l'autisme') was published in the *Journal officiel* on 12 December 1996. For a summary of the functions of the Centres Ressources Autisme, see Regis Brunod, 'Le Centre Ressources Autisme Île-de-France (CRAIF)', *Annales Médico-psychologiques, revue psychiatrique*, 170:7 (2012), 491–3.

32 Cour des comptes, *Évaluation de la politique en direction des personnes présentant des troubles du spectre de l'autisme. Enquête demandée par le Comité d'évaluation et de contrôle des politiques publiques de l'Assemblée nationale Décembre 2017*, www.ccomptes.fr/sites/default/files/2018–01/20180124-rapport-autisme.pdf, accessed 29 January 2021.

33 See also Richard Bates, 'France's Autism Controversy and the Historical Role of Psychanalysis in the Diagnosis and Treatment of Autistic Children', *Nottingham French Studies*, 59:2 (2020), 221–35.

34 Jeffrey A. Lieberman with Ogi Ogas, *Shrinks: The Untold Story of Psychiatry* (London: Weidenfeld & Nicolson, 2015), pp. 154, 192.

35 However, because of demographic growth and declining death rates, numbers did not fall in absolute terms. See France Meslé and Jacques Vallin, 'La Population des établissements psychiatriques: évolution de

la morbidité ou changement de stratégie médicale?', *Population*, 36:6 (1981), 1035–68.

36 See Lieberman, *Shrinks*, pp. 176–93.

37 The term 'antipsychiatry', coined by David Cooper in 1967, has long been recognised as unsatisfactory. In practice, many thinkers and practitioners associated with it argued for psychiatry's reform, not its abolition. Following John Foot's work on Franco Basaglia, this chapter understands 'antipsychiatry' as a radical movement within psychiatry, critiquing the theories, diagnoses and practices employed in psychiatry before the 1960s. John Foot, *The Man Who Closed the Asylums: Franco Basaglia and the Revolution in Mental Health Care* (London: Verso, 2015).

38 R. D. Laing and Aaron Esterson, *Sanity, Madness and the Family* (first published 1964) (London: Tavistock, 1970), pp. 11–12.

39 Thomas Szasz, *The Myth of Mental Illness: Foundations of a Theory of Personal Conduct* (New York: Hoeber-Harper, 1961).

40 Erving Goffman, *Asylums. Essays on the Social Situation of Mental Patients and Other Inmates* (New York: Doubleday, 1961).

41 Michel Foucault, *Folie et déraison: Histoire de la folie à l'âge classique* (Paris: Plon, 1961).

42 Foot, *The Man Who Closed the Asylums*, Ch. 7.

43 See Richard Weisman, 'Reflections on the Oak Ridge Experiment with Mentally Disordered Offenders, 1965–1968', *International Journal of Law and Psychiatry*, 18:3 (1995), 265–90. Twenty-eight former patients at Oak Ridge successfully sued the Ontario government for the treatment they received from Barker and Dr Gary Meier, which they argued amounted to 'inhumane treatment and psychological and physical abuse'. See 'Psychiatrists, Ontario government liable for horrific patient abuse at mental health facility', *World News*, 2 July 2020.

44 Hale, *Rise and Crisis*, p. 277.

45 Cited in Mijolla, *La France et Freud 1954–1964*, p. 74.

46 Sherry Turkle, 'French Anti-Psychiatry', in David Ingleby (ed.), *Critical Psychiatry: the Politics of Mental Health* (Harmondsworth: Penguin, 1981), pp. 150–83.

47 Marcelle Marini, *Jacques Lacan: The French Context*, trans. Anne Tomiche (New Brunswick, NJ: Rutgers University Press, 1992).

48 Jacques Lacan, *Autres écrits* (Paris: Seuil, 2001), p. 229.

49 Roudinesco, *Jacques Lacan*, p. 449.

50 Oury's early career is described in Camille Robcis, *Disalienation: Politics, Philosophy, and Radical Psychiatry in Postwar France* (Chicago: University of Chicago Press, 2021), Ch. 3; Julian Bourg, *From Revolution to Ethics: May 1968 and Contemporary French*

Thought (Montreal: McGill-Queen's University Press, 2007), Ch. 10; and François Dosse, *Gilles Deleuze and Félix Guattari: Intersecting Lives*, trans. Deborah Glassman (New York: Columbia University Press, 2011), Ch. 2–3. On La Borde's connection to the wider history of French antipsychiatry, see also Jacques Postel and David F. Allen, 'History and Anti-Psychiatry in France', in Mark S. Micale and Roy Porter (eds), *Discovering the History of Psychiatry* (Oxford: Oxford University Press, 1994), pp. 384–414.

51 See Pierre Bailly-Salin, 'The Mentally Ill Under Nazi Occupation in France', *International Journal of Mental Health*, 35:4 (2006–7), 11–25.

52 On Tosquelles, Saint-Alban and Lacan see Robcis, *Disalienation*, Ch. 1.

53 Dosse, *Intersecting Lives*, p. 26.

54 *Ibid.*, p. 36; Jacques Lacan, 'Propos sur la causalité psychique', *L'Évolution psychiatrique* (1947), 123–65.

55 Cited in Dosse, *Intersecting Lives*, p. 37.

56 On Lacan's intellectual influence on Oury, see Robcis, *Disalienation*, pp. 82–6.

57 Dosse, *Intersecting Lives*, p. 70.

58 *Ibid.*, p. 71.

59 Antoine de Gaudemar, 'Maud Mannoni dans la nuit. La psychanalyste spécialiste des enfants est morte dimanche à 74 ans', *Libération*, 17 March 1998.

60 Octave Mannoni's best-known work, *Psychologie de la colonisation* (Paris: Seuil, 1950), drew on his colonial experience in Madagascar. It provoked sharp criticism from Aimé Césaire and Frantz Fanon for its racist assumptions. See François Vatin, 'Octave Mannoni (1899–1989) et sa *Psychologie de la colonisation.* Contextualisation et décontextualisation', *Revue du MAUSS*, 37:1 (2011), 137–78.

61 Maurice Dugautiez to Dolto, 28 February 1949, *Une vie de correspondances*, p. 175.

62 On the Lacan-Mannoni relationship, see Laure Razon, Olivier Putois and Alain Vanier, 'The Lacanian Concept of Cut in Light of Lacan's Interactions with Maud Mannoni', *Frontiers in Psychology*, 8:2177 (December 2017).

63 Roudinesco, *Jacques Lacan*, pp. 491–4.

64 Maud Mannoni, *Le Psychiatre, son 'fou' et la psychanalyse* (Paris: Seuil, 1970); *L'Enfant arriéré et sa mère: étude psychanalytique* (Paris: Seuil, 1964). English edition: *The Retarded Child and the Mother*, trans. A. M. Sheridan Smith (London: Tavistock, 1973).

65 Jacques Lacan, *Écrits* (Paris: Seuil, 1966); *Le Séminaire de Jacques Lacan, livre XI – Les quatre concepts fondamentaux de la*

psychanalyse, 1964, ed. Jacques-Alain Miller (Paris: Seuil, 1973), seminar of 10 June 1964. Mannoni arranged for a French translation of David Cooper's *Psychiatry and Anti-Psychiatry* to be published in the same collection.

66 Mannoni, *Retarded Child*, pp. xi–xii (from Mannoni's original English-language preface to this edition).

67 *Ibid.*, p. 61.

68 *Ibid.*, p. 62.

69 *Ibid.*, pp. 124–31.

70 *Ibid.*, p. 63.

71 *Ibid.*, p. xxiii.

72 *Ibid.*, p. xxii.

73 *Ibid.*, p. 23.

74 *Ibid.*, p. 61.

75 Françoise Dolto, *Le Cas Dominique* (1971) (Paris: Seuil, 1985), p. 246, original emphasis.

76 Silberman, *Neurotribes*, p. 190.

77 Maud Mannoni, *Le Premier Rendez-vous avec le psychanalyste* (Paris: Denoël/Gonthier, 1965), p. 56.

78 *Ibid.*, pp. 61–3.

79 Dolto, preface to Mannoni, *Premier Rendez-vous*, pp. 5–49, 22–3.

80 *Ibid.*, p. 23.

81 Mannoni, *Premier Rendez-vous*, p. 65.

82 *Ibid.*, p. 67, original emphasis.

83 Mannoni, *Retarded Child*, p. 128.

84 Laing and Esterson, *Sanity, Madness*, p. 13.

85 Nina Sutton, *Bettelheim, A Life and Legacy* (Boulder, CO: Westview, 1997), p. x.

86 Bettelheim, *Empty Fortress*, p. 99.

87 On Deligny and autism, see Damian Milton, 'Tracing the Influence of Fernand Deligny on Autism Studies', *Disability & Society*, 31:2 (2016), 285–9.

88 Dominique Provost and Andrée Bauer, 'Trends and Developments in Public Psychiatry in France since 1975', *Acta Psychiatrica Scandinavica*, 104 (2001), 63–8.

89 Maud Mannoni, 'Introduction', *Recherches*, 8 (1968), 13.

90 On *Recherches* see Dosse, *Intersecting Lives*, Ch. 4. As well as her case study of Dominique, Dolto co-wrote a text with Jean Oury for this publication, on 'L'Enfant, la psychose et l'institution' ('The Child, Psychosis, and the Institution'), *Recherches*, 8 (1968), 115–30.

91 Françoise Dolto, 'Clinique psychanalytique', *Recherches*, 8 (1968), 155–242.

92 Four volumes of extracts from Dolto's seminars were subsequently published: *Séminaire de psychanalyse d'enfants 1* (Paris: Seuil, 1982); *Séminaire de psychanalyse d'enfants 2* (Paris: Seuil, 1985); *Inconscient et destins. Séminaire de psychanalyse d'enfants 3*, ed. Jean-François de Sauverzac (Paris: Seuil, 1989); *La Vague et l'océan: Séminaire sur les pulsions de mort (1970–1971)*, ed. Colette Manier (Paris: Gallimard, 2003).
93 Dolto, *Dominique*, p. 40.
94 *Ibid.*, p. 14.
95 *Ibid.*, p. 19.
96 *Ibid.*, p. 13.
97 *Ibid.*, p. 20.
98 *Ibid.*, p. 33.
99 *Ibid.*, p. 34.
100 *Ibid.*, p. 62.
101 *Ibid.*, p. 68.
102 *Ibid.*, pp. 63–4.
103 *Ibid.*, p. 72.
104 *Ibid.*, p. 124.
105 *Ibid.*, p. 75
106 *Ibid.*, pp. 78, 73.
107 *Ibid.*, pp. 95, 98.
108 *Ibid.*, pp. 105, 189.
109 *Ibid.*, p. 97.
110 *Ibid.*, p. 144.
111 *Ibid.*, pp. 152, 140.
112 *Ibid.*, p. 189.
113 Françoise Dolto, 'Les Mères, entretien réalisé et réécrit par J.-B. Pontalis', *Les Temps modernes*, January 1963, reprinted in Dolto, *CdE*, pp. 59–75, 75.
114 Dolto, *Dominique*, pp. 168–9.
115 *Ibid.*, p. 166.
116 *Ibid.*, p. 175.
117 Gerry A. Stefanatos, 'Regression in Autistic Spectrum Disorders', *Neuropsychology Review*, 18:4 (2008), 305–19.
118 Dolto, *Dominique*, pp. 80, 188.
119 E.g. 'Léon' case, in Dolto, *L'Image inconsciente*, pp. 288–328; Dolto, *Cause des enfants*, p. 491.
120 Sauverzac, *Françoise Dolto*, p. 177.
121 Jacques Hochmann, 'La Bataille de l'autisme. Réflexions sur un phénomène social contemporain', *PSN Psychiatrie Sciences Humaines Neurosciences*, 7:3 (2009), 99–111, 105.

122 *Sociologie politique*, February 1972, 10.
123 *Témoignage chrétien*, 10 February 1972.
124 *Nouvelles littéraires*, 31 January 1972, 13. Review by Jacques Brosse.
125 *Magazine littéraire*, March 1972, 59–60. Review by Raymond Bellour.
126 *Le Nouvel Observateur*, 357 (September 1971). Review by Philippe Nemo.
127 *Chronique sociale de France*, July 1972, 76–9. Review by Jean-François Skrzypczak. Original emphasis.
128 *Réforme*, 18 March 1972, 12–14. Review by Marianne Roland-Michel.
129 *La Croix*, 1 February 1972. Review by Olivier Cotinaud.
130 *Le Mur* (dir. Sophie Robert, France, 2011).
131 *Ibid.*
132 E.g. Sophie Callat, 'Autisme: le documentaire "Le Mur" condamné par la justice', *Le Nouvel Observateur*, 26 January 2012; David Jolly and Stephane Novac, 'A French Film Takes Issue With the Psychoanalytic Approach to Autism', *New York Times*, 19 January 2012.
133 'Documentary filmmaking threatened by court ruling on autism documentary', 7 February 2012, https://rsf.org/en/news/documentary-filmmaking-threatened-court-ruling-autism-documentary, accessed 29 January 2021.
134 Catherine Vincent, '"Le Mur, la psychanalyse à l'épreuve de l'autisme" à nouveau libre de diffusion', *Le Monde*, 16 January 2014.
135 Interview with Ségolène Neuville on French parliamentary TV, 1 April 2016, www.lcp.fr/la-politique-en-video/segolene-neuville-la-psychanalyse-ne-fait-pas-partie-des-methodes-recommandees, accessed 8 May 2020.
136 Gwendal Rouillard, 'Question au Gouvernement – Autisme – 5 avril 2016', www.youtube.com/watch?v=EO5OzhWSkl8, accessed 8 May 2020.
137 Jacques Lacan, *The Seminar of Jacques Lacan vol. XVII: The Other Side of Psychoanalysis*, trans. Russell Grigg (London: W. W. Norton, 2006), p. 129. In *Le Mur*, analyst Geneviève Loison is shown employing a toy crocodile in her work with children, as a method of assessing whether they are in danger from 'the mother-crocodile'.
138 Sauverzac, *Françoise Dolto*, p. 265.
139 *Ibid.*, pp. 277–9.
140 *Ibid.*, p. 278, n. 43.

6

Radio star: psychoanalysis in the public sphere, 1968–88

The publication of *Le Cas Dominique* in 1971, and the simultaneous reissuing by Éditions du Seuil of *Psychanalyse et pédiatrie*, her thesis written in the 1930s, reinforced Dolto's public status as an expert in child psychology and added her to the growing list of French psychoanalysts enjoying a degree of publishing success in the years after 1968. Dolto made it into *Who's Who in France* in 1975. But it was her radio career that was principally responsible for making her a household name, especially the *Lorsque l'enfant paraît* ('When the baby comes' or 'When the child appears') broadcasts on France Inter in 1976–78. These broadcasts transformed her public profile and occasioned her retirement as an analyst, since her fame, she felt, affected her ability to be a neutral presence for clients. The *Lorsque l'enfant paraît* recordings, and the letters sent in by listeners, open a window onto both how Dolto sought to use the media to disseminate certain messages, and more broadly onto the concerns of French parents and young people in the 1970s. They show Dolto definitively assuming a position in the cultural mainstream, with all of the engagement with and contestation of her ideas that this implies, and in ways that highlight some of the political and social complexities and uncertainties of 1970s France.

This chapter analyses these broadcasts along with several other examples of Dolto's public interventions and impacts in the decade or so after 1968. Beginning with a separate series of broadcasts that Dolto made for the Europe 1 station in 1968–69 (of which transcripts were published under the title *S.O.S. Psychanalyste!*), it situates Dolto in the context of the history of French radio, with particular reference to other broadcasters who used radio to create a sense of intimacy and community around discussions of personal-yet-public issues. The chapter goes on to examine Dolto's interventions on homosexuality and education, situating these with regard to contemporary political debates.

The final section analyses the Maison Verte children's centres that Dolto and her colleagues created after 1978. The proliferation of these centres across France is a particularly important example of Dolto's success in disseminating psychoanalytic thinking into everyday life and institutions, representing perhaps the most extensive long-term project for taking psychoanalysis 'beyond the couch' anywhere in the world in recent decades. The MV project achieved an unusually extensive integration between psychoanalysis and state educational priorities. These 'structures Dolto', as they were called, went further than any other institution in France – and arguably anywhere – to insert psychoanalysis into the everyday lives of thousands of families, and to convert it into a form of common sense.

S.O.S. Psychanalyste!

The growing psychologisation of western society in the twentieth century occurred in tandem with the development of the broadcast media. Cultural historian Maggie Andrews has described how the emergence of radio in the interwar period 'dramatically changed men and women's experience of domesticity, offering education and reducing isolation through a shared listening experience and a sense of belonging to wider imagined communities'.[1] Radio blurred the boundary between public and private, bringing world affairs and politics into the home, and domestic affairs into public debate. It was a new platform from which expertise about everyday life could be disseminated, including psychological and psychoanalytic expertise. A prominent exemplar of how it could be used in this way was the British child psychoanalyst Donald Winnicott, who used series of 1940s BBC broadcasts to address the psychical effects of World War II on children, especially evacuees and those living apart from their parents.[2]

France's relationship with radio was transformed by the country's experience of World War II. In the 1930s, the main attractions of French broadcasting were music and drama; coverage of news and current affairs was generally disappointing, especially on the somewhat ponderous public networks.[3] Vichy's public radio, though it became infamous for its pro-Nazi propaganda during the last phase of the Occupation, implemented certain innovations in its earlier years. It created the first station aimed at young people, Radio-Jeunesse, featuring readings from Charles Péguy, poetry and choral singing. Its family-based soap, *L'Alphabet de la famille* (*The Family Alphabet*), became the most popular programme on the flagship Radio Nationale station. Philip Nord argues that this show, which followed the lives of a mother and three children (the father being absent in a POW camp), struck a chord through its 'emotional intimacy at a moment of national difficulty'.[4]

For Vichy's opponents, the Free French and BBC broadcasts from London created a different kind of emotional intimacy – a precious, furtive connection to the wider world beyond Vichy's moral universe. De Gaulle's war experience convinced him of radio's importance in shaping national politics, and – once in power – the consequent need to bring it under close state management. The postwar Radiodiffusion Française, and its successor Radiodiffusion-Télévision Française (RTF, later Office de Radiodiffusion-Télévision Française – ORTF), had a mandate to promote social cohesion and French identity.[5] Its directors came under political pressure to equate the nation's interests with the government's, and to keep political debate within restricted parameters. *La Tribune de Paris*, which hosted the sex education debate featuring Dolto discussed in Chapter 4, was the successor show to the Free French's *Les Français parlent aux français* ('The French speak to the French'), and carried a certain social and cultural weight as a result.[6] As Rebecca Scales has shown, the association of radio with social responsibility in the Liberation context also provided an opportunity for the medium to be used to advocate for better treatment of disabled people, via the 1947 show *La Tribune de l'invalide*.[7]

In a (tacitly accepted) breach of the state monopoly, the 'peripheral' stations Europe 1, Radio Monte-Carlo and Radio Luxembourg (later Radio-Télévision Luxembourg – RTL) emerged as competitors in the 1950s, offering what Raymond Kuhn describes as 'less hidebound, more informal and unashamedly more commercial and populist' content.[8] In the 1960s, these stations were well placed to foster new communities reflecting France's changing cultural landscape. The Europe 1 youth-oriented show *Salut les copains*, broadcast in the afternoons as teenagers were leaving school, functioned as the focal point for an imagined community of young musical '*copains*' based on camaraderie and equality. It featured and helped develop the careers of new stars including Johnny Hallyday, Françoise Hardy and Sylvie Vartan.[9] Dolto's son Jean-Chrysostome (1943–2008), now known as 'Carlos' and building a career as a singer and *bon viveur*, became an important part of this radio-based community. He worked on *Salut les copains* from 1962, and then as an assistant and vocalist to Vartan and Hallyday, before releasing his first solo record in 1969. By the mid-1970s he was a fully fledged pop star in his own right, with moderately risqué hits such as *Tout nu et tout bronzé* ('*Naked and Tanned All Over*', 1973), *Papayou* (1975) and *Big Bisous* ('*Big Kisses*', 1977), and a glamorous wedding featured in *Paris Match*.[10] While Carlos's success had no discernible impact on his mother's career, it was a first-hand reminder of radio's potential to launch careers and bring about broader cultural change. Radio in the 1960s was still the leading broadcast medium. In 1961, only 20 per cent of French households had a television (rising to 40 per cent by 1964 and 79 per cent by 1973) – but 80 per cent had a radio, rising to 95 per cent by the mid-1970s.[11]

French broadcasting was profoundly affected by the events of May 1968, not just in terms of reporting them but because the ORTF's own staff went on strike, with many strikers subsequently sacked.[12] In the longer term, the cultural changes associated with 1968 led to public radio becoming more responsive to its audiences and less of a governmental mouthpiece. Programming aimed at young people and women was redesigned, for example through the new, ultimately short-lived stations Inter Variétés and Inter Jeunesse (1966–72). French state radio in the 1970s attempted to reconcile what politicians thought a state broadcaster should do – President Georges Pompidou affirmed in 1970 that 'like it or not, the ORTF is the voice of France' – with the idea that radio should be a service for its listeners.[13] Dolto's *Lorsque l'enfant paraît* can be thought of as a successful attempt to reach a middle ground between these two imperatives.

Dolto had already, in 1968–69, hosted a lesser-known programme on Europe 1, consisting of a weekly series of 'on-air consultations' directed at parents and children who phoned or wrote in with 'emergency' psychological or personal issues. This show was unusual in its focus on children's problems, and in the large proportion (over 50 per cent) of callers who were themselves aged under eighteen. It also differed from comparable programmes, such as those of Madame Soleil and Ménie Grégoire (discussed below), in that the responder was a qualified medical professional – in theory an anonymous one, since Dolto went by the name 'Docteur X', though her identity was well known in medical and psychoanalytic circles. Some 187 transcripts from these broadcasts were later published as a (still-anonymous) book, under the title *S.O.S. Psychanalyste!*[14]

Since a telephone remained something of a luxury item in late-1960s France, the child callers to Dolto's programme likely skewed towards wealthier families.[15] Sixty per cent were girls, and the average age was twelve. Most frequently, they wished to discuss a conflict with their parents, over subjects ranging from the right to read comics, or be allowed out with members of the opposite sex, to having contact with a divorced parent. Difficulties with siblings and problems at school were also prominent concerns, as were friendships, issues with body image or weight, or compulsive actions such as thumb sucking or nail biting. Two callers mentioned the recent May 1968 events as causing familial conflicts: 'since then, my parents can't understand at all that I've changed a bit, and they stop me from getting involved in any collective thing at college', complained one, while another reported that since the events his parents treated him 'like a stranger' and falsely suspected him of involvement in (presumably revolutionary) 'committees' and 'groups'.[16] Dolto told these callers to talk things over with their parents, and show them that they still loved them despite any political differences. She welcomed the self-actualisation that the students appeared to have achieved through political involvement: 'it took this social event to show you that you were more mature than you thought'.[17] Dolto's responses to the young callers were not obviously drawn from psychoanalytic theory; often her advice was simply to talk more and empathise with their parents, siblings or friends. She encouraged children to take personal responsibility for their circumstances and aim for greater behavioural maturity. She told one nine-year-old girl who still sucked her thumb to work at self-mastery and not succumb to infantile temptations.[18] She told children to acknowledge their desires and accept realities that they could not easily change.

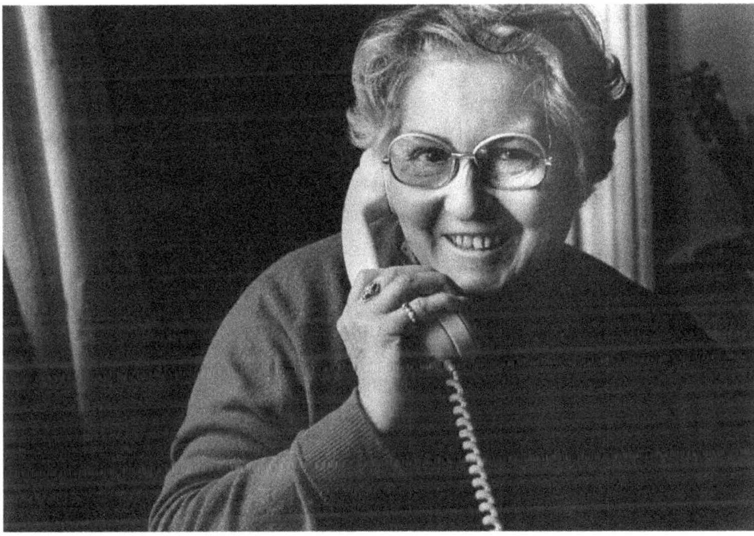

Figure 6.1 Dolto posing with a telephone, 1970s

Girls worried about being overweight were told to 'accept it. Accept, I say ... it's of no importance. What drives a woman is her heart.'[19]

Among the parents who called the programme, the most frequent subjects of concern were jealousies, sibling rivalries, toilet training, phobias, separation anxiety and issues around eating, sleeping or discipline. Several raised issues of a sexual nature, such as puberty, how to tell children the facts of life or the question of parental nudity around children. Two single mothers asked Dolto how to broach the question of their children's paternity without 'traumatising' them.[20] Many of Dolto's responses combined reassurance, plausible psychological insight and liberal attitudes. She reassured parents that certain issues, such as the psychological consequences of being born left-handed, were nothing to be worried about. One mother of a five-year-old girl who liked playing doctors with her male cousin – a game involving some evidently pleasurable physical intimacy – wondered if she should put a stop to this, 'by saying that it was ugly, that it was wrong'. Dolto told her to leave the children be. 'Why do you say that the body is ugly? Don't get yourself worked up about children's awakening sexuality.'[21]

Dolto was more willing to offer psychoanalytic interpretations to parents than to the child callers. Though she did not use the words 'Oedipus complex', a father concerned about his three-year-old son's aggression was told that 'it's the moment when the small boy starts to feel a bit manly [*mâle*], he wants to keep his mummy just for himself and attempts to exclude you'.[22] Similarly, Dolto explained to a pregnant mother that her three-year-old daughter's jealousy towards the unborn baby was because the daughter would herself like to be having her daddy's baby.[23] Dolto communicated such ideas without explaining their origin in Freudian theory. Although the show's title made the psychoanalytic link explicit, Dolto's pseudonym of 'Docteur X' blurred the lines between psychoanalytic and medical knowledge. Her interpretations were thus presented as established medical wisdom, even though they were in some cases quite idiosyncratic. On the subject of toilet training, for example, Dolto issued stark warnings about the risks of attempting to train a child 'too soon', by which she meant before twenty-five to twenty-six months. A younger child 'can't stay out of nappies [*ne peut être propre*] except in order to please its mother, which has to be paid for later with another kind of dependence … a very large personality defect … difficulties in writing and reading … problems in speaking well'.[24] By attempting to toilet train a fourteen-month-old child 'you're taking a big risk with that child's future'. Ideally, Dolto wanted mothers to enable children to become continent in their own time. But if they left it too late, Dolto might equally accuse them of enclosing the child in a 'fusional relationship', with all the dark consequences that that was supposed to entail. Dolto's insistence on perilous infant determinism in this domain diverged substantially from other psychoanalytically informed parenting advisors; Benjamin Spock, for example, predicted no comparable terrors for children toilet trained before age two, and 'found that waiting for the child to take the initiative didn't work for some parents at all'.[25]

In addition to this mixture of often pragmatic, often reassuring, occasionally anxiety-inducing advice, Dolto used the show to promote her vision of the family, in particular stressing paternal authority and heteronormative gender divisions. The nine-year-old thumb-sucker mentioned above was advised to throw herself into housework, so as to 'really acquire the qualities of a woman in a house'.[26] She dismissed one mother-daughter dispute with the comment 'I think that, if there's a father there, he could put things in order!'[27] A mother of two boys called to express her concern about their desire to play with toy guns, despite her husband having no problem with it. Dolto response was 'so why are you asking me? … *When it comes to raising boys, listen above all to your husband and ask him to take care of his children*, and don't run the risk of Docteur X saying something contrary to your husband … The mother should be first and foremost for girls' things, and the father, it's very important, for boys' things.'[28] Occasionally forced to choose between a liberal parenting attitude and paternal power, Dolto sided with the latter. One mother explained how she sought to bring up her children 'very freely, that's to say I don't spank them much and I let them roam around all of the apartment'. She felt that this worked well, resulting in children who were 'pretty active, noisy and who aren't scared of much'. Her problem was that her mother, mother-in-law and husband all predicted that 'dire troubles' would result from her methods. Dolto told the caller that while she was completely correct in her approach, she should nonetheless give way on the grounds that '*your husband is the master in the house*'.[29] If he decided to confine the children to one room rather than let them roam across the flat, the mother must not demur.

Dolto's stance on valorising and not challenging paternal power could sometimes tip over into acceptance of abuse, including sexual abuse, throwing the responsibility for such behaviour back onto the victims. One woman was warned against referring to her son's father, from whom she was separated, as an 'unscrupulous individual': 'you have to hold yourself at fault [in the child's eyes] and not his progenitor'.[30] A girl complaining that her father was 'very hard on me' was told to accept this since 'you chose this father to be born to'.[31] As Dolto explained to a Canadian judge in 1983, she believed that children were generally complicit in cases of abuse:

> The educator … can indeed explain [to a victim of sexual abuse] that the child was complicit in their father's excitement, perhaps without having sought it. I believe that these children are more or less complicit in what happens.[32]

She had similarly little sympathy with victims of bullying: 'When a child tells you how they've been assaulted, you must always praise the aggressor. You must say: "He wanted to make contact with you, and you weren't capable of responding."'[33] If a child was aggressive towards others, this should be seen as 'an attempt to make contact with them and not something naughty'. Dolto felt it was generally the victims, not the perpetrators of bullying, who were manifesting 'neurotic reactions' and may need psychotherapy.

Mothers, meanwhile, were expected to dedicate themselves extensively to their children. In several cases, Dolto hinted that a child's problems originated in insufficient maternal devotion of time and energy. One mother, requesting advice on how to reduce her young son's thumb sucking, was told that the habit most likely derived from boredom: 'It's not his brother that he needs, it's conversations with Mum. Do you let them play with water enough? At least an hour a day, you know.'[34] Another mother, worried that her baby cried a lot despite her competence in '*puériculture*', was told that 'perhaps the fact of having studied childcare has taken away from you the natural reactions of mums who, in fact, ought to have their babies in their arms almost constantly'.[35]

This last comment illustrates Dolto's nostalgic tendency to idealise rural life and the pre-industrial past, and deplore 'unnatural' book-based learning in ways that call to mind the right-wing nostalgia of the interwar period. In earlier times (she wrote in a 1973 essay), 'life was more psychologically healthy, before the Pasteurian discoveries and their application to household hygiene'.[36] She regretted the invention of formula milk on the grounds that 'it produced a generation of the civilised ... who no longer benefit from the heat and comforting odour of the maternal breast'.[37] 'Civilised', for Dolto here, was a dirty word. Societal and technological change had reduced children's opportunities for social interactions beyond the nuclear family; the twentieth-century child 'has a larger material space, but a smaller one in terms of emotional relations'.[38] None of these views is especially surprising in the light of Dolto's experiences and orientation in the 1930s and 1940s, but her status as a senior cultural presence imbued them with authority in the 1970s. By that time, she was a clinician with decades of experience, an associate of figures from radical psychiatry and psychoanalysis who were enjoying a cultural ascendency and an established media expert on children's psychology. If she was repeating ideas that sounded like old Pétainist tropes, mustn't it be because they had, in some sense, been proven to be true?

Ménie Grégoire's painful problem

To further situate Dolto within the French media landscape it is worth briefly pausing over three other female presenters who used radio to create communities of emotional intimacy. Clara Candiani, Madame Soleil and – especially – Ménie Grégoire helped to establish the radio as a place where emotional distress and personal dilemmas could be shared with a reassuring mediator and a sympathetic public. Introducing psychological (in Grégoire's case, psychoanalytic) expertise or terminology into their conversations, they embodied the idea that airing such issues on the radio could lead to some form of public as well as personal benefit.

Candiani (1902–96) was a pioneering female journalist, reporting for *Le Figaro* from 1927, and a left-wing Catholic with a strong interest in social issues. Her husband was a founder of the Secours Catholique charity. From 1947 to 1982 she presented a six-minute weekly broadcast on France Inter entitled, with unmissable Free French echoes, *Les Français donnent aux Français* ('The French give to the French'). The programme appealed to listeners to help fellow citizens in need by highlighting individual cases of distress. Those whose stories were covered included elderly people living in isolation, adolescents battling addictions, parents of severely disabled children and unemployed people threatened with eviction. Candiani's show confronted its audience with the emotional, financial and psychological suffering of people living around them and invited reflection on how such suffering could be ameliorated. It generated a large correspondence, receiving around forty letters per day. The community and solidarity it appealed to were national, as befitting its place on the state broadcaster.

'Madame Soleil' (Germaine Moritz, 1913–96) was an astrologer who became a national celebrity thanks to her show on Europe 1 from 1970 to 1993. At her peak, to obtain a private consultation with Madame Soleil acquired a certain cachet; her clients from the business, arts and political worlds reportedly included President François Mitterrand.[39] Her show's switchboard often received thousands of calls per day. Madame Soleil acquired a reputation for psychological insight, as someone who could not merely read the stars but help resolve personal problems; listeners described her as 'very much a psychologist' (*très psychologue*).[40] Her show's success demonstrated a strong popular demand to have one's personal issues listened to respectfully, along with a relative lack of public concern for the scientific or academic credentials of the interlocutor so long as they seemed sincere and effective. One listener told Sherry Turkle in the 1970s that 'Soleil does an honest astrology, which I prefer to pseudo-psychoanalysis'.[41]

This last comment was a reference to Ménie Grégoire (1919–2014), a journalist and writer whose show *Allô Ménie* ran on RTL (which broadcast only in the northern half of France) from 1967 to 1981.[42] On the programme, which went out daily from 3.00 p.m. to 3.30 p.m., Grégoire responded to listeners' personal problems and dilemmas. Potential participants sent in letters which were screened by the production team, and those selected would then speak to Grégoire (who was not told their content in advance) by phone during the broadcast. In the show's peak years (1968–78), Grégoire's daily listenership was in the region of 1.3 million people, representing 40 per cent of the national radio audience for its time slot. Researching French public perceptions of psychoanalysis in the mid-1970s, Turkle found that 'everyone had an opinion on Ménie Grégoire'.[43] In 1973, Grégoire launched a second show, *Responsabilité sexuelle*, which focused on sexual problems. On this programme Grégoire was always joined by a male expert, usually a psychoanalyst, sexologist or priest. *Responsabilité sexuelle* was notable for the frankness with which Grégoire discussed sexual issues, such as inability to reach orgasm, using a directness of vocabulary not previously employed on air.[44]

Contemporaries described Grégoire's broadcasts as occupying a space in between the confessional and the analyst's couch. Though not a psychoanalyst, Grégoire had spent some ten years in analysis with René Laforgue – Dolto's analyst – and regularly used psychoanalytic terminology in her programmes.[45] She tried to create a close bond between herself and her audience, empathising and sharing in her correspondents' distress. She referred to her audience as a 'community of hearts', to the programme as a kind of 'collective psychoanalysis' and to herself as 'the confidante'.[46] Turkle argued that Grégoire's goal was to 'educate [her listeners] into a new way of talking about their problems'.[47] Over time, the letters Grégoire received became more detailed and emotionally revealing, as listeners responded to her expectations and placed trust in her 'community of hearts'.[48]

Grégoire's views on gender roles, sexuality and the family were similar to Dolto's, and drawn from similar sources. Grégoire sometimes expressed them forcefully, most notably in a famous debate held at the Salle Pleyel in Paris on 10 March 1971 and broadcast live on RTL, under the rubric 'homosexuality, this painful problem'. The panel of respondents included a priest, a psychoanalyst and André Baudry, director of the homosexual rights group Arcadie. During the debate, Grégoire argued that 'there is a norm for life, and there is a negation of life or of the laws of life in homosexuality … you know that happy women are those who've met men who have satisfied them'.[49] She was supported by the psychoanalyst and priest, who concurred that homosexuality was both psychogenetic and a (curable) form of suffering. This discourse was strongly disputed by homosexual rights activists who attended the debate, including Christine Delphy, Guy Hocquenghem and Pierre Hahn, who stressed that homosexuals were not 'suffering', or, if so, only because of societal repression. The activists eventually stormed the stage with cries of '*liberté!*', at which point RTL cut the live feed. The Salle Pleyel event has come to be seen as a foundational moment in the history of the French homosexual rights movement.[50] John Mowitt's account emphasises the radiophonic aspect: the protesters' interruption of the transmission ruptured Grégoire's illusion of having created a tolerant, supportive, inclusive community, making her prejudices explicit. By contesting Grégoire's control of her media platform, they challenged implicitly accepted notions of what could and could not be said on radio.[51] By directly confronting Grégoire's familialist, Laforguian discourse, they also demonstrated the divergence between radical (sexual) politics and one version – Dolto's version – of psychoanalysis.

In Dolto's theorising, homosexuality was a psychical structure that could be provoked during early childhood by parental attitudes. She stated in 1978 that

> There's nothing physiological about homosexuality. It's a psychological structure. And certain children are led into this psychological structure when they're young by the hostile attitude of their father towards their feminine side (for boys) or to their masculinity (for girls).[52]

Despite this assertion that homosexuality did not have a physiological cause, Dolto did concede that it was possible to be 'truly homosexual ... [where it's] not possible to behave differently'. She did not think that this was the case for many people, and also thought that 'in certain cases', homosexuality was 'treatable ... by psychoanalysis'. Often, a child 'who seems to be becoming homosexual' could be 'brought back' to heterosexuality by emphasising the unhappy, childless future that awaited homosexuals – 'in telling them that being homosexual is an unhappy state, because a homosexual can't have descendants as their sexuality is not oriented towards the other sex'.[53]

If children could be influenced towards either heterosexuality or homosexuality by their social environment, and if the former was preferable (as Dolto certainly believed), then it followed that the environment should be watched for influences that might encourage an undesirable outcome. In 1972, Dolto launched an attack on the Franco-American children's publishing company Harlin Quist, in an interview in *L'Express* under the headline 'Littérature enfantine, attention danger' ('Children's literature: danger signs'). She objected in particular to illustrations by Nicole Claveloux in an American children's book – Richard Hughes's *Gertrude and the Mermaid* (1971) – that had recently been translated into French.[54] The book tells the story of a wooden doll who, feeling ignored by her owner, goes exploring and befriends a mermaid. Claveloux's somewhat psychedelic illustrations represented the characters as disembodied, floating in a surreal landscape. Dolto described the images as 'frankly dangerous, [because they] express the fantasies of infantile oral and anal sexuality':

> the bodies of the characters are non-existent. Only the legs, hands and faces are drawn ... the trees are mineralised, the animals vegetalised, the men can be one or the other interchangeably. Nothing is more harmful for a child than this confusion of realms. It's important that a man should be a man, that a tree should be a tree.

Though the images might appear inoffensive to adult eyes, 'children find something different in them: an echo of the chaotic and terrifying world that populates their nightmares'. Dolto accused the publishers of using the book to revolutionary ends: 'it's perhaps an effective method of attacking a society which one contests, by targeting its descendants' (*d'attaquer dans sa descendance une société qu'on conteste*).[55]

Dolto's criticisms were all the more devastating in this case because her opinion had been directly sought by the publishers, François Ruy-Vidal and Harlin Quist. Ruy-Vidal, who was interested in psychoanalysis, had thought that by using innovative, polysemic, psychoanalytically informed imagery he could 'de-banalise' children's literature – 'give it a poetic and psychological function capable of underpinning profound pedagogical actions'.[56] Dolto's very public denunciation, which affected sales of the publisher's entire catalogue in the 1972 Christmas season, was thus particularly humiliating, and left a lasting mark. In a 2003 letter to the editors of Dolto's correspondence, Ruy-Vidal refused permission for his exchanges with Dolto to be published, stating that her intervention had an immediate and sustained negative impact on his career. In the short term, Quist had forced Ruy-Vidal out of the company, accusing him of ruining its reputation. In the longer term, 'a sort of rumour became established according to which, since the article was titled "Attention danger!" I was dangerous and all my books were too'.[57]

Why did Dolto make such devastating criticisms of a book which – she later admitted – she hadn't even read?[58] She had long believed in the power of images to cause negative effects on children's developing psyches: in a 1952 talk for the École des Parents, she had argued that watching films (any films) caused nightmares, and that children under nine shouldn't be allowed to go to the cinema.[59] But Dolto's insinuations that the book was designed to attack society's descendants by sowing gender confusion among children show that the main factor was surely her concern to eliminate any cultural influences that might (according to her assumptions about children's psychological development) undermine conventional gender identities. The rumours that were circulating about Ruy-Vidal and Quist being in a homosexual relationship would hardly have reassured her on this point. The episode shows just how strongly Dolto believed in the necessity of policing conventional norms around gender and sexuality, for Ruy-Vidal's aim to give children's literature an added 'poetic and psychological function' was something that she would, had her homophobia not got in the way, have enthusiastically welcomed.

Educational utopias

In the 1960s and 1970s, the French education system experienced major changes. Demographic growth necessitated the proliferation of new large schools, and changing conceptions of adolescence created demands for teenagers to spend longer in formal education.[60] Many teachers, parents and pupils believed – especially after May 1968 – that state schools had become too rigid and authoritarian, prioritising rote learning and *dictées* to the detriment of a holistic education of mind and body.[61] A 1969 circular from the Ministry of Education explained that 'education can no longer be limited to instruction through the acquisition of knowledge'.[62] New timetables stipulated six hours of physical activity per week and a further six hours for *activités d'éveil* – i.e. discovery-based learning in history, geography, art and music.[63] *Lycées* abandoned dress codes and punishment regimes, and tolerated students smoking, wearing makeup and using informal pronouns with teachers.

Governments of the 1970s halted this liberalising trend. Arguing that pedagogical innovation had gone too far, René Haby, Education Minister from 1974 to 1978, withdrew support for innovative teacher training programmes and reduced the ability of parents and pupils to influence school management. Haby's 1975 reform created a standardised secondary system for all eleven- to sixteen-year-olds, deferring the age at which pupils were streamed by ability.[64] This prompted an uptick of interest in private schools, which frequently espoused child-centred, active-learning pedagogies to a greater extent than state schools.[65] A subsequent 1984 proposal to integrate private schools fully into the state system provoked large public protests, not only from religious conservatives worried about the implications for religious education but also from a wider public concerned that the reform would limit academic freedom and end parents' ability to exercise choice over their children's schooling.

This was the background to the ideas on education that Dolto developed in the later part of her career, which she set out in her 1985 book *La Cause des enfants*. Dolto argued that, despite the spread of more liberal approaches to pedagogy and a more relaxed school etiquette, the standardised system had created 'sheep pens' in which children's creativity was stifled: 'a programme in which all the children have to be homogeneous, all at the same level of knowledge, is absolutely inhumane … We are eliminating talent, inspiration, desire, because we have sought to bring this whole mass into a system.'[66] She criticised the full timetables and extensive homework demanded by state *lycées*, contrasting them unfavourably with the long stretches of time left free for intellectual exploration during her own experience of private and home-schooling.[67] The modern *lycée* 'appears to have become the most boring place in existence … it's not even a day-hospital [used for psychiatric patients] … it's more like a day-prison'.[68] The whole Éducation Nationale edifice, 'inherited from Jules Ferry, should be closed down and something different rebuilt'.[69]

Dolto's suggestion, which she described as utopian, was that schools be reconceived as youth centres ('*Maisons des jeunes*'), with the roles of youth club and holiday camp added to their educational function. In her idealised scheme, each school day would end at 4.00 p.m., when a team of activity leaders would arrive to manage the evening's entertainment and supervise homework. This team would be tasked with holistic educational functions that the existing system supposedly neglected: 'the formation of character, physical skills, coordination and manual dexterity, initiation, memory, and sensory control'.[70] Children would have the right to sleep in schools (which would provide appropriate facilities) as and when they wished.[71] Academic education would no longer follow a standard pattern, instead becoming personalised, '*à la carte*', allowing children to begin studying subjects at different ages according to their desires and abilities.[72] Examination centres would conduct assessments on demand, as and when pupils felt they had reached the appropriate level. Class attendance would be optional. Teaching recruitment would be widened to include industry experts without formal teaching qualifications. The education ministry would be folded into a larger 'Ministry of Youth and Sport', 'tasked with shaping bodies and minds'.[73]

In 1975, Dolto was offered an opportunity to implement some of her ideas on a small scale, when three young educationists, Fabienne d'Ortoli, Michel Amram and Pascal Lemaître, asked her advice on a project for a new private boarding school, at La Neuville-du-Bosc in Normandy. D'Ortoli, Amram and Lemaître were interested in the pedagogy of Célestin Freinet and the impact of the educational environment. They intended to 'create a place where children and adults would live, and each work according to their level – and not necessarily at traditional subjects'.[74] They contacted Dolto on the recommendation of another advisor to the scheme, the pedagogue Fernand Oury, Félix Guattari's former *lycée* teacher, who knew Dolto through the radical psychiatry circles (including his brother Jean) described in Chapter 5. Oury believed that the state school system had become 'school-as-barracks' (*l'école caserne*) – a phrase Dolto borrowed – in which 'the instructor is above all the children's caretaker or watchman [*gardien*]'.[75] La Neuville, by contrast, was envisaged as a holistic space for children to develop. Its founders (who had little to no teaching experience) told Dolto that 'even the word "school" disturbs us, seems reductive to us ... so we don't use it. We want to do the cooking ourselves, go to the market with the children, get them to participate in all sorts of activities at the same time ... not to artificially separate sports, games, performance, and lessons as if these were all different things.'[76] Dolto was enthused by their overall approach, especially their emphasis on making students responsible for their own learning and activities, their stress on extra-curricular activities, and by the school's rural location – telling the founders that 'the countryside is very important for an educational project', allowing for easy contact with nature and space to explore.[77] In addition, La Neuville could become a refuge for children with mental health problems and learning disabilities who did not thrive in mainstream schools. D'Ortoli, Amram and Lemaître emerged from their initial discussions with Dolto with a reinforced conviction that they were on the right path – that 'the project was possible, viable ... because our utopian vision was responding to a need, to a necessity'. Their encounter with Dolto transformed the project from 'a sketch' into 'a work in progress' (*chantier*).[78] Once La Neuville was up and running, Dolto became a significant patron, referring several of her child patients there and using her contacts and reputation to support the school, including by helping with publicity for fundraising and recruitment. The school remains in existence in 2021, with around 40 children attending.

Dolto was probably correct to describe her ideas on education as 'utopian', in that they would have been impractical to implement on a national scale. They stood the best chance of being enacted in small, well-funded private schools like La Neuville, where there was no need to (in Dolto's words) 'bring in this whole mass'.[79] That phrase betrayed a current of elitism in her thinking, an apparent echo of her upper-class family's interwar disdain for universalist republican institutions. Dolto's educational vision of the 1970s and 1980s indeed aligned significantly with the educational principles that Pétain articulated in August 1940:

> At the base of our educational system was a profound illusion: the belief that academic instruction suffices to form the heart and forge the character … The French school of tomorrow will teach with regard to the human person, family, society, nation [*patrie*] … a much bigger place will be given to manual work, the educative value of which too often goes unrecognised.[80]

Dolto expressed enthusiasm for such ideas at the time, as shown in Chapter 3. While her published vision in *La Cause des enfants* avoided Vichy's overtly national-racial aspects, her private correspondence hinted at a concern for France's national and ethnic future if education were not reformed. In one 1970 letter she wrote of a 'sort of generalized septicaemia of the French, who appear like an organism afflicted with an obsessive neurosis'. This affliction she attributed to 'French institutions [which] have created petty and lazy minds. I don't see how our race [*ethnie*], with its specific values, will be able to emerge from this without some profound upheavals.'[81] A kind of national revolution was still required, with education at the forefront.

Lorsque l'enfant paraît

A further result of the post-1968 educational reforms was that renewed attention was paid to nursery and primary schooling. Jacques Chirac's 1974 government appointed Annie Lesur, a doctor, to the newly created post of secretary of state for pre-school education. Some 84 per cent of French children aged between two and four attended *écoles maternelles* (nursery schools) by the early 1970s, with the state aiming to enrol three million pupils by 1975 and recruit an additional 30,000 teachers.[82] Comprehensive provision of *écoles maternelles*, it was hoped, would be an important tool for reducing educational inequalities. To redress geographical imbalances in the meantime, the government promoted the use of television and radio programmes to supplement formal nursery education in more remote areas of France.

This context helps to explain the decision in 1976 by Pierre Wiehn, director of France Inter from 1975 to 1981, and his programmes advisor Jean Chouquet, to invite Dolto to participate in a new series of broadcasts on the psychology and parenting of small children. Dolto had already received an official seal of approval from the education ministry in 1973, when it circulated to all school directors the text of an interview on sex education that she had given to a parenting magazine.[83] Dolto shared the government's aim to use the programme to help people in rural areas, hoping that it would fill 'the very large gap between people in cities, where there are very varied and specialised educational facilities, and those who live in the country ... so that everyone feels supported'.[84] Undertaking the new programme was a significant moment in Dolto's career. Her ideas were now to be distributed via the authority of the state broadcaster, still to some extent 'the voice of France', with the explicit aim of ensuring some degree of universal national access to her parenting and pedagogical expertise.

Lorsque l'enfant paraît differed in important respects from Dolto's 1968–69 '*consultations sur les ondes*' on Europe 1. Unlike in the earlier show, Dolto would not take phone calls, but only respond to letters. This fitted with the aim of maximising access, since universal access to telephones could not be assumed. Dolto argued that the very act of writing a letter was therapeutically beneficial, something that would in itself help people to solve their problems. It was perhaps also in part a defensive measure: the peremptory nature of Dolto's phone conversations on Europe 1 had been criticised by the EdP and the Ordre des Médecins, which forbade her to publish the *S.O.S. Psychanalyste!* transcripts under her own name.[85] The new format gave Dolto more control. She could pre-select the themes for discussion and the specific letters to which she would respond. She hired her daughter and future executor Catherine (b. 1946), a doctor and psychotherapist, to assist in the task of narrowing down the 100–150 letters received in a typical week to the handful discussed in each broadcast. The selected correspondents were sent a letter informing them in advance of the day on which their question would be aired.

Dolto's remarks were broadcast daily at 3.00 p.m. and lasted fifteen minutes.[86] This slot, the same one used by Ménie Grégoire, targeted mothers by being timed to fit between the end of lunch and the return of children from school. On air, Dolto was accompanied by Jacques Pradel (b. 1947), the host of the daily afternoon show *Le Temps de vivre* within which Dolto's short broadcast was incorporated. *Le Temps de vivre* was intended as 'a calm series peppered with interviews with popular educators' – it had regular sections on history and classical music, but few female voices.[87] Dolto's segments were not broadcast live. Instead, Pradel went to Dolto's apartment on Rue Saint-Jacques once a week to record a series of programmes. Like Grégoire on *Responsabilité sexuelle*, Dolto thought it important to have a male voice alongside hers, to represent the idea of a father and a mother: 'I don't want the responses to come from one authority. Raising a child is a two-person job' (*ça se fait à deux*).[88] Pradel, a recent recruit to the station, was Dolto's junior by forty years; he had a young child.

In this show, Dolto's patriarchal vision of the family and of gender roles came to the fore somewhat less than in her previous broadcasts. Dolto wanted *Lorsque l'enfant paraît* to at least appear to be driven by listeners' concerns, and mostly refrained from doctrinaire pronouncements or the appearance of moral judgement. A clear strength of the programme was the sincerity and seriousness with which Dolto treated the correspondents, making a readily apparent effort to engage empathetically and imaginatively with their problems and emotions. A large proportion of the letters not discussed on air later received a written reply. 'I think that the public could feel our commitment', her daughter Catherine later commented.[89] The letters selected were chosen so as to be emblematic of, or an entry point into, common parenting issues – a typical early example was how to approach leaving a young child at nursery for the first time – but also because they could illustrate how Dolto's parenting principles could be applied in practice.[90] For example, Dolto advised families in which the father was frequently absent because of work commitments to ensure his continued symbolic presence in the home by speaking of him often, writing letters and making a minor celebration of each return.[91] Part of Dolto's appeal was that she had precise suggestions to hand for every difficult situation: what food to prepare for a child who would not eat, how to deal with an older child's jealousy at the birth of a sibling, how to explain divorce or parental separation. That these suggestions would not have been applicable to all cases was not the point: her prescriptions indicated the kinds of practical outcomes her line of thinking could have, and encouraged parents to devise their own solutions in the same spirit.

The archive of letters sent to the show – around 6,000 were received over two years – makes it clear that, for many listeners, Dolto was a revelation. 'I appreciate in particular your good sense, the strength of your love of children', wrote one woman from Aix.[92] 'I'm really struck by the clarity and simplicity of the things you say!' wrote a mother of two from Poitou-Charentes.[93] Other letters praised Dolto's 'warmth', 'understanding' and 'vast intelligence covering all these key issues'.[94] Some young children also liked the show: one amused mother wrote in to share her four-year-old's pronouncement that 'grandma must listen to Dolto to learn how to speak to children'.[95] In the first months, the letters mostly came from mothers, and raised direct questions of child-rearing such as toilet training, sibling rivalry, breastfeeding or how to broach the subjects of sex and death. Over time, the number of letters received per week rose, as did their average length. Doctors, teachers, nurses, civil servants and other professionals wrote offering their perspectives. Dolto received hundreds of requests: students seeking help with their essays; parents wanting suggestions of books to read or psychotherapists to consult; organisations hoping she might attend their conferences.

Increasing numbers of letters also began to arrive from adolescents and young adults regarding their own existential problems, seeing Dolto as someone who would understand their issue and be able to help. Some of these letters described the more commonplace sufferings of adolescence, such as loneliness, parental incomprehension or yearning for love. 'I can no longer work at college, I don't care about the Future, I think only of being Loved, loved truly and profoundly', wrote one correspondent in May 1977.[96] Others raise more serious problems, such as eating disorders or unwanted pregnancies. 'I think you are the only person who could help me', wrote one seventeen-year-old girl suffering from severe depression and alcoholism. 'Talking to friends does nothing and it is very difficult to ask people for such profound assistance.'[97] These correspondents were not necessarily keen to have their case discussed on air, with many hoping instead for a written response. For some the act of writing was in itself enough: 'I'm not expecting you to respond … but I had to confide my suffering [*chagrin*] to someone, and my parents and my teachers are too stupid and foolish', wrote one eighteen-year-old.[98] Social distress was a recurrent theme in these letters: their authors wrote to Dolto because they felt ill at ease in the world, had no one to confide in or were having difficulty overcoming a traumatic experience. A fifteen-year-old girl wrote about having been raped the previous year; her current problem, however, was that her parents, shaken by having been unable to protect her, were now no longer willing to let her out of the house. 'They shout at me and make me work harder than my brothers and sisters. I almost have the impression that they no longer love me.'[99] One sixteen-year-old described the health problems he had suffered throughout his childhood, as a result of which he now appeared younger and more feminine than his male classmates, who bullied him ceaselessly. 'For the last seven years my life has been a nightmare … am I a social misfit [*un inadapté*], or have I been traumatised by the disease that's blighted me?' he asked.[100] There were enough of these kinds of letters that Dolto set aside one programme per week, on Wednesdays, to respond to some of them on air, and thereafter began referring to them as 'Wednesday letters'.[101]

Letters from writers over eighteen were generally not discussed on air if they concerned personal problems. Dolto often responded to these in writing, but apparently not systematically, and in only some of the cases where the surviving archive material suggests that she responded is her answer preserved. These letters are often among the most interesting in terms of demonstrating how personal distress overlapped with wider social and political attitudes. For example, a twenty-five-year-old man from Rennes, unemployed and an alcoholic, wrote of his difficult childhood in a rural family and his mother's early death from lung cancer. But above all, 'I am gay, a homo [*pédé*] and I think it's that that's made me ill and a drunkard […] It's not easy being a homo in Rennes […] I drink in order to be able to tell guys that I like them and that I want them.'[102] Another striking letter came from a thirty-eight-year-old man from the Auvergne, who wrote in asking Dolto to help clarify 'a very obscure point for me regarding my own behaviour':

> In 1974, my wife looked after a baby for a few months on behalf of social services; this child is of Arab race [*de race arabe*] … this baby

> awakened some very strange feelings and reactions in me. It sometimes happened that I rejected him with all my strength, found myself thinking that he smelled bad, or was even tempted to mistreat him.[103]

Given Dolto's own difficulties in keeping pace with changing social attitudes towards questions of race and homosexuality (discussed further in the Afterword), she was hardly the ideal interlocutor for such questions – and indeed there is no evidence in the archive that she responded to either of these letters. The fact that the writers chose to write to her indicates, as much as anything, the paucity of other options for finding advice in the 1970s. As many of Dolto's correspondents made clear to her, they felt they had nowhere else to turn.

Overall, three-quarters of the letter-writers were female, and an even higher proportion of those who wrote in with a parenting dilemma were women – most men who wrote did so in a professional capacity or from intellectual interest rather than as fathers. Letters arrived from all parts of France and sometimes beyond – around 7 per cent came from abroad, mostly Germany, Belgium and Switzerland. The numbers from each French region were mostly in proportion to their populations, but with some exceptions. Wealthier regions such as those around Paris and Lyon, the Pays de la Loire, Midi-Pyrénées and Auvergne were over-represented; disproportionately few letters came from poorer regions such as Lorraine, Burgundy, Picardy and Languedoc. This pattern was repeated in letters from Paris: most correspondents lived in the wealthy western districts, not the working-class areas of the north and east.

The concept of childhood determinism pervades much of the correspondence from parents.[104] Many accepted the assumption that by making parenting mistakes they could permanently traumatise their offspring, and wrote for advice either on avoiding this fate or on repairing the already-inflicted damage. Mothers enquired about the potential long-term psychological repercussions of a difficult weaning, or allowing children to sleep in the parental bedroom, and frequently raised concerns about sex education.[105] A number of parents, perhaps prompted by Dolto's conviction on this point, worried that their children might have suffered significant traumas before they had even been born.[106] The very first letter the show ever received asked whether children who were obliged to repeat a year of school 'would be forever scarred' by the experience, and whether the parents might be to blame.[107] Another mother blamed her liberal parenting style for her child's exclusion from school.[108] There was also a striking example of a mother blaming herself for her son's autism diagnosis:

> One day [when he was two] he soiled himself [*il n'avait pas été propre*] and received a spank from me, saying mummy didn't love him at all ... [after] that his toilet habits were exemplary ... [but] maybe that was one of the causes of his great backwardness! ... I've always worked, and our youngest has been raised in an atmosphere of nervousness, tiredness and anxiety! I think that this child has suffered 'on my account' from a lack of tenderness, and because of this has withdrawn into himself. I regret it with all my heart.[109]

Dolto responded by private letter, saying that the mother should not blame herself because 'you couldn't have done otherwise – I think that at each moment you did what you could'. She did not, however, challenge the mother's explanation of the origin of her son's condition, and encouraged her to 'attempt once again a psychoanalytic psychotherapy'.[110]

This letter was not broached on air. Nor were those letters – a small but significant proportion – that contested Dolto's views. The objections fell into a few different categories. Social conservatives took issue with Dolto's liberal line on adolescent sexuality and masturbation, accusing her of disrespecting 'morality' and 'honour' or expressing disappointment that Dolto did not promote official Catholic doctrine.[111] Some writers attacked Dolto's fundamental assumptions on childhood determinism, such as the Parisian single mother who wrote that '[according to you] whatever I [now] do, as of today, the psychosexual development of my son is equally compromised, correct? "All the cards have been played" [*tout est joué*]. I can't think of anything more discouraging, less inspiring, less "positive" than this aspect of psychoanalysis.'[112] Several women criticised Dolto's view of gender roles and gendered parenting. 'Why must the little boy copy what his father does, why from a certain age must he have especially close relationships with men, and why must he reject, ignore and disdain women? Why is a woman saying this?', wrote an engineering student in 1977.[113] A woman from Lille accused Dolto of perpetuating outdated ideas: 'You have a tendency to emphasise the boy's strength, so as to make him a man, and to return the girl to her mother to develop her femininity, as was taught 20–30 years ago.'[114] A Lyon mother disparaged Dolto's preference for large families: 'You seem, in effect, to be an evangelist for large families ... I find this particularly inappropriate for our era ... an only child is capable of having sufficient social relations!'[115]

Dolto's views on education also provoked challenges. A primary school head in Champagne thought that Dolto's presentation of public-sector schools as monolithic and authoritarian was a straw man: 'you must know that traditional classes where children are fixed to their benches no longer exist ... children today are happy: they move, are active, express themselves'.[116] Other teachers were suspicious of Dolto's motives in criticising the republican education system: 'who is hiding [behind you], who are you, what are your qualities, what university degrees qualify you to criticise and make solemn appeals on the airwaves to those "responsible" for education?', asked one.[117] Another contested Dolto's suggestion that teachers should see themselves at the service of parents, rather than the state: 'it would be serious if parents came to believe that teachers were their employees ... You would be depriving the civil community of its true political dimension.'[118] These teachers, not unreasonably, suspected that Dolto's views on education were linked to the politics of educational provision – that Dolto was using her psychoanalytic prestige and media platform to mount a surreptitious attack on the entire public service ethos of republican education.

These examples demonstrate that Dolto's listeners engaged critically with her pronouncements and often did not take them on trust. In particular, the objection that Dolto was perpetuating outdated stereotypes around gender, education and family roles seems to have become more common as the months progressed. Nonetheless, such criticism remained rare in the overall correspondence – much less common than praise for Dolto's ideas as progressive and enlightened. Overall, the correspondence shows that for thousands of people, Dolto's broadcast was a site of intense engagement. It was variously a source of knowledge and counsel, solace, consolation – and contestation. Letter-writers took the opportunity to share problems, pour out emotions and debate ideas. The intensity of the correspondence was communicated on air, thanks to Pradel's habit of reading out sections of the letters, but little of the contestation that emerges from the archive was broadcast. This seems in fact to have been a reason why, despite its enormous popularity, *Lorsque l'enfant paraît* ceased to air in 1978. Producers at France Inter raised objections to Catherine Dolto's methods of selecting letters for broadcast, sensing that the selections were not a representative cross-section but were being chosen to fit certain agendas – but Dolto refused to continue without her daughter, fearing that she would thereby lose the ability to control the content. 'She wanted someone very close to her at her side to make sure that questions that didn't suit her weren't chosen', recalled Pradel in 2013.[119] As with *Le Cas Dominique*, Dolto needed to be able to control the narrative, especially if there was a risk that she might be publicly challenged on positions that increasing numbers of people felt to be outdated or offensive.

The Maison Verte

Following the show's cessation Dolto threw her energies into a new venture. The MV was conceived as a new kind of psychoanalytically informed institution: a space for children to play and spend time, staffed by medical, psychoanalytic and educational professionals. In planning from 1975–76, the project came to fruition in 1979, assisted by public funds and exploiting the prestige Dolto had acquired on France Inter. It was developed by a working group of practitioners at the CMPP at Étienne Marcel in central Paris, who initially wanted to explore new ways to communicate the CMPP's approach to medical professionals and the general public.[120] The working group included Pierre Benoit, Colette Langignon and Bernard This – paediatricians and psychoanalysts trained by Dolto and sharing her theoretical orientation. The project that emerged was a children's centre, but one with a less explicitly medical purpose than the CMPPs. Rather, Dolto's group proposed to create a centre for young children and their parents or carers to attend, where children could play and meet others without being aware of any medical or psychotherapeutic oversight. That oversight would still be present, in the form of trained staff, but these professionals would intervene only occasionally, and would have no formal responsibility for the children's care.

In developing this project, Dolto and her group had specific medical, ideological and political goals in mind. They imagined the MV not just as somewhere new for children to go, but as a response to parenting needs and anxieties that (they felt) were not being met by the existing provision of crèches, daycare centres and *écoles maternelles*. Their solution was to create a new type of institution, which eventually became known by the term Lieux d'Accueil Enfants-Parents (LAEPs – Parent and Child Welcome Spaces), and which remain an important feature of the French state's provision for young children today. The MV was not quite the first LAEP: a somewhat similar initiative, without the psychoanalytic aspect, had been set up by the Institut de Recherche Appliqué pour l'Enfant et pour le Couple (Institute of Applied Research for the Child and for the Couple) in Paris in 1976.[121] But the MV and its subsequent imitator institutions – sometimes referred to as 'les structures Dolto' – became the model for hundreds of LAEPs nationwide. As the MV's intellectual driving force and media figurehead, Dolto was, and remains, closely associated with LAEPs in general. The French state's 2014 definition of LAEPs bore considerable resemblance to the concept for original MV as defined in 1977 by Dolto, Benoît, Langignon and This:

> A place of meeting and welcome for all children, a space that is neither medical, nor pedagogical, nor psychotherapeutic, but essentially attractive, lively ... an attractive place of socialisation and stimulation for children from 0 to 3 years old, but also a place of welcome, listening and interaction for parents and adults.
>
> *(Dolto et al., 1977)*[122]

> A place which welcomes, informally and without pre-registration, young children (0–5 years old) accompanied by a responsible adult, for a limited time ... The staff provide a convivial space for play and interaction ... a space to talk [and] meet with a view to providing support to the parental function, separate from any therapeutic aims.
>
> *(Caisse nationale des allocations familiales, 2014)*[123]

The idea was thus for the MV to be mainly a site for play and socialisation, brightly coloured and filled with toys and play areas. What neither of these definitions acknowledge, however, is the centrality of psychoanalysis to these institutions. Although it was officially 'neither medical, nor pedagogic, nor psychotherapeutic', the MV's creators also understood it as a site of early intervention and identification of cases suitable for medico-psychological treatment, as their 1977 project document made clear:

> Experience shows that it is not prudent to wait for parents to bring their children for consultations at CMPPs. By the time that personality problems or somatic troubles have appeared, or that problems at school have developed, it's often too late. Precious time has been lost. It would be preferable to intervene at the first flare-ups of jealousy, or when the child's first separation anxieties appear.[124]

From the perspective of Dolto and her colleagues, a drawback of the CMPP model was that children were only referred there once their psychological problems were relatively advanced and a parent or teacher had identified a need for expert intervention. Ordinary parents were unlikely to consult a psychoanalyst or CMPP when their child was in the early stages of a neurosis, either because they did not have the ability to recognise the warning signs, or – like Turkle's working-class interviewees described in Chapter 4 – did not have a great deal of trust in the system. Therefore, incipient psychological problems – or as Dolto termed them, 'micro-neuroses' – could never be nipped in the bud.[125] Psychoanalysts had no means of staging early interventions. The CMPPs were merely 're-education' centres.[126]

The great hope for the MV was thus that it would be a preventative institution. Psychoanalysts would be placed in regular contact with children in a relaxed setting designed for play, where they could observe children's behaviour without needing to open a case file. They would get access to a much wider section of the child population than that which they encountered in their clinics, and be able to identify and rectify psychological issues before they became fully fledged neuroses or psychoses. Psychoanalysts' full power to improve the psychological health of the nation would only be realised if they were able to insert themselves more often into children's daily lives:

> We thought that in order to palliate problems before they worsen, we needed a place where parents would come with their child without a requirement to highlight any particular symptom.
>
> In order to do this, it makes sense to put in place an organic structure which allows us to meet with parents or childminders, as part of their social life: they need to be helped in the course of the daily difficulties they have with their children.[127]

While the MV announced itself as a 'non-medical' and 'non-psychological' institution, this was only true in the sense that no formal consultations took place there. A central intention of the project was, in fact, to advance the psychoanalytic education of parents and guardians of children, to introduce more psychoanalytic thinking into everyday parenting and to build psychoanalytic oversight seamlessly into children's everyday experience such that parents barely noticed its presence. In creating this scheme, Dolto and her group literally took psychoanalysts 'beyond the couch', to borrow Michal Shapira's term – embedding them in places that parents would want to attend for other reasons, rather than sitting in their consulting rooms waiting for clinical referrals.

Dolto's views, especially those on infant determinism and on trauma and its unconscious transmission from a very early age, were at the heart of the project. The MV would aim to prevent 'the harmfulness of pre- and postnatal traumas, which can in most cases be avoided'.[128] Parents could, for example, be taught the importance of not toilet training their children too soon.[129] The MV would be a place where people could put words and meanings to symptoms: instead of being given medication, they would be encouraged to 'recognise the specific human dimension of the speaking-beings [*parlêtres*] that we are'.[130] The staff would treat the children as the most important people present, addressing the children directly and recording only the (first) name of the child who attended, not the parent. The centre would thereby 'help with separation from the parents', preventing 'fusional' mother-child relationships by occupying 'the place of a third party' – that is, performing a 'paternal function'.[131] Dolto's belief in the reality of antenatal psychological traumas, and their potential to occur from the very moment of conception, implied that the centres should also try to attract pregnant women, and from as early as possible in their pregnancy.[132]

Dolto contended that in the long run, there would be major public health benefits, and thus major cost savings for the state, from such interventions. The 1977 proposal document argued that 'the *effects of the unconscious* constantly make themselves felt in the body' and that 'the quality of parent-child relationships is essential for the future of our country'.[133] Having formed an 'Association Lieu de Petite Enfance et de Parentalité' ('Association for a Space for Small Children and Parenthood') to manage the project, the working group set about applying for public funding on this basis. The association put its case to Bertrand Fragonard, an official working for Health Minister Simone Veil, who approved a grant of 250,000 francs in October 1978 with a further 250,000 to follow.[134] This allowed the MV to open on 6 January 1979, at Place St Charles in the fifteenth arrondissement of Paris.

According to the association's records, in its first year, 455 separate families attended the centre, and visited on average eight times each.[135] By 1985 the number of visits had doubled, and the centre had also had 677 visits from pregnant women.[136] Seventy-three per cent of the 1979 attendees lived in the fifteenth arrondissement. Eighty-three per cent of the parents/guardians attending were mothers and only 12 per cent fathers, though the latter figure was increasing: fathers appeared more likely to attend on subsequent, rather than initial, visits. Of the children who came, 87 per cent were aged between six months and four years – in other words, the centre mostly catered to the birth to three years age group that was too young for *écoles maternelles*. Initially open only in the mornings, it ultimately settled on a daily 2.00 p.m. to 7.00 p.m. timetable (plus two hours on Saturday mornings). Fifty-one per cent of children attending stayed between one and two hours, 20 per cent under an hour and 29 per cent over two hours.

As for the staff, half consisted of the 'animation' team, which welcomed the children and led activities. The other half consisted of psychoanalysts, divided equally between those who were and were not medically qualified (Dolto herself accounting for a large proportion of the hours contributed by the former group). The rota was constructed such that at any one time there would be at least one activity leader and one psychoanalyst present. As Dolto wrote in 1979, the idea was that while the activity leaders were organising games and running group activities, the psychoanalyst 'is there and doesn't do anything but be there' – but simply by being there, 'drinks in the anxiety of these mothers, who from one day to the next after they've given birth no longer interest anyone'.[137] By acting as a sponge to soak up maternal anxiety, the psychoanalysts would prevent its pathogenic transmission to the children.

Once Dolto's group had paved the way and persuaded the French state of the merits of funding the scheme, LAEPs on the MV model began to appear nationwide in the 1980s, supported by local and national public funds from the Allocations Familiales, the Fonds d'Action Sociale and the Fondation de France. Dolto's hope that private sector sponsorship might ultimately suffice, thus avoiding the 'educational dogmatism and the administrative and bureaucratic sickness that oversees anything collective', was not realised.[138] However, her ambition that the centres 'should exist in every city neighbourhood and every village town hall' was substantially fulfilled.[139] The MV's success led to Dolto being invited to contribute to a 1982 Ministry of Health working group on the 'fight against inequality through prevention and family education'.[140] In 1985 the Ministry for Social Affairs and National Solidarity, launching a campaign to 'Open Up France to Children', argued in a circular that the MV 'should serve as an example and be replicated [*démultiplié*] everywhere'.[141] From the point of view of President François Mitterrand's Socialist government, the LAEPs appeared to be a promising tool for improving the lives of mothers and children from poorer areas, who lacked places they could easily take their children. This social policy angle was reflected in proposals for centres modelled on the MV, such as the Maison de la Petite Enfance in Lille-Moulins, which sought to 'lead parents from deprived areas to become aware of their young children's potential' and promised to offer 'professional and social reintegration internships' to long-term unemployed people.[142] The project for the 'La Petite Planète' centre in Pontivy, Morbihan, included a library of parenting guidance literature.[143] This was in keeping with Dolto's vision. In 1977 she had foreseen a role for the MVs as civic centres, suggesting that they might for example become a place for retired people to volunteer and thereby rediscover a sense of social purpose.[144]

The MV had another spurt of popularity in 1987, after Dolto discussed it in a lengthy interview on the popular cultural affairs television programme *Apostrophes*, and further centres on the MV model continued to appear. By 1996, a protected national fund was reserved for them in the Allocations Familiales budget, and by 2004 there were over 200 MV-affiliated institutions in France, plus thirty-one in other countries.[145] While each centre had its own character and local priorities, they were largely faithful to Dolto's original concept – including the psychoanalytic aspects. For example, according to a 1987 article, La Maisonnée in Strasbourg 'indisputably contributes to preventing children's problems ... it addresses the difficulties encountered in the early stages of life without dramatising them'.[146] According to evaluations from the 1990s, the team at La Marouette (Nantes) 'underlines the indispensable paternal function in the formation of the child', while La Petite Planète (Morbihan) sought to 'avoid the severe disturbances seen in specialised consultations … proceeding on the basis that talking can cure'.[147] Further growth saw the number of state-funded LAEPs (not all affiliated to the original MV) reach 850 by 2010, with a disproportionately large number built in urban areas and deprived neighbourhoods (*quartiers défavorisés*).[148]

Despite funding these centres and encouraging their spread, the French state collected relatively little empirical evidence as to their effectiveness. In particular, the evidence that would be needed to evaluate Dolto's claims of long-term public health benefits, such as a longitudinal study comparing families using the centres with those that did not, does not exist. Two qualitative reports on the MVs/LAEPs were, however, compiled in 1995 and 2011 – the latter commissioned by a children's association in Strasbourg and based on surveys and interviews with parents and LAEP staff.[149] This report found that the main benefit of the centres was 'socialisation'. They had become a first space for children to interact with strangers secure in the presence of a parent/guardian – 'a first approach to other children, a first contact which facilitates integration into daycare'.[150] According to one parent, the centres allowed children to 'learn the basic rules of life, socialise with people, develop their behaviours and reactions'.[151] Parents also benefited from the social contact provided by the centres. One mother stated that 'meeting other mums allowed me to feel less isolated'; 'I enjoy coming in to talk and not feel alone in the role of mum'.[152] Notably, the centres could help parents of immigrant backgrounds to feel more integrated in their local community: the centres were like a 'French language bath' helping them to feel 'more open towards life in France'.[153] The study's authors also contended, more nebulously, that the centres promoted democratic attitudes, transmitting 'an ideal of familial dialogue … this model reflects the progress of family democracy … by democratic and egalitarian values which [the centres] reference, and the respect for difference'.[154]

The LAEP staff, too, spoke of the 'richness' of their exchanges with parents and children. They were often enthused to be able to

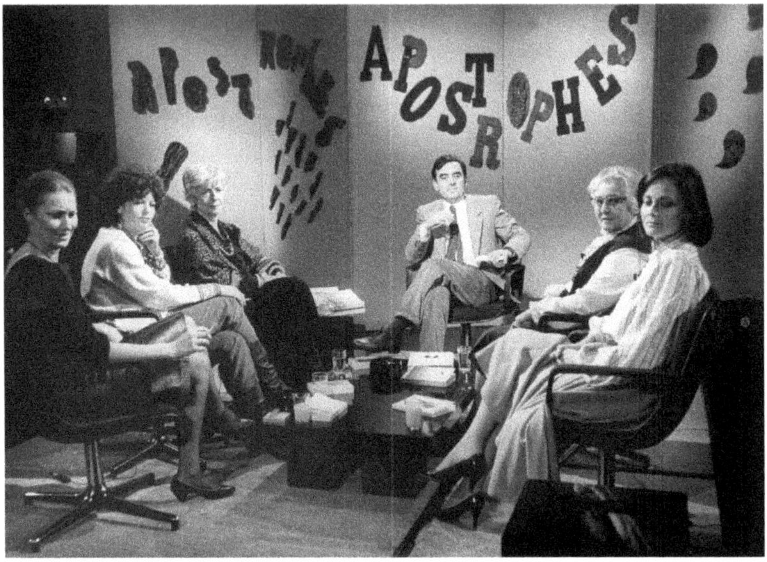

Figure 6.2 Dolto on the cultural affairs television programme *Apostrophes*, 14 January 1983

transmit Dolto's wisdom to a wider audience: 'I'm from a generation which was cradled by Dolto, as mothers we grew up with Dolto ... we're convinced by [her approach], we know it, we can do it.'[155] The centres' ability to spread psychoanalytic ideas could occasionally be glimpsed in the comments of parents, such as one mother who believed that attending an LAEP had helped to prevent a 'fusional' relationship between her and her child:

> He saw that he could be several metres away from me and live his life as a little boy, play with others while feeling secure ... I also learnt to be less attached [*fusionnelle*], as when I distanced myself [from my son], I could share the task of watching him with others.[156]

The issue of how to use the centres to disseminate psychoanalytic thinking to parents was a delicate one, however, and attempts to do so were not always successful. Sandrine Garcia, an education academic who attended MVs both as a parent and as a researcher before writing her 2011 book *Mères sous influence* (*Mothers Under Pressure*), noted a gulf between 'the uses parents made of the place and the rhetoric of preventing "embryonic relational neuroses"'.[157]

Garcia felt that the parents in the centre she attended mainly used it as a place to rest, talk or read while their children played, and that the psychoanalysts' interventions were often an unwelcome intrusion. Rather than simply observing and listening, Garcia reported, the analysts had 'deliberate strategies for approaching parents, which led, after a certain time, to advising them … they didn't simply listen to things parents said to them, they actively solicited speech from them, sometimes in a very aggressive way'. She discerned 'a paternalist social relationship between the mothers and the staff, which could lead to a clearly prescriptive tone'.[158] Some parents stated that the staff could be judgemental or make unwelcome pointed comments, for example if they felt that a child was clinging to its mother too much. Despite the concentration on *quartiers défavorisés*, Garcia found that the middle classes were overrepresented among MV users, something also observed in 1995 by Gérard Neyrand.[159] Garcia further reported that the staff dropped hints that it would be better for her child if she gave up full-time work: '"You're not part-time?" … "It's not too tiring?" The questioning had a suggestive quality.'[160]

The impact of the MV and the broader LAEP scheme is thus contested in similar ways to that of Dolto's radio work. Many parents clearly found, and find, much of value there, without necessarily accepting the full psychoanalytic rationale – while a minority dispute some of the underlying assumptions and particularly their implications for gender relations. In view of this, it seems very possible that, over time, the psychoanalytic element of the LAEPs will diminish, and indeed this may already have happened: the 2011 report indicated that compared with the 1980s, more attention was being focused on parental well-being and socialisation than on children's psychological structures, suggesting a slight move away from Dolto's initial vision.

Nonetheless, as of the early 2020s, Dolto's name and child-rearing approach remain closely associated with the scheme, which could plausibly claim to be the most extensive long-term project for taking psychoanalysis 'beyond the couch' anywhere in the world in recent decades.[161] The MV and its imitator centres built the idea of infant determinism and other psychoanalytic concepts into the institutional fabric of the French welfare state. The MV's success in this regard lay in the subtlety of the unofficial and ambiguous way in which it brought psychoanalysts and children into contact. Rather than parents having actively to seek out a relationship with an analyst, the latter were present in LAEPs by default, able to stage frequent, small-scale interventions with children and parents without being subject to the bureaucracy or accountability of a formal medical or psychotherapeutic engagement. In the apt words of the title of a (celebratory) 2013 book by two psychoanalysts, 'Freud s'invite dans les lieux d'accueil enfants-parents' – Freud *invites himself* into the LAEPs.[162] While other western countries have built comparable networks of children's centres, these generally do not have psychoanalysts on hand to 'drink in the anxiety of mothers'. This aspect is unique to France, and Dolto and her ideas are at its heart.

Dolto as 'star'

With the twenty-first century waning of the cultural influence of psychoanalysis in France, the 'structures Dolto' may stand as the apogee of its transformation into a form of common sense, and its implantation into the everyday lives of many thousands of families. Dolto was able to achieve such large-scale social impacts by aligning psychoanalytic objectives with broader social goals. The LAEPs filled a real gap in provision for sociable spaces for young children and their parents/carers; psychoanalysts were present in them, but their presence was not the main need being met. Dolto's radio broadcasts, similarly, responded to evident demand from parents, children and the wider public for clear, empathetic advice in difficult situations, in an era of social dislocation and during a decline of older (community- or religion-based) channels of knowledge transmission. Dolto's offer chimed with a governmental aim to offer such assistance in a way that could reach all homes, not just those in major urban areas. Her shows, like those of Ménie Grégoire, provided a new sense of community for people undergoing similar experiences. Dolto's psychoanalytic orientation was incidental to her appeal for many listeners – and indeed some of them actively objected to some of her theoretical ideas, while continuing to treat her as a potential source of wisdom and advice.

In their book *Stardom in Postwar France*, John Gaffney and Diana Holmes argued that 'stars' arise because they 'capture ... the preoccupations, values, conflicts and contradictions of a particular culture, its "climate of feeling"'. Stars are a window into an era or culture – especially a culture in flux – who can 'restate, often in new and modern forms, old identities and values, as well as calling a society towards newer, and perhaps confused, emergent values'.[163] In a similar vein, David Looseley has written of Édith Piaf as 'a rhetorical figure' whose popularity fulfilled key symbolic functions for wider French culture.[164] Dolto's popularity should be seen from this perspective. She embodied a transition, already well advanced, from authoritarian parenting based on a culture of honour, tradition and deference to elders, to one oriented around libertarian, child-centred, discovery-based pedagogies. She was perhaps especially well placed to do this because she appeared to have something of a foot in both camps – while being professionally associated with radical philosophical and psychoanalytic currents, her persona was that of a maternal, reassuring, Christian broadcaster who opposed feminism and defended the heteronormative social order. A lifelong Parisian, but who idealised life in the French countryside, she attracted the attention of the state broadcaster, gaining a platform to disseminate her psychoanalytic ideas – understood as modern, scientific and metropolitan – to all corners of the nation. Liberal in some regards, reactionary in others, a pioneering woman who opposed advances in women's rights, Dolto's focus on practical everyday issues held broad appeal, perhaps especially to people who were daunted by the abstract, radical direction both of Lacanian psychoanalysis and of French feminism after the abortion reform of 1975. By turns a utopian dreamer and a staunch social conservative, Dolto was an appropriate symbol of mid-1970s France: aware that the post-1968 cultural upheavals must lead to permanent change, but nervous about social dislocations in a time of economic uncertainty – nostalgic for a world in which men were men and trees were trees.

Notes

1 Maggie Andrews, *Domesticating the Airwaves: Broadcasting, Domesticity and Femininity* (London: Continuum, 2012), p. xi.

2 See Shapira, *War Inside*, Ch. 4; Lisa Farley, 'Analysis on Air: A Sound History of Winnicott in Wartime', *American Imago*, 69:4 (2012), 449–71.

3 Nord, *France's New Deal*, pp. 241–53.
4 *Ibid.*, pp. 304–6.
5 See Jean Chalaby, 'One Nation, One State, One Television: Making Sense of De Gaulle's Broadcasting Policy', in Jessica Wardhaugh (ed.), *Paris and the Right in the Twentieth Century* (Newcastle-upon-Tyne: Cambridge Scholars, 2007), pp. 86–103; Chaplin, *Turning on the Mind*, introduction; Raymond Kuhn, *The Media in France* (London: Routledge, 1994), pp. 89ff.
6 Nord, *France's New Deal*, p. 353.
7 Rebecca Scales, 'Radio, Broadcasting, Disability Activism, and the Remaking of the Postwar Welfare State', *French Politics, Culture & Society*, 37:3 (2019), 53–78.
8 Kuhn, *Media*, p. 93.
9 Jonathyne Briggs, *Sounds French: Globalization, Cultural Communities, and Pop Music, 1958–1980* (New York: Oxford University Press, 2015), Ch. 1; Chris Tinker, *Mixed Messages: Youth Magazine Discourse and Sociocultural Shifts in Salut les copains (1962–1976)* (Oxford: Peter Lang, 2010).
10 *Paris Match*, 1518, 30 June 1978.
11 Kuhn, *Media*, pp. 77–80; Chaplin, *Turning on the Mind*, pp. 50, 115.
12 Christian Brochand, *Histoire générale de la radio et de la télévision en France 2, 1944–1974* (Paris: La Documentation française, 1994), pp. 154–5.
13 Cited in Robert Prot, *Précis d'histoire de la radio et de la télévision* (Paris: L'Harmattan, 2007), p. 181.
14 Françoise Dolto ('Docteur X'), *S.O.S. Psychanalyste! Des consultations sur les ondes* (Paris: Fleurus, 1976).
15 Eighty per cent of the homes of senior managers and members of liberal professions contained a telephone in 1967, but only 2 per cent of industrial working-class households. Duchen, *Women's Rights*, p. 88.
16 Dolto, *S.O.S. Psychanalyste!*, pp. 343–7.
17 *Ibid.*, p. 345.
18 *Ibid.*, p. 143.
19 *Ibid.*, pp. 282–6.
20 *Ibid.*, pp. 117–22.
21 *Ibid.*, pp. 55–6.
22 *Ibid.*, p. 46.
23 *Ibid.*, p. 47.
24 *Ibid.*, pp. 33–6.
25 Benjamin Spock, *The Common Sense Book of Baby and Child Care* (New York: Duell, Sloan & Pearce, 1946), p. 256.
26 Dolto, *S.O.S. Psychanalyste!*, p. 147.

27 *Ibid.*, p. 113.
28 *Ibid.*, pp. 56–7. Original emphasis.
29 *Ibid.*, pp. 74–5. Original emphasis.
30 *Ibid.*, pp. 120–1. Original emphasis.
31 *Ibid.*, p. 187.
32 Françoise Dolto and Andrée Ruffo, *Entretiens III: L'Enfant, le juge et la psychanalyste* (Paris: Gallimard, 1999), p. 81.
33 Françoise Dolto, 'L'Agressivité chez le jeune enfant', *Pratique des mots* (December 1981), reprinted in Dolto, *EME*, pp. 245–59, quote p. 248.
34 Dolto, *S.O.S. Psychanalyste!*, pp. 21–2.
35 *Ibid.*, p. 23.
36 Françoise Dolto, 'Repenser l'éducation des enfants: à propos du dressage à la propreté sphinctérienne' (1973), reprinted in *Les Étapes majeures de l'enfance*, pp. 260–310, quote p. 267.
37 *Ibid.*
38 Dolto, *Cause des enfants*, p. 34.
39 'Madame Soleil, Astrologer, 83' [obituary], *New York Times*, 30 October 1996.
40 Edgar Morin (ed.), *La Croyance astrologique moderne* (Lausanne: L'Age d'Homme, 1981), pp. 165ff.
41 Turkle, *Psychoanalytic Politics*, p. 207.
42 On Ménie Grégoire, see Coffin, 'From Interiority to Intimacy'; Claire Blandin, 'Médias: paroles d'experts/paroles de femmes', *Histoire@Politique. Politique, culture, société*, 14 (2011); Anne-Marie Sohn, 'Les Individus-femmes entre négation du moi et narcissisme. Les auditrices de Ménie Grégoire (1967–1968)', in Geneviève Dreyfus-Armand, Robert Frank, Marie-Françoise Lévy and Michèle Zancarini-Fournel (eds), *Les Années 68: le temps de la contestation* (Brussels: Editions Complexe, 2008), pp. 179–97; Guy Robert, 'RTL: le divan radiophonique de Ménie Grégoire', *Cahiers d'histoire de la radiodiffusion*, 55 (1998), 88–154; Dominique Cardon, '"Chère Ménie …". Émotions et engagements de l'auditeur de Ménie Grégoire', *Réseaux*, 13:70 (1995), 41–78; Turkle, *Psychoanalytic Politics*, Ch. 8.
43 Turkle, *Psychoanalytic Politics*, p. 207.
44 Dominique Cardon, 'Droit au plaisir et devoir d'orgasme dans l'émission de Ménie Grégoire', *Le Temps des Médias*, 1 (2003), 77–94.
45 Pierre Haski, 'Mort de Ménie Grégoire: quand la France parlait de sexe à son micro', *Le Nouvel Observateur*, 16 August 2014; Catherine Mallaval, 'Ménie mémoire', *Libération*, 25 January 2001.
46 Cardon, '"Chère Ménie"', 54; Blandine Schmidt, 'La radio de tous les maux', *Recherches en communication*, 37 (2012), 97–109, 100.
47 Turkle, *Psychoanalytic Politics*, p. 207.

48 *Ibid.*
49 On this episode, see John Mowitt, *Radio: Essays in Bad Reception* (Berkeley, CA: University of California Press, 2011), Ch. 4; Scott Gunther, *The Elastic Closet: A History of Homosexuality in France, 1942–present* (Basingstoke: Palgrave, 2008), Ch. 2. A transcript can be downloaded from http://semgai.free.fr/doc_et_pdf/Gregroie_douloureux_prob.pdf, accessed 30 June 2020.
50 Gunther, *Elastic Closet*, p. 48.
51 Mowitt, *Radio*, pp. 105ff.
52 Françoise Dolto, *Lorsque l'enfant paraît 2* (Paris: Seuil, 1978), p. 155.
53 *Ibid.*, p. 156.
54 Françoise Dolto, 'Littérature enfantine, attention danger', *L'Express*, 11 December 1972, 139, interview by Janick Jossin. Richard Hughes, *Gertrude et la sirène* (Paris: Editions Quist-Vidal, 1971); a translation of *Gertrude and the Mermaid* (New York: Harlin Quist, 1971).
55 Dolto, 'Littérature enfantine, attention danger'.
56 Cited in Michèle Piquard, 'François Ruy-Vidal et Harlin Quist, nouveaux concepteurs dans l'édition pour la jeunesse des années 1970. Étude de cas: Les Contes de Ionesco', *Communication et histoire: Écritures et espaces – temps pluriels, journées d'étude organisées les 9 et 10 mars 2001 par le Centre d'Histoire et des Récits de l'Information et des Médias-Réseaux en Europe, Université Paris III-La Sorbonne Nouvelle et le Centre d'Étude de l'Écriture (CEE), Université Paris 7-Denis Diderot* (Paris, 2002), 74–82, 80. (Thanks to Sophie Heywood for this reference.)
57 François Ruy-Vidal to Annie Trassaert/Éditions Gallimard, 22 April 2003, Archives de François Ruy-Vidal at Le Fonds patrimonial jeunesse Heure Joyeuse, Paris: Carton 15: Correspondances et échanges sur publications. (Thanks to Sophie Heywood for this reference.)
58 'Une histoire Dolto – table tournante organisé par R. Boquié et M. Bernand', *Postscriptum* (1973), 20–1.
59 Dolto, 'Les Troubles du sommeil', *EME*, pp. 157–8.
60 Antoine Prost, *Éducation, société et politiques: une histoire de l'enseignement en France de 1945 à nos jours* (Paris: Seuil, 1997), pp. 156–60.
61 *Ibid.*, p. 161.
62 Quoted in W. D. Halls, *Education, Culture and Politics in Modern France* (Oxford: Pergamon, 1976), p. 24.
63 Prost, *Éducation*, p. 163.
64 On Haby's reforms, see André Robert, *L'École en France de 1945 à nos jours* (Grenoble: Press universitaires de Grenoble, 2010), Ch. 4.
65 Gabriel Langouet and Alain Leger, 'Public and Private Schooling in France: An Investigation into Family Choice', *Journal of Education Policy*, 15:1 (2000), 41–9.

66 Dolto, *Cause des enfants*, pp. 405–7. Dolto followed up this successful book with a further volume, *La Cause des adolescents* (Paris: Robert Laffont, 1988).
67 *Ibid.*, pp. 399–400.
68 *Ibid.*, p. 424.
69 *Ibid.*, p. 423.
70 *Ibid.*, p. 405.
71 *Ibid.*, p. 433.
72 *Ibid.*, p. 406.
73 *Ibid.*, p. 410.
74 Fabienne d'Ortoli and Michel Amram, *L'École avec Françoise Dolto* (Paris: Hatier, 1990), p. 25.
75 Cited in *ibid.*, p. 22.
76 *Ibid.*, p. 26.
77 *Ibid.*, p. 25.
78 *Ibid.*, pp. 32–3.
79 Dolto, *Cause des enfants*, pp. 405–7.
80 Philippe Pétain, 'L'Éducation nationale', *Revue des Deux Mondes*, 15 August 1940.
81 Dolto to Arturo Prat, October 1970, *Une vie de correspondances*, p. 476.
82 Halls, *Education*, pp. 77–8.
83 Françoise Dolto, 'L'Homme quittera son père et sa mère', *Parents et maîtres*, 81 (1973) 365–87; 'Circulaire no. 73–299 du juillet 1973 aux Recteurs, aux Inspecteurs d'académie, aux Chefs d'établissement, aux Inspecteurs départementaux de l'Éducation nationale', AFD, box 29: Éducation/La famille, fiche A9.
84 Dolto, 'Le Métier des parents', *CdE*, pp. 11–13.
85 See Dolto to Ursula Huber, 17 August 1969, *Une vie de correspondances*, pp. 448–50. Dolto suspected that behind the criticism lay 'a lot of jealousies' and 'a cabal ranged against the Europe 1 station, which the Pompidou government has it in for, finding it too left-wing'.
86 In June 1978, towards the end of its run, the programme was moved to a morning slot.
87 Anne-Marie Gustave, 'Françoise Dolto, la voix qui sauve', *Télérama*, 6 November 2008.
88 As recalled by Pradel, interviewed in *ibid.* See also Françoise Dolto, 'Françoise Dolto et la radio', *Psychiatrie Française*, 2 (1984), 160–3.
89 Catherine Dolto, 'Anthologie radiophonique', sleeve notes to the CD audio release of *Lorsque l'enfant paraît, Intégrale de l'anthologie radiophonique 1976–1977* (Paris, 2009).
90 Françoise Dolto, *Lorsque l'enfant paraît 1* (Paris: Seuil, 1977), pp. 48–54.

91 *Ibid.*, pp. 34–6.
92 AFD, LLP 9, week 11, letter 61, November 1977.
93 AFD, LLP 1, week 2, October 1976.
94 AFD, LLP 12, week 31, letter 98, July 1977; AFD, box labelled 'LLP divers', letter 24.
95 AFD, LLP 13, week 34, letter 17, April 1978.
96 AFD, LLP 6, week 35, letter 2, May 1977.
97 AFD, LLP 11, week 20, letter 11, January 1978.
98 AFD, LLP 6, week 30, letter 9, July 1977.
99 AFD, LLP 13, week 34, letter 39, April 1978.
100 AFD, LLP 3, week 18, February 1977.
101 See Dolto, *Lorsque l'enfant paraît 2*, pp. 169–87.
102 AFD, LLP 13, week 34, letter 92, April 1978.
103 AFD, LLP 16, week 43, letter 3, July 1978.
104 See Richard Bates, 'Trauma and Anxiety in 1970s Parenting: Letters to Françoise Dolto, 1976–1978', *Journal of Medical Humanities* 42:2 (2021), 269–76.
105 AFD, LLP 7, week 3, letter 2, September 1977; Box LLP 1, week 1, letter 10, October 1976.
106 E.g. AFD, LLP 1, week 2, letter 15, October 1976; LLP 13, week 34, letter 90, April 1978; LLP 12, week 31, letter 28, April 1978; LLP 1, week 2, letter 4, October 1976.
107 AFD, LLP 1, week 1, letter 1, September 1976.
108 AFD, LLP 14, week 39, letter 6, June 1978.
109 AFD, LLP 4, week 25, letter 44, March 1977.
110 AFD, LLP 4, week 25, letter 44, March 1977. Copy of Dolto's response attached to the listener's letter.
111 AFD, LLP 4, week 25, letters 5 and 17, March 1977.
112 AFD, LLP divers; fiche 'FD ne répond pas "exprès"', letter dated 21 November 1978.
113 AFD, LLP 4, week 25, letter 11, March 1977.
114 AFD, LLP 15, week 43, letter 57, June 1978.
115 AFD, LLP 11, week 20, letter 29, January 1978.
116 AFD, LLP 4, week 25, letter 50, March 1977.
117 AFD, LLP 16, week 46, letter 19, July 1978.
118 AFD, LLP 6, week 35, letter 4, May 1977.
119 Éric Favereau, 'Dolto, comment te dire radio. Et si la psychanalyste n'avait pas parlé sur les ondes?', *Libération*, 11 July 2013.
120 Françoise Dolto, Pierre Benoit, Colette Langignon and Bernard This, 'Projet de Centre de l'enfance, 6 juillet 1977', in Marie-Hélène Malandrin (ed.), *Une psychanalyste dans la cité: l'aventure de la Maison verte* (Paris: Gallimard, 2009), pp. 110–17, 112.

121 Garcia, *Mères sous influence*, p. 292.
122 Dolto et al., 'Projet de Centre', p. 110.
123 'Lieux d'accueil enfants-parents: guide à l'usage des partenaires, Édition 2014', www.caf.fr/sites/default/files/caf/493/Laep2014Def.pdf, accessed 29 January 2021.
124 Dolto et al., 'Projet de Centre', p. 110.
125 Françoise Dolto, 'Conférence au congrès de l'ANPASE, Bordeaux, Avril 1980', in Malandrin (ed.), *Psychanalyste dans la cité*, pp. 209–10.
126 Dolto et al., 'Projet de Centre', p. 111.
127 *Ibid.*, pp. 110–11.
128 *Ibid.*, pp. 112–13.
129 Dolto, 'Réflexions de Françoise Dolto concernant le projet d'un Centre de petite enfance et de parentalité, 6 juillet 1977', in Malandrin (ed.), *Psychanalyste dans la cité*, pp. 118–21.
130 Dolto et al., 'Projet de Centre', pp. 112–13.
131 Cited in Henriette Scheu and Nathalie Fraoli (eds), *Lieux d'accueil enfants-parents et socialisation(s)* (Strasbourg: Le Furet, 2011), pp. 23, 106.
132 Dolto et al., 'Projet de Centre', p. 114.
133 *Ibid.*, pp. 114, 117. Original emphasis.
134 See documents reproduced in Malandrin (ed.), *Psychanalyste dans la cité*, pp. 123–32. The association also obtained a 60,000-franc grant from the Fondation de France, and 15,000 francs in contributions from local parents.
135 All figures in this paragraph from AFD, MV I, fiche '1979'.
136 Typed report dated April 1986, AFD, MV II, fiche '1986'.
137 Dolto to Suzanne Gasiglia, 14 August 1979, *Une vie de correspondances*, p. 641.
138 Dolto, 'Réflexions', p. 120.
139 *Ibid.*, pp. 118–21.
140 Jean-François Nguyen, Médecin Inspecteur de la Santé, to Dolto, 26 February 1982. AFD, box labelled 'Droits de l'enfant – la loi'.
141 Circular dated 11 June 1985. AFD, MV II, fiche '1985'.
142 Letter from Lille-based association 'Action, Formation, Étude, Recherche', undated, to Dolto at the MV. AFD, MV II, fiche '1986'.
143 'Pontivy: La planète des tous-petits', *Le Télégramme de Brest*, 13 September 1994.
144 'Dolto, 'Réflexions', p. 118.
145 The international centres included eleven in Switzerland, four in Belgium, three in Italy and Québec, two in Brazil and Russia and one in New York. An MV opened in London in 2013.

146 From a review in *Le Journal des psychologues*, 45 (1987) 29–31, AFD, MV II.
147 AFD, MV III. La Marouette: fiche 127, typed document, undated (1998); 'Pontivy: La planète des tous-petits'.
148 Scheu and Fraoli, *Lieux d'accueil*, p. 13.
149 *Ibid.*; Gérard Neyrand, *Sur les pas de la Maison Verte. Des lieux d'accueil pour les enfants et leur parents* (Paris: Syros, 1995).
150 Scheu and Fraoli, *Lieux d'accueil*, p. 108.
151 *Ibid.*, p. 105.
152 *Ibid.*, p. 103.
153 *Ibid.*, pp. 114–15.
154 *Ibid.*, pp. 139, 134, 140.
155 *Ibid.*, p. 124.
156 *Ibid.*, p., 59.
157 Garcia, *Mères sous influence*, 299.
158 *Ibid.*, p. 294.
159 Neyrand, *Sur les pas*, p. 151.
160 Garcia, *Mères sous influence*, p. 298.
161 For example, as of 2020 the website of the Allocations familiales named Dolto at the top of its introductory page on LAEPs. www.caf.fr/allocataires/vies-de-famille/futur-parent/garde-d-enfant/les-lieux-d-accueil-enfants-parents, accessed 29 January 2021.
162 Françoise De Grandt-Gauliard and Radu Turcanu, *Freud s'invite dans les lieux d'accueil enfants-parents* (Paris: Erès, 2013).
163 John Gaffney and Diana Holmes, *Stardom in Postwar France* (New York: Berghahn, 2007), p. 1.
164 Looseley, *Édith Piaf*, p. 16.

Afterword: Dolto in the twenty-first century

While certain aspects of Dolto's legacy, such as the MV/LAEPs, have had long-term impacts on French society, 'Doltomania' was primarily a phenomenon of the last quarter of the twentieth century. Since 2000, her ideas have increasingly come to seem out of touch with modern life – while nonetheless remaining thoroughly French.

A vignette from the film *2 Days in New York* (2012), Julie Delpy's sequel to her 2007 bilingual comedy *2 Days in Paris*, gives a sense of her shifting reputation. The comedy in these films substantially derives from cultural misunderstandings: between Delpy's French character 'Marion' and her American boyfriend 'Jack', and between the two of them and Marion's stereotypically French family. The main dividing line in the films is not nationality, but rather that between worldly metropolitan characters and others with narrower horizons. Marion, an artist, gets into arguments with racist taxi drivers; Jack, a photographer, gives misleading directions to provincial American tourists in baseball caps because 'they voted for Bush'.[1] The relationship between Marion and her sister 'Rose', played by Alexia Landeau, is part of this opposition. Rose, a child psychotherapist who wrote her thesis on Dolto, is depicted as much less of a global citizen than Marion, and possessed of a strong but not necessarily justified sense of her own psychological perspicacity. At one point, Rose takes Marion to task over her parenting, insinuating that Marion's son might become autistic because she (Marion) is too 'taciturn' and has an unresolved anger management problem (*problème de rage*).[2] This scene is presented in such a way as to suggest that Rose's ideas are not to be taken fully seriously – Delpy exploits them for comedic value and as a site of tension between the sisters. Rose's mother-blaming approach to autism comes across as comically unfounded, out of place in twenty-first-century families. In the context of the broader opposition between global-metropolitan and national-parochial mindsets running through these films, there is a sense in which Rose's – Dolto's – approach to psychology appears as a particularly 'French' – which in the context of the films, also means outdated and provincial – way of thinking, out of sync with modern cosmopolitan life.

Even in the 1980s, at the height of her fame, Dolto was beginning to appear out of touch with the modern world. Her 1983 trip to a psychiatry conference in Fort-de-France, Martinique, proved 'disconcerting' to her.[3] Most of the conference participants took an ethno-psychiatric perspective, analysing the effects of racial and colonial dominance on mental illness. 'The issue of race hits you in the face here [*ce problème noir ici vous saute à la gorge*], whereas in France, [people think that] Martinique is just France', Dolto commented. 'The psychoanalytical point of view is completely absent … the sense of personal or internal family conflict isn't among their categories.'[4] Dolto felt intimidated.[5] Notwithstanding the influence of the Martinique-born Frantz Fanon on the radical psychiatry of the 1960s with which she associated, she was not well versed in the psychology of race and colonialism, and had not interrogated the racist assumptions that she had carried with her from her interwar right-wing origins.[6] To be confronted with these issues in a place where she was a genuine outsider, and lacked her usual cultural authority, made the experience even more disturbing. However, this moment of dissonance did not cause Dolto to rethink her orientation. Speaking at a 1984 conference in Tunis on 'the child, family and the environment', Dolto, unlike most of the other speakers, made no reference to local circumstances, instead presenting the case of a French child whose suffering and cure were explained in terms of the unconscious transmission of maternal anxiety.[7] Her conclusion that 'the psychical balance of a child is tightly linked to its ancestral past, even to [events] more than two generations distant' was not intended to refer to socio-political issues, and might easily have come from René Laforgue's casebook of 'family neurosis' patients from fifty years earlier.

This Laforguian way of thinking, with some adaptations, had propelled Dolto to a national platform in the 1970s. But after 2000,

Dolto was no longer seen as a unifying national expert, but rather as someone linked to a particular ideological outlook. Discussion of her began to polarise. In 2008, her centenary, the television channel TF1 ran a hagiographical feature-length drama about Dolto, with Josiane Balasko in the starring role.[8] The same year, however, cognitive-behavioural therapist Didier Pleux published the first of two sharply critical books, castigating Dolto's theories as 'outdated and very often inappropriate, even toxic'.[9] Pleux's attacks formed part of a broader cultural battle in the 2000s over the scientific validity, and political implications, of psychoanalysis in France. This anti-Freudian wave notably produced the 2005 *Livre noir de la psychanalyse* (*Black Book of Psychoanalysis*), a collection of texts mainly by cognitive-behavioural therapists, taking aim at the epistemological foundations of psychoanalytic knowledge and the Freudian legacy in France. Several chapters condemned Dolto in particular.[10]

Other critics took issue less with Dolto personally so much as the use made of her ideas, methods and reputation by her successors, imitators and disciples – the sort of people denounced by Élisabeth Roudinesco on Dolto's centenary in 2008 as the 'idolaters [who] keep on sanctifying her'.[11] For Dominique Mehl, Dolto's major legacy was to inaugurate an entire genre of mass media intervention by psychoanalysts, while legitimising a fussy and superior tone of 'concrete and prescriptive interventions, guiding parental words and consciences in minute detail'.[12] Mehl's criticism underscores that made of MV staff by Sandrine Garcia, who was repulsed by their 'highly-affected manner of addressing children ... the body leaning towards the child, voice extremely soft, taking particular care to articulate and separate each syllable'.[13] A number of critics have associated Dolto's followers with a certain kind of Parisian bourgeois condescension. Guy Baret in *Allô maman Dolto* mocked '*Doltomaniaques*' by giving their children absurdly pretentious double-barrelled names like 'Pierre-Sosthène' or 'Marie-Guenièvre'. An animated short comedy film produced by students at the École Supérieure des Métiers Artistiques in 2016, since viewed over 200,000 times on YouTube, features an argument about child-rearing between several Paris metro passengers, set off by a young girl loudly demanding that her father buy her a pony. One haughty passenger, copy of *La Cause des enfants* in hand, chimes in with 'this situation illustrates the perfect decadence and failure of the education system' and 'but haven't you read Dolto?', only to be told 'Dolto, Dolto, you know where you can shove your Dolto!'[14]

An example of a Dolto-imitator in a political and media context is Edwige Antier, who in 2005–06 published a two-volume work titled *Dolto en héritage* (*Dolto's Legacy*).[15] Antier also had a show on France Inter ('*Enfances*'), modelled on Dolto's programmes from the 1970s.[16] She embraced the two key strands of Dolto's approach, liberal educational attitudes and traditional-patriarchal gender roles, as the subtitles of the two book volumes – 'understand everything, not permit everything', and 'boy or girl: the birth of sexual identity' – indicate. As a member of Parliament for the centre-right UMP party, Antier sought to ban the smacking of children by parents. In 2005, in a direct echo of Dolto's intervention over the supposedly dangerous imagery in *Gertrude and the Mermaid*, she took issue with the children's book *Jean a deux mamans* (*Jean's Got Two Mums*) by Ophélie Texier, aimed at three- to five-year-olds.[17] The book formed part of a collection which presented various kinds of family situation to young children, with titles including *Albert Lives at his Grandma's* and *Barnaby is Adopted*. For Antier, *Jean a deux mamans* was 'rubbish' (*n'importe quoi*) because lesbian parenting was 'a marginal occurrence [which] communicates … anti-values'; such a book should 'by no means' be stocked in a municipal library because 'at that age, the structuring of the psyche is in the middle of building the Oedipus complex … reading or recounting that type of story upsets everything and can damage [a child's] psychical construction'.[18]

Whereas the Mitterrand administration of the 1980s saw possibilities for using Dolto's ideas to advance socialist goals, after 2000 Dolto's legacy more frequently appeared aligned with conservative and Catholic positions on family policy. In 2012, during debates over the 'mariage pour tous' – i.e. broadening the marriage contract to include homosexual couples – a number of psychoanalysts protested in *Le Monde* that allowing lesbian and gay couples to marry and raise children risked 'obliterating sex difference … The birth of all children would be disrupted by it.'[19] Several of the psychoanalysts who signed the letter in *Le Monde* were working in areas that Dolto's work helped to establish, such as researching 'prenatal transference', or promoting preventive interventions in psychical health. While psychoanalysts in general were divided over the questions of gay marriage and parenting, opponents deployed language reminiscent of Dolto's arguments, claiming that 'all the world's children have the right to sexually differentiated parenting, which confers on them a psychical foundation' (*une origine psychique fondatrice*).[20] Adoption of children by gay couples 'would lead to the disappearance of fathers and mothers from the foundation of family life', according to Christian Flavigny, director of child and adolescent psychoanalysis at the Salpetrière hospital.[21] Dolto's daughter, Catherine Dolto-Tolitch, champion of her mother's legacy, was also quoted by opponents of the gay marriage bill.[22] Dolto-Tolitch has spoken in support of elements of the agenda of La Manif Pour Tous, a political campaign group based around opposition to gay marriage and defence of the 'traditional family'. In 2015 she claimed that legalising surrogate pregnancies would lead to 'barbarism' and 'violence', because of unconscious psychological transmissions occurring during the pregnancy.[23] La Manif Pour Tous itself, as an organisation centrally concerned with what Scott Gunther terms the 'sanctity of filiation' and with opposing what it sees as the erosion of traditional gender roles, can only be understood in the context of the importance given to these topics by twentieth-century French psychoanalysis, not least by Dolto.[24]

While a huge amount of good feeling towards Dolto remains at a popular level, changing social attitudes mean that there is also considerable empathy with the experience of people such as the writer and gay activist Lionel Labosse (b. 1966), whose upbringing was negatively affected by Dolto's ideas. During his adolescence, Labosse recalled in his 2005 book, *Altersexualité, éducation & censure*, '[my] mother was a devoted reader of Dolto, and it was to her books that I went in secret to try and dig up some information about what was happening to me; and obviously, since it was printed, I believed that it was true … this visceral homophobia was even more insidious as Françoise Dolto was felt to be an anticonformist and a destroyer of received ideas'.[25] For Labosse, and doubtless for other people in similar situations, it was not just Dolto's ideas themselves that were harmful, but the fact that her reputation as progressive and enlightened made it so much harder to dismiss them as outdated and reactionary. Attacking Dolto's national treasure status has thus arguably been somewhat necessary, in order to diminish the credibility of such prejudices.

In this book I have sought not so much to judge Dolto's work as to historicise it, working from the premise that the lack of such historical contextualisation in discussion of Dolto's ideas and psychoanalysis more broadly has hampered France's ability to know quite what to do with Dolto's legacy. As Dolto's life recedes into history, it becomes easier to see her ideas as products of a particular set of historical circumstances, rather than – as she and her followers believed – timeless truths about the human condition. This book has argued that Dolto's ideas were largely formed in the 1930s. In that decade Dolto, helped by René Laforgue and Édouard Pichon in particular, learned how to combine the social and political values of the French Right and the Parisian bourgeoisie with a holistic view of human health, a libertarian approach to education and a particularly anti-feminist strain of psychoanalysis that focused on family neuroses, penis envy and the role of mothers in pathologising children. This combination, packaged in the unusual form of a female, medically qualified psychoanalyst specialising in the treatment of children – and with a flair for anecdote and media engagement – proved attractive in the post-war years, as France became more open to psychological thinking. It was already somewhat divisive – as Dolto's role in the 1953 split in the SPP showed – owing to its association with Catholic intellectual currents and with people with collaborationist or antisemitic wartime records. Dolto's appeal and charisma reached a zenith in the 1970s following the social and economic upheavals of 1968 and the years immediately following, during which psychoanalysis had taken off as a mainstream French phenomenon. Under these circumstances, Dolto's combination of psychoanalysis and nostalgic social conservatism proved reassuring to broadcasters, government and the public alike. With the weakening of traditional family and religious structures, but without the peer-to-peer networks that would replace them in later decades, a public hungry for sources of advice and reassurance on personal and family problems found solace in Dolto's confident dispensation of wisdom that appeared simultaneously homespun and scientifically credible. As Dolto's fame progressed, however, more people started to contest what now seemed to be the outdated premises of some of her advice, notably on childhood determinism, gender roles and sexuality. This contestation has slowly but inexorably increased in the years following her death.

Given that French society as a whole still seems reluctant to move on from Dolto entirely, the kind of historical contextualisation of her ideas that I have set out in this book feels particularly essential. There are good reasons for wishing to retain some of what Dolto contributed: even her most vehement critics admit her capacity for psychological insight, for understanding the dynamics of individual families and for imagining ways to alter those dynamics through specific actions, speech or attitudinal changes. Many people have found (and continue to find) her books to be important sources of inspiration in finding solutions to problems within their families. Her emphasis on treating children with the same respect as adults, and on taking care to explain important events to them in terms that they can make sense of, are rightly celebrated. Separating these valuable aspects of her work from her time-bound prejudices on gender roles, fusional mothers, race and homosexuality is, however, not straightforward. There are no simple dividing lines that can be drawn – yet it is necessary to delineate them if Dolto is to be retained in today's literature of child-rearing without, for example, causing more mothers needlessly to castigate themselves for having produced a child with autism or a learning disability. The work of historical contextualisation that I have offered here may help to draw such lines. Ultimately, it will be up to the parents of the future to decide whether it is worth the effort.

Notes

1 *2 Days in Paris* (dir. Julie Delpy, France, 2007).
2 *2 Days in New York* (dir. Julie Delpy, France, 2012).
3 Dolto to Frosso Carapanos, 9 April 1983, *Une vie de correspondances*, p. 750.
4 *Ibid.*
5 According to the Martiniquais doctor Michel Boussat. *Une vie de correspondances*, p. 750, n. 26.
6 On Fanon's relationship to radical psychiatry, see Robcis, *Disalienation*, Ch. 2.
7 'Tunisie – Actualités', *Le Temps Tunisie*, 10 March 1984; 'Sciences et médecine', *La Presse de Tunisie*, 21 March 1984, 7. (Cuttings in AFD, box labelled 'Étranger – Tunisie'.)

8 Serge Le Péron, *Françoise Dolto, le désir de vivre*, TF1, 20 October 2008.
9 Pleux, *Génération Dolto*, p. 10.
10 Catherine Meyer and Mikkel Borsch-Jacobsen (eds), *Le Livre noir de la psychanalyse: vivre, penser et aller mieux sans Freud* (Paris: Arènes, 2010 (2005)). Chapters by Jacques van Rillaer, Jean Cottraux, Violaine Guéritault and Didier Pleux attacked Dolto directly. The book provoked responses from prominent psychoanalysts, notably Jacques-Alain Miller, *L'Anti-livre noir de la psychanalyse* (Paris: Seuil, 2006).
11 Baret, *Comment rater…*, p. 137; Élisabeth Roudinesco, 'La Cause des enfants', *Le Monde*, 21 October 2008.
12 Mehl, *La Bonne Parole*, p. 56.
13 Garcia, *Mères sous influence*, p. 298.
14 *Méli-Métro – ESMA 2016*, dir. Alexandre Blain, Lucas Germain, Christophe Gigot, Jade Guilbault, Andreas Muller and Simon Puculek. www.youtube.com/watch?v=RdEKcogdCMs, accessed 29 January 2021.
15 Edwige Antier, *Dolto en héritage 1: tout comprendre, pas tout permettre* (Paris: Robert Laffont, 2005); *Dolto en héritage 2: fille ou garçon: la naissance de l'identité sexuelle* (Paris: Robert Laffont, 2006).
16 Caroline Constant, 'Retrouver le chemin de son enfance', *L'Humanité*, 27 October 2004.
17 Ophélie Texier, *Jean a deux mamans* (Paris: École des loisirs, 2004).
18 Delphine de Mallevoüe, 'L'Homoparentalité racontée aux tout-petits' and 'Entretien avec Edwige Antier, pédiatre', *Le Figaro*, 9 September 2005.
19 Collective article, 'Touche pas à père et mère', *Le Monde*, 8 November 2012.
20 *Ibid.*
21 Christian Flavigny, 'L'Enfant bientôt privé de "père et mère"?', *Le Monde*, 8 November 2012.
22 E.g., Hervé Mariton, 'Rapport UMP sur la famille durable: droit de réponse', 27 July 2011, http://leplus.nouvelobs.com/contribution/176776-rapport-ump-sur-la-famille-durable-mon-droit-de-reponse.html, accessed 29 January 2021.
23 Catherine Dolto, 'GPA: Nous préparons la barbarie à venir', *La Manif pour tous*, 51, 6 May 2015, http://la-manif-pour-tous-51.blogspot.co.uk/2015/05/cdolto-gpa-nous-preparons-la-barbarie.html, accessed 29 January 2021.
24 Scott Gunther, 'Making Sense of the Anti-Same-Sex-Marriage Movement in France', *French Politics, Culture & Society*, 37:2 (2019), 131–58.
25 Lionel Labosse, *Altersexualité, éducation & censure* (Paris: Publibook, 2005), pp. 114–15.

Bibliography

Dolto's archives

I consulted Dolto's archives when they were held by the Association Françoise Dolto, rue Cujas, Paris. They have since moved to the Archives Nationales under the classification 752AP.

A selection of material from Dolto's personal archive was published as Yann Potin (ed.), *Françoise Dolto, archives de l'intime* (Paris: Gallimard, 2008).

Newspapers and periodicals

Archives de neurologie
Chronique sociale de France
Elle
Études carmélitaines
Femmes françaises
Huffington Post
Journal médical français
L'Année biologique
L'École des parents
L'Évolution psychiatrique
L'Express
Le Figaro
L'Humanité
La Croix
La Manif pour tous
Le Monde

Le Nouvel Observateur
La Nouvelle Revue française
La Presse de Tunisie
Le Télégramme de Brest
Le Temps Tunisie
Libération
Magazine littéraire
New York Times
Nouvelles littéraires
Parents et maîtres
Postscriptum
Psyché
Psychiatrie française
Psychoanalytic Review
Recherches
Réforme
Revue des deux mondes
Revue française de psychanalyse
Sciences humaines
Sociologie politique
Télérama
Témoignage chrétien
Vrai
World News

Published works

Abraham, Karl, 'Manifestations of the Female Castration Complex', *International Journal of Psycho-Analysis*, 3:1 (1922), 1–29.

Adler, Karen H., *Jews and Gender in Liberation France* (Cambridge: Cambridge University Press, 2003).

Anderson, Warwick; Jenson, Deborah; and Keller, Richard C. (eds), *Unconscious Dominions: Psychoanalysis, Colonial Trauma, and Global Sovereignties* (Durham, NC: Duke University Press, 2011).

Andrews, Maggie, *Domesticating the Airwaves: Broadcasting, Domesticity and Femininity* (London: Continuum, 2012).

Antier, Edwige, *Dolto en héritage 1: tout comprendre, pas tout permettre* (Paris: Robert Laffont, 2005).

———, *Dolto en héritage 2: fille ou garçon: la naissance de l'identité sexuelle* (Paris: Robert Laffont, 2006).

Asperger, Hans, 'Die "Autistischen Psychopathen" im Kindesalter', *Archiv für Psychiatrie und Nervenkrankheiten*, 117:1 (1944), 132–5.

Aublet, Yves, *Dans la tourmente de la Grande guerre: 1914–1918: Deauville, Trouville et le canton* (Cabourg: Cahiers du Temps, 2001).

Bailly-Salin, Pierre, 'The Mentally Ill Under Nazi Occupation in France', *International Journal of Mental Health*, 35:4 (2006–7), 11–25.

Barbas, Jean-Claude (ed.), *Philippe Pétain: Discours aux Français: 17 juin 1940 – 20 août 1944* (Paris: Albin Michel, 1989).

Baret, Guy, *Allô maman Dolto: Halte à la doltomania!* (Paris: R. Deforges, 1992).

———, *Comment rater l'éducation de votre enfant avec Françoise Dolto* (Paris: Ramsay, 2003).

Bates, Richard, 'Democratic Babies? Françoise Dolto, Benjamin Spock and the Ideology of Postwar Parenting Advice', *Journal of Political Ideologies*, 24:2 (2019), 201–19.

———, 'France's Autism Controversy and the Historical Role of Psychanalysis in the Diagnosis and Treatment of Autistic Children', *Nottingham French Studies*, 59:2 (2020), 221–35.

———, 'Trauma and Anxiety in 1970s Parenting: Letters to Françoise Dolto, 1976–1978', *Journal of Medical Humanities*, 42:2 (2021), 269–76.

Beale, Marjorie, *The Modernist Enterprise: French Elites and the Threat of Modernity, 1900–1940* (Stanford, CA: Stanford University Press, 2000).

Beauvoir, Hélène de, *Souvenirs*, ed. Marcelle Routier (Paris: Séguier, 1987).

Beauvoir, Simone de, *Le Deuxième Sexe I: Les faits et les mythes* (Paris: Gallimard, 1949). English edition: *The Second Sex*, trans. Constance Borde and Sheila Malovany Chevallier (New York: Vintage, 2010 (1949)).

———, *Mémoires d'une jeune fille rangée* (Paris: Gallimard, 1958). English edition: *Memoirs of a Dutiful Daughter* (1958), trans. James Kirkup (London: Penguin, 2001).

Bellos, David, *Georges Perec: A Life in Words* (London: Harvill, 1995).

Berenson, Edward, and Giloi, Eva (eds), *Constructing Charisma: Celebrity, Fame, and Power in Nineteenth-Century Europe* (New York: Berghahn, 2010).

Bertin, Célia, *Marie Bonaparte, A Life* (New York: Harcourt, 1982).

Bettelheim, Bruno, *The Empty Fortress: Infantile Autism and the Birth of Self* (New York: Free Press, 1967).

Binet, Alfred, and Simon, Théodore, *Les Enfants anormaux: guide pour l'admission des enfants anormaux dans les classes de perfectionnement* (Paris: Colin, 1907).

Blandin, Claire, 'Médias: paroles d'experts/paroles de femmes', *Histoire@ Politique. Politique, culture, société*, 14 (2011), www.histoire-politique.fr/index.php?numero=14&rub=dossier&item=134, accessed 12 September 2020.

Bonnafé, Lucien; Follin, Sven; Kestemberg, Evelyne; Kestemberg, Jean; Le Guillant, Louis; Lebovici, Serge; Monnerot, Émile; and Shentoub, Salem, 'La psychanalyse, idéologie réactionnaire', *La Nouvelle Critique* (1949), 57–72.

Bourdieu, Pierre, 'L'illusion biographique', *Actes de la recherche en sciences sociales*, 62–3 (1986), 69–72.

Bourg, Julian, *From Revolution to Ethics: May 1968 and Contemporary French Thought* (Montreal: McGill-Queen's University Press, 2007).

Boverat, Fernand, 'Il faut faire naître', *Revue de l'alliance nationale pour l'accroissement de la population française*, 143 (1924), 163–71.

Brejon de Lavergnée, Matthieu, *Le Temps des cornettes: Histoire des Filles de la Charité XIXe–XXe siècle* (Paris: Fayard, 2018).

Briggs, Jonathyne, *Sounds French: Globalization, Cultural Communities, and Pop Music, 1958–1980* (New York: Oxford University Press, 2015).

———, 'The Enduring Fortress: The Influence of Bruno Bettelheim in the Politics of Autism in France', *Modern Intellectual History*, 17:4 (2020), 1163–91.

Brochand, Christian, *Histoire générale de la radio et de la télévision en France, Tome 2 1944–1974* (Paris: La Documentation française, 1994).

Brower, M. Brady, 'Science, Seduction, and the Lure of Reality in Third Republic France', *History of the Present*, 1:2 (2011), 170–93.

Brunet, Luc-André, *Forging Europe: Industrial Organisation in France, 1940–1952* (London: Palgrave, 2017).

Bruno de Jésus-Marie, *La Belle Acarie, bienheureuse Marie de l'Incarnation* (Paris: Desclée de Brouwer, 1942).

Buhle, Mari Jo, *Feminism and Its Discontents: A Century of Struggle with Psychoanalysis* (Cambridge, MA: Harvard University Press, 1998).

Burgess, Greg, 'The Demographers' Moment: Georges Mauco, Immigration and Racial Selection in Liberation France, 1945–46', *French History & Civilization*, 4 (2011), 166–77.

Cardon, Dominique, '"Chère Ménie…". Émotions et engagements de l'auditeur de Ménie Grégoire', *Réseaux*, 13:70 (1995), 41–78.

———, 'Droit au plaisir et devoir d'orgasme dans l'émission de Ménie Grégoire', *Le Temps des médias*, 1 (2003), 77–94.

Carrel, Alexis, *L'Homme, cet inconnu* (Paris: Plon, 1935).

Carroy, Jacqueline; Ohayon, Annick; and Plas, Régine, *Histoire de la psychologie en France: XIXe–XXe siècles* (Paris: La Découverte, 2006).

Célestin, Emmanuel, *Essor ou déclin de l'Église: Lettre pastorale, Carême de l'an de grâce 1947* (Paris: A. Lahure, 1962).

Chalaby, Jean, 'One Nation, One State, One Television: Making Sense of De Gaulle's Broadcasting Policy', in Jessica Wardhaugh (ed.), *Paris and the Right in the Twentieth Century* (Newcastle-upon-Tyne: Cambridge Scholars, 2007), pp. 86–103.

Chamak, Brigitte, 'Autism as Viewed by French Parents', in Vinood B. Patel, Victor R. Preedy and Colin R. Martin (eds), *Comprehensive Guide to Autism* (New York: Springer, 2014), 2533–43.

Chamak, Brigitte, and Bonniau, Béatrice, 'Changes in the Diagnosis of Autism: How Parents and Professionals Act and React in France', *Culture, Medicine, & Psychiatry*, 37:3 (2013), 405–26.

Chanson, Paul, *Art d'aimer et la continence conjugale* (Paris: Éditions familiales de France, 1950).

Chaperon, Sylvie, *Les Années Beauvoir (1945–1970)* (Paris: Fayard, 2000).

Chaplin, Tamara, *Turning on the Mind: French Philosophers on Television* (Chicago: University of Chicago Press, 2007).

———, 'Lesbians Online: Queer Identity and Community Formation on the French Minitel', *Journal of the History of Sexuality*, 23:3 (2014), 451–72.

Chérer, Sophie, *Ma Dolto* (Paris: Stock, 2008).

Childers, Kristen Stromberg, *Fathers, Families, and the State in France, 1914–1945* (Ithaca, NY: Cornell University Press, 2003).

Choisy, Maryse, *Le Chrétien devant la psychanalyse* (Paris: Téqui, 1955).

Chrysostom, St John, *On Marriage and Family Life*, trans. Catherine P. Roth and David Anderson (Crestwood, NY: St Vladimir's Seminary Press, 2003).

Clark, Linda, *Schooling the Daughters of Marianne: Textbooks and the Socialization of Girls on Modern French Primary Schools* (New York: State University of New York Press, 1984).

Clarke, Jackie, *France in the Age of Organization: Factory, Home and Nation from the 1920s to Vichy* (New York: Berghahn, 2011).

Cobb, Richard, *Promenades: A Historian's Appreciation of Modern French Literature* (Oxford: Oxford University Press, 1980).

Coffin, Judith G., 'Beauvoir, Kinsey, and Mid-Century Sex', *French Politics, Culture & Society*, 28:2 (2010), 18–37.

———, 'From Interiority to Intimacy: Psychoanalysis and Radio in Twentieth-Century France', *Cultural Critique*, 91 (2015), 114–49.

———, *Sex, Love, and Letters: Writing Simone de Beauvoir* (Ithaca, NY: Cornell University Press, 2020).

Colvin, Kelly Ricciardi, *Gender and French Identity after the Second World War, 1944–1954: Engendering Frenchness* (London: Bloomsbury, 2017).

Coutrot, Jean, *De quoi vivre* (Paris: Grasset, 1935).

Dalbiez, Roland, *La Méthode psychanalytique et la doctrine freudienne* (Paris: Desclée de Brouwer, 1936).

Damousi, Joy, 'Representations of the Body and Sexuality in Communist Iconography, 1920–1955', *Australian Feminist Studies*, 12:25 (1997), 59–75.

Damousi, Joy, and Plotkin, Mariano Ben (eds), *Psychoanalysis and Politics: Histories of Psychoanalysis Under Conditions of Restricted Political Freedom* (New York: Oxford University Press, 2012).

Darrow, Margaret H., *French Women and the First World War: War Stories of the Home Front* (Oxford: Berg, 2000).

Dean, Carolyn, *The Self and Its Pleasures: Bataille, Lacan, and the History of the Decentered Subject* (Ithaca, NY: Cornell University Press, 1992).

Deleuze, Gilles, and Guattari, Félix, *L'Anti-Oedipe: Capitalisme et schizophrénie* (Paris: Minuit, 1972).

Desmazières, Agnès, *L'Inconscient au paradis: comment les catholiques ont reçu la psychanalyse, 1920–1965* (Paris: Payot, 2011).

Diamond, Hanna, *Fleeing Hitler: France 1940* (Oxford: Oxford University Press, 2007).

Dolto, Boris, *Le Corps entre les mains* (Paris: Vuibert, 2006).

Dolto, Françoise, *Psychanalyse et pédiatrie* (Paris: Seuil, 1971 (1939)). English edition: *Psychoanalysis and Paediatrics: Key Psychoanalytic Concepts with Sixteen Clinical Observations of Children*, trans. Françoise Hivernel and Fiona Sinclair (London: Karnac, 2013).

———, 'Ayez votre médecin de famille', *Vrai*, 3, 15 November 1941, 28–9.

———, 'Nos enfants ... Savez-vous leur parler?', *Vrai*, 4, 1 December 1941, 23.

———, 'Introduction à une page d'éducation', *Femmes françaises*, 18 January 1946, 14.

———, 'La Psychanalyse chez les enfants atteints des troubles du comportement', in *Ve Congrès international des Médecins Catholiques, Paris 6–9 juillet 1951* (Paris: l'Expansion scientifique française, 1952), 71–89.

———, 'Les Mères, entretien réalisé et réécrit par J.-B. Pontalis', *Les Temps modernes*, January 1963.

———, 'Clinique psychanalytique', *Recherches*, 8 (1968), 155–242.

———, *Le Cas Dominique* (Paris: Seuil, 1971).

———, 'Littérature enfantine, attention danger', *L'Express*, 11 December 1972, 139.

———, 'L'Homme quittera son père et sa mère', *Parents et maîtres*, 81 (1973), 365–87.

———, [as Docteur X] *S.O.S. Psychanalyste! Des consultations par les ondes* (Paris: Fleurus, 1976).
———, *Lorsque l'enfant paraît 1* (Paris: Seuil, 1977).
———, *Lorsque l'enfant paraît 2* (Paris: Seuil, 1978).
———, *Lorsque l'enfant paraît 3* (Paris: Seuil, 1979).
———, *Au jeu du désir* (Paris: Seuil, 1981).
———, *Séminaire de psychanalyse d'enfants 1* (Paris: Seuil, 1982).
———, *L'Image inconsciente du corps* (Paris: Seuil, 1984).
———, 'Françoise Dolto et la radio', *Psychiatrie française*, 2 (1984), 27–32.
———, *Séminaire de psychanalyse d'enfants 2* (Paris: Seuil, 1985).
———, *La Cause des enfants* (Paris: Robert Laffont, 1985).
———, *La Difficulté de vivre* (Paris: Paris: Vertiges-Carrère, 1986).
———, *Enfances* (Paris: Seuil, 1986).
———, *Tout est langage* (Paris: Gallimard, 1987).
———, *La Cause des adolescents* (Paris: Robert Laffont, 1988).
———, *Autoportrait d'une psychanalyste*, ed. Alain and Colette Manier (Paris: Seuil, 1989).
———, *Inconscient et destins. Séminaire de psychanalyse d'enfants 3*, ed. Jean-François de Sauverzac (Paris: Seuil, 1989).
———, *Les Étapes majeures de l'enfance*, ed. Claude Halmos (Paris: Gallimard, 1994).
———, *Les Chemins de l'éducation*, ed. Claude Halmos (Paris: Gallimard, 1994).
———, *La Vague et l'océan: séminaire sur les pulsions de mort (1970–1971)*, ed. Colette Manier (Paris: Gallimard, 2003).
———, *Lettres de jeunesse, correspondance 1913–1938*, ed. Colette Percheminier (Paris: Gallimard, 2003).
———, *Une vie de correspondances 1938–1988*, ed. Muriel Djéribi-Valentin (Paris: Gallimard, 2005).
Dolto, Françoise, and Oury, Jean, 'L'Enfant, la psychose et l'institution', *Recherches*, 8 (1968), 115–30.
Dolto, Françoise, and Ruffo, Andrée, *L'Enfant, le juge et la psychanalyste* (Paris: Gallimard, 1999).
Dolto, Françoise, and Séverin, Gérard, *L'Évangile au risque de la psychanalyse 1* (Paris: Seuil, 1977).
———, *L'Évangile au risque de la psychanalyse 2* (Paris: Seuil, 1979).
———, *La Foi au risque de la psychanalyse* (Paris: Seuil, 1981).
Dolto, Jean-Chrysostome, *Je m'appelle Carlos* (Paris: Ramsay, 1996).
Dosse, François, *Gilles Deleuze and Félix Guattari: Intersecting Lives*, trans. Deborah Glassman (New York: Columbia University Press, 2011).
Downs, Laura Lee, *Childhood in the Promised Land: Working-Class Movements and the Colonies de Vacances in France, 1880–1960* (Durham, NC: Duke University Press, 2002).

Drouard, Alain, *Une inconnue des sciences sociales: la Fondation Alexis Carrel, 1941–1945* (Paris: Éditions de la Maison des sciences de l'homme, 1992).

———, *Alexis Carrel (1873–1944): De la mémoire à l'histoire* (Paris: L'Harmattan, 1995).

Duché, Didier-Jacques, *Histoire de la psychiatrie de l'enfant* (Paris: Presses universitaires de France, 1990).

Duchen, Claire, *Women's Rights and Women's Lives in France, 1944–1968* (London: Routledge, 1994).

Ellis, Jack D., *The Physician-Legislators of France: Medicine and Politics in the Early Third Republic, 1870–1914* (Cambridge: Cambridge University Press, 1990).

Evans, Bonnie, *The Metamorphosis of Autism: A History of Child Development in Britain* (Manchester: Manchester University Press, 2017).

Evans, Richard I., *Jean Piaget: The Man and His Ideas*, trans. Eleanor Duckworth (New York: E. P. Dutton, 1973).

Evleth, Donna, 'The Ordre des Médecins and the Jews in Vichy France, 1940–1944', *French History*, 20:2 (2006), 204–24.

Farley, Lisa, 'Analysis on Air: A Sound History of Winnicott in Wartime', *American Imago*, 69:4 (2012), 449–71.

Fette, Julie, *Exclusions: Practicing Prejudice in French Law and Medicine, 1920–1945* (Ithaca, NY: Cornell University Press, 2012).

Ffytche, Matt, and Pick, Daniel (eds), *Psychoanalysis in the Age of Totalitarianism* (London: Routledge, 2016).

Fishman, Sarah, *The Battle for Children: World War II, Youth Crime, and Juvenile Justice in Twentieth-Century France* (Cambridge, MA: Harvard University Press, 2002).

———, *From Vichy to the Sexual Revolution: Gender and Family Life in Postwar France* (Oxford: Oxford University Press, 2017).

Foot, John, *The Man who Closed the Asylums: Franco Basaglia and the Revolution in Mental Health Care* (London: Verso, 2015).

Foucault, Michel, *Histoire de la folie à l'âge classique. (Folie et déraison)* (Paris: Plon, 1961).

Fouilloux, Étienne, *Une église en quête de liberté: la pensée catholique française entre modernisme et Vatican II (1914–1962)* (Paris: Desclée de Brouwer, 1998).

Fox, Robert, *The Savant and the State: Science and Cultural Politics in Nineteenth-Century France* (Baltimore, MD: Johns Hopkins University Press, 2012).

Freud, Sigmund, 'Sexuality in the Aetiology of the Neuroses' (1898), in James Strachey (ed.), *The Standard Edition of the Complete Psychological Works of Sigmund Freud, Vol. 3 (1893–1899): Early Psycho-Analytic Publications* (London: Hogarth, 1962), pp. 263–86.

———, 'Three Essays on the Theory of Sexuality' (1905), in James Strachey (ed.), *The Standard Edition of the Complete Psychological Works of Sigmund Freud, Vol. 7 (1901–1905): A Case of Hysteria, Three Essays on Sexuality and Other Works* (London: Hogarth, 1953), pp. 123–245.

———, '"Civilized" Sexual Morality and Modern Nervous Illness' (1908), in James Strachey (ed.), *The Standard Edition of the Complete Psychological Works of Sigmund Freud, Vol. 9 (1906–1908): Jensen's 'Gradiva' and Other Works* (London: Hogarth, 1959), pp. 181–204.

———, 'On the History of the Psycho-Analytic Movement' (1914), in James Strachey (ed.), *The Standard Edition of the Complete Psychological Works of Sigmund Freud Vol. 14 (1914–1916): On the History of the Psycho-Analytic Movement, Papers on Meta-Psychology and Other Works* (London: Hogarth, 1957), pp. 7–66.

Fromm, Erich, *Psychoanalysis and Religion* (New Haven, CT: Yale University Press, 1950).

Gaffney, John, and Holmes, Diana, *Stardom in Postwar France* (New York: Berghahn, 2007)

Garcia, Sandrine, *Mères sous influence: de la cause des femmes à la cause des enfants* (Paris: La Découverte, 2011).

Geissmann, Claudine, and Geissmann, Pierre, *A History of Child Psychoanalysis*, trans. The Melanie Klein Trust (London: Routledge, 1998).

Gildea, Robert, *France Since 1945* (Oxford: Oxford University Press, 2002).

———, *Empires of the Mind: The Colonial Past and the Politics of the Present* (Cambridge: Cambridge University Press, 2019).

Girginov, Vassil, 'Totalitarian Sport: Towards an Understanding of its Logic, Practice and Legacy', *Totalitarian Movements and Political Religions*, 5:1 (2004), 25–58.

Goffman, Erving, *Asylums. Essays on the Social Situation of Mental Patients and Other Inmates* (New York: Doubleday, 1961).

Golsan, Richard, 'Ideology, Cultural Politics and Literary Collaboration at *La Gerbe*', *Journal of European Studies*, 23:89–90 (1993), 27–47.

Gorrara, Claire, 'Crises of Witnessing: Édith Thomas and the War Years', *Modern & Contemporary France*, 4:3 (1996), 361–3.

Graham, Philip J., 'Susan Isaacs and the Malting House School', *Journal of Child Psychotherapy*, 34:1 (2008), 5–22.

———, *Susan Isaacs: A Life Freeing the Minds of Children* (London: Karnac, 2009).

Grandt-Gauliard, Françoise de, and Turcanu, Radu, *Freud s'invite dans les lieux d'accueil enfants-parents* (Paris: Erès, 2013).

Greenwald, Lisa, *Daughters of 1968: Redefining French Feminism and the Women's Liberation Movement* (Lincoln, NE: University of Nebraska Press, 2018).

Grégoire, Ménie, *Le Métier de femme* (Paris: Plon, 1965).

Grellet, Isabelle, and Kruse, Caroline, *Des jeunes filles exemplaires: Dolto, Beauvoir et Zaza* (Paris: Hachette, 2004).

Grenard, Fabrice, *La France du marché noir (1940–1949)* (Paris: Payot, 2008).

Gunther, Scott, *The Elastic Closet: A History of Homosexuality in France, 1942–present* (Basingstoke: Palgrave, 2008).

———, 'Making Sense of the Anti-Same-Sex-Marriage Movement in France', *French Politics, Culture & Society*, 37:2 (2019), 131–58.

Hale, Nathan G., *The Rise and Crisis of Psychoanalysis in America: Freud and the Americans 1917–1985* (New York: Oxford University Press, 1995).

Hall, Guy; Hivernel, Françoise; and Morgan, Siân (eds), *Theory and Practice in Child Psychoanalysis: An Introduction to the Work of Francoise Dolto* (London: Karnac, 2009).

Halls, W. D., *Education, Culture and Politics in Modern France* (Oxford: Pergamon, 1976).

Herzog, Dagmar, *Cold War Freud: Psychoanalysis in an Age of Catastrophes* (Cambridge: Cambridge University Press, 2017).

Hess, Antoine, *Les Analystes parlent* (Paris: Belfond, 1981).

Heuyer, Georges, *Enfants anormaux et délinquants juvéniles: nécessité de l'examen psychiatrique des écoliers* (Paris: G. Steinheil, 1914).

Heuyer, Georges, and Vervaeck, Paul, *Délinquance et criminalité de l'enfance* (Paris: Masson, 1935).

Heywood, Colin, *Growing up in France: From the Ancien Régime to the Third Republic* (Cambridge: Cambridge University Press, 2007).

———, 'Innocence and Experience: Sexuality among Young People in Modern France, c. 1750–1950', *French History*, 21:1 (2007), 44–64.

Hivernel, Françoise, '"The Parental Couple": Françoise Dolto and Jacques Lacan: Contributions to the Mirror Stage', *British Journal of Psychotherapy*, 29:4 (2013) 505–18.

Hochmann, Jacques, 'La Bataille de l'autisme. Réflexions sur un phénomène social contemporain', *PSN Psychiatrie Sciences Humaines Neurosciences*, 7:3 (2009), 99–111.

Hughes, Richard, *Gertrude and the Mermaid* (New York: Harlin Quist, 1971).

Inglis, Fred, *A Short History of Celebrity* (Princeton, NJ: Princeton University Press, 2010).

Isaacs, Susan, *The Nursery Years: The Mind of the Child from Birth to Six Years* (London: Routledge, 1929).

Jaccard, Roland (ed.), *Histoire de la psychanalyse* (Paris: Hachette, 1982).

Jackson, Julian, *Living in Arcadia: Homosexuality, Politics, and Morality in France from the Liberation to AIDS* (Chicago: University of Chicago Press, 2009).

Josset, Patrice, *Hôpital d'enfants Armand-Trousseau* (Paris: Assistance Publique, 1999).

Jury, Paul, *Journal d'un prêtre* (Paris: Gallimard, 1956).

Kanner, Leo, *Child Psychiatry* (Springfield, IL: C. C. Thomas, 1935).

———, 'Autistic Disturbances of Affective Contact', *Nervous Child*, 2 (1943), 217–50.

———, 'Early Infantile Autism', *Journal of Pediatrics*, 25:3 (1944), 211–17.

———, 'Emotional Interference with Intellectual Functioning', *American Journal of Mental Deficiency*, 56:4 (1952), 701–7.

Kaufmann, Dorothy, 'Uncovering a Woman's Life: Edith Thomas (Novelist, Historian, *Résistante*)', *The French Review*, 67:1 (1993), 61–72.

Kuhn, Raymond, *The Media in France* (London: Routledge, 1994).

Labosse, Lionel, *Altersexualité, éducation & censure* (Paris: Publibook, 2005).

Lacan, Jacques, *Écrits* (Paris: Seuil, 1966).

———, *Le Séminaire de Jacques Lacan, livre XI – Les quatre concepts fondamentaux de la psychanalyse, 1964*, ed. Jacques-Alain Miller (Paris: Seuil, 1973).

———, *Le Séminaire de Jacques Lacan, livre XVII – L'Envers de la psychanalyse*, ed. Jacques-Alain Miller (Paris: Seuil, 1991). English edition: *The Seminar of Jacques Lacan vol. XVII: The Other Side of Psychoanalysis*, trans. Russell Grigg (London: W. W. Norton, 2006).

———, *Autres écrits* (Paris: Seuil, 2001).

Laing, R. D., and Esterson, Aaron, *Sanity, Madness and the Family* (London: Tavistock, 1970).

Langouet, Gabriel, and Leger, Alain, 'Public and Private Schooling in France: An Investigation into Family Choice', *Journal of Education Policy*, 15:1 (2000), 41–9.

Lee, R. S., *Freud and Christianity* (London: James Clark, 1948).

Lieberman, Jeffrey A., with Ogi Ogas, *Shrinks: The Untold Story of Psychiatry* (London: Weidenfeld & Nicolson, 2015).

Liebman, Joshua L., *Peace of Mind* (New York: Bantam, 1946).

Looseley, David, *Édith Piaf: A Cultural History* (Liverpool: Liverpool University Press, 2015).

Lumbroso, Daniela, *Françoise Dolto, la vie d'une femme libre* (Paris: Plon, 2007).

Macknight, Elizabeth C., 'Faiths, Fortunes and Feminine Duty: Charity in Parisian High Society 1880–1914', *Journal of Ecclesiastical History*, 58:3 (2007), 482–506.

Makari, George, *Revolution in Mind: The Creation of Psychoanalysis* (New York: Gerald Duckworth, 2008).

Malandrin, Marie-Hélène (ed.), *Une psychanalyste dans la cité: l'aventure de la Maison verte* (Paris: Gallimard, 2009).

Mannoni, Maud, *L'Enfant arriéré et sa mère: étude psychanalytique* (Paris: Seuil, 1964). English edition: *The Retarded Child and the Mother. A Psychoanalytic Study*, trans. Alan M. Sheridan Smith (London: Tavistock, 1973).

———, *Le Premier Rendez-vous avec la psychanalyste* (Paris: Denoël/Gonthier, 1965).

———, *Le Psychiatre, son 'fou' et la psychanalyse* (Paris: Seuil, 1970).

———, *Ce qui manque à la vérité pour être dite* (Paris: Denoël, 1988).

Marini, Marcelle, *Jacques Lacan: The French Context*, trans. Anne Tomiche (New Brunswick, NJ: Rutgers University Press 1992).

Maritain, Jacques, *Primauté du spirituel* (Paris: Plon, 1927).

———, *Humanisme intégral: problèmes temporels et spirituels d'une nouvelle chrétienté* (Paris: Le Cerf, 1936).

Marshall, P. David, *Celebrity and Power: Fame in Contemporary Culture* (Minneapolis, MN: University of Minnesota Press, 2014).

Mauco, Georges, *Les Étrangers en France: leur rôle dans l'activité économique* (Paris: A. Colin, 1932).

———, *Vécu 1899–1982: Histoire de l'apparition de la psychanalyse en France* (Paris: Émile Paul, 1982).

Mayer, Arno J., *The Persistence of the Old Regime: Europe to the Great War* (London: Croom Helm, 1981).

Maza, Sarah C., *Violette Nozière: A Story of Murder in 1930s Paris* (Berkeley, CA: University of California Press, 2011).

Mehl, Dominique, *La Bonne Parole: Quand les psys plaident dans les médias* (Paris: La Martinière, 2003).

Meissner, W. W., 'Psychoanalysis and Catholicism – Dialogues in Transformation', *Psychoanalytic Inquiry*, 28:5 (2008), 580–9.

Mension-Rigau, Éric, *L'Enfance au château: l'éducation familiale des élites françaises au vingtième siècle* (Paris: Rivages, 1990).

Meslé, France, and Vallin, Jacques, 'La Population des établissements psychiatriques: évolution de la morbidité ou changement de stratégie médicale?', *Population*, 36:6 (1981), 1035–68.

Metzl, Jonathan M., '"Mother's Little Helper": The Crisis of Psychoanalysis and the Miltown Resolution', *Gender & History*, 15:2 (2003), 228–55.

Meyer, Catherine, and Borch-Jacobsen, Mikkel, *Le Livre noir de la psychanalyse: vivre, penser et aller mieux sans Freud* (Paris: Arènes, 2010).

Micale, Mark S., 'On the "Disappearance" of Hysteria: A Study in the Clinical Deconstruction of a Diagnosis', *Isis*, 84:3 (1993), 496–526.

Micale, Mark S., and Lerner, Paul Frederick, *Traumatic Pasts: History, Psychiatry, and Trauma in the Modern Age, 1870–1930* (Cambridge: Cambridge University Press, 2001).

Mijolla, Alain de, 'La Psychanalyse en France (1893–1965)', in Roland Jaccard (ed.), *Histoire de la psychanalyse, tome 1* (Paris: Hachette, 1982), pp. 9–105.

———, *Freud et la France: 1885–1945* (Paris: Presses universitaires de France, 2010).

———, *La France et Freud Tome 1 1946–1953: Une pénible renaissance* (Paris: Presses universitaires de France, 2012).

———, *La France et Freud Tome 2: D'une scission à l'autre 1954–1964* (Paris: Presses universitaires de France, 2012).

Miller, Jacques-Alain (ed.), *L'Anti-livre noir de la psychanalyse* (Paris; Seuil, 2006).

Milton, Damian, 'Tracing the Influence of Fernand Deligny on Autism Studies', *Disability & Society*, 31:2 (2016), 285–9.

Morgenstern, Sophie, *La Psychanalyse infantile: symbolisme et valeur clinique des créations imaginatives chez l'enfant* (Paris: Denoël, 1937).

Morin, Edgar (ed.), *La Croyance astrologique moderne* (Lausanne: L'Age d'Homme, 1981).

Moscovici, Serge, *La Psychanalyse: son image et son public. Étude sur la représentation sociale de la psychanalyse* (Paris: Presses universitaires de France, 1961).

Mowitt, John, *Radio: Essays in Bad Reception* (Berkeley, CA: University of California Press, 2011).

Muel-Dreyfus, Francine, *Vichy et l'éternel féminin. Contribution à une sociologie politique de l'ordre des corps* (Paris: Seuil, 1996).

Nettelbeck, Colin W., 'The Eldest Daughter and the Trente Glorieuses: Catholicism and National Identity in Postwar France', *Modern & Contemporary France*, 6:4 (1998), 445–62.

Neyrand, Gérard, *Sur les pas de la Maison Verte. Des lieux d'accueil pour les enfants et leur parents* (Paris: Syros, 1995).

Nord, Philip G., *The Republican Moment: Struggles for Democracy in Nineteenth-Century France* (Cambridge, MA: Harvard University Press, 1995).

———, *France's New Deal: From the Thirties to the Postwar Era* (Princeton, NJ: Princeton University Press, 2010).

Offen, Karen, *Debating the Woman Question in the French Third Republic, 1870–1920* (Cambridge: Cambridge University Press, 2018).

Ohayon, Annick, *L'Impossible Rencontre: psychologie et psychanalyse en France, 1919–1969* (Paris: La Découverte, 2006 (1999)).

———, 'L'École des parents ou l'éducation des enfants éclairée par la psychologie (1929–1946)', *Bulletin de psychologie*, 449 (2000), 635–42.

———, 'Édouard Pichon, psychanalyste français', in Michel Arrivé, Valelia Muni Toke and Claudine Normand (eds), *De la grammaire à l'inconscient: dans les traces de Damourette et Pichon: actes du colloque de Cerisy-la-Salle du 1er au 11 août 2009* (Limoges: Lambert-Lucas, 2009), pp. 141–8.

———, 'Psychoanalysis under the Vichy Regime', in Joy Damousi and Mariano Ben Plotkin (eds), *Psychoanalysis and Politics: Histories of Psychoanalysis Under Conditions of Restricted Political Freedom* (New York: Oxford University Press, 2012), pp. 35–56.

Oraison, Marc, *Vie chrétienne et problèmes de la sexualité* (Paris: Lethielleux, 1952).

d'Ortoli, Fabienne, and Amram, Michel, *L'École avec Françoise Dolto: le rôle du désir dans l'éducation* (Paris: Hatier, 1990).

Paxton, Robert O., *Vichy France; Old Guard and New Order, 1940–1944* (New York: Knopf, 1972).

Pedersen, Susan, *Family, Dependence, and the Origins of the Welfare State: Britain and France, 1914–1945* (Cambridge: Cambridge University Press, 1993).

Perec, Georges, *W ou le souvenir de l'enfance* (Paris: Denoël, 1975).

Pichon, Édouard, *Le Développement psychique de l'enfant et de l'adolescent. Évolution normale, pathologie, traitement. Manuel d'étude* (Paris: Masson, 1936).

Piquard, Michèle, 'François Ruy-Vidal et Harlin Quist, nouveaux concepteurs dans l'édition pour la jeunesse des années 1970. Étude de cas: Les Contes de Ionesco', *Communication et histoire: Écritures et espaces – temps pluriels, journées d'étude organisées les 9 et 10 mars 2001 par le Centre d'Histoire et des Récits de l'Information et des Médias-Réseaux en Europe, Université Paris III-La Sorbonne Nouvelle et le Centre d'Étude de l'Écriture (CEE), Université Paris 7-Denis Diderot* (Paris, 2002), 74–82.

Pleux, Didier, *Génération Dolto* (Paris: Odile Jacob, 2008).

———, *Françoise Dolto, la déraison pure* (Paris: Autrement, 2013).

Pollard, Miranda, *Reign of Virtue: Mobilizing Gender in Vichy France* (Chicago: University of Chicago Press, 1998).

Postel, Jacques, and Allen, David F., 'History and Anti-Psychiatry in France', in Mark S. Micale and Roy Porter (eds), *Discovering the History of Psychiatry* (Oxford: Oxford University Press, 1994), pp. 384–414.

Potin, Yann (ed.), *Françoise Dolto, archives de l'intime* (Paris: Gallimard, 2008).

Potts, John, *A History of Charisma* (Basingstoke: Palgrave, 2009).

Prost, Antoine, *Histoire de l'enseignement en France, 1800–1967* (Paris: Colin, 1968).

———, *Éducation, société et politiques: une histoire de l'enseignement en France de 1945 à nos jours* (Paris: Seuil, 1997).

Prot, Robert, *Précis d'histoire de la radio et de la télévision* (Paris: L'Harmattan, 2007).

Provost, Dominique, and Bauer, Andrée, 'Trends and Developments in Public Psychiatry in France since 1975', *Acta Psychiatrica Scandinavica*, 104 (2001), 63–8.

Pulju, Rebecca, *Women and Mass Consumer Society in Postwar France* (Cambridge: Cambridge University Press, 2011).

Quinn, Susan, *A Mind of Her Own: The Life of Karen Horney* (London: Macmillan, 1988).

Racamier, Paul-Claude (ed.), *Le Psychanalyste sans divan: la psychanalyse et les institutions de soins psychiatriques* (Paris: Payot, 1970).

Razon, Laure; Putois, Olivier; and Vanier, Alain, 'The Lacanian Concept of Cut in Light of Lacan's Interactions with Maud Mannoni', *Frontiers in Psychology*, 8:2177 (December 2017).

Reggiani, Andrés Horacio, *God's Eugenicist: Alexis Carrel and the Sociobiology of Decline* (Oxford: Berghahn, 2006).

Rennes, Juliette, 'The French Republic and Women's Access to Professional Work: Issues and Controversies in France from the 1870s to the 1930s', *Gender & History*, 23:2 (2011), 341–66.

Reynolds, Siân, *France Between the Wars: Gender and Politics* (London: Routledge, 1996).

Richards, Graham, 'Britain on the Couch: The Popularization of Psychoanalysis in Britain 1918–1940', *Science in Context*, 13:2 (2000), 183–230.

Rimland, Bernard, *Infantile Autism: The Syndrome and its Implications for a Neural Theory of Behavior* (London: Methuen, 1964).

Robcis, Camille, *The Law of Kinship: Anthropology, Psychoanalysis, and the Family in France* (Ithaca, NY: Cornell University Press, 2013).

———, 'Frantz Fanon, Institutional Psychotherapy, and the Decolonization of Psychiatry', *Journal of the History of Ideas*, 81:2 (2020), 303–25.

———, *Disalienation: Politics, Philosophy, and Radical Psychiatry in Postwar France* (Chicago: University of Chicago Press, 2021).

Robert, André D., *L'École en France de 1945 à nos jours* (Grenoble: Presses universitaires de Grenoble, 2010).

Robert, Guy, 'RTL: le divan radiophonique de Ménie Grégoire', *Cahiers d'histoire de la radiodiffusion*, 55 (1988), 88–154.

Roberts, Mary Louise, *Civilization without Sexes: Reconstructing Gender in Postwar France, 1917–1927* (Chicago: University of Chicago Press, 1994).

Ross, Kristin, *Fast Cars, Clean Bodies: Decolonization and the Reordering of French Culture* (Cambridge, MA: MIT Press, 1995).

Roudebush, Marc, 'A Patient Fights Back: Neurology in the Court of Public Opinion in France during the First World War', *Journal of Contemporary History*, 35:1 (2000), 29–38.

Roudinesco, Élisabeth, *La Bataille de cent ans: histoire de la psychanalyse en France (tome 1)* (Paris: Ramsay, 1982).

———, *La Bataille de cent ans: histoire de la psychanalyse en France (tome 2)* (Paris: Seuil, 1986).

———, 'René Laforgue et la collaboration manquée Paris/Berlin, 1939–1942. Documents concernant l'histoire de la psychanalyse en France durant l'Occupation', *Cahiers confrontation*, 16 (1986), 243–78.

———, *Jacques Lacan & Co.: A History of Psychoanalysis in France, 1925–1985*, trans. Jeffrey Mehlman (London: Free Association, 1990).

———, 'Georges Mauco (1899–1988): Un psychanalyste au service de Vichy. De l'antisémitisme à la psychopédagogie', *L'Infini*, 51 (1995), 69–84.

Rudolph, Nicole C., *At Home in Postwar France: Modern Mass Housing and the Right to Comfort* (New York: Berghahn, 2015).

Sanos, Sandrine, *Simone de Beauvoir: Creating a Feminist Existence in the World* (New York: Oxford University Press, 2016).

Sauverzac, Jean-François de, *Françoise Dolto: Itinéraire d'une psychanalyste: essai* (Paris; Flammarion, 1995).

Scales, Rebecca, 'Radio, Broadcasting, Disability Activism, and the Remaking of the Postwar Welfare State', *French Politics, Culture & Society*, 37:3 (2019), 53–78.

Schauder, Claude (ed.), *Lire Dolto aujourd'hui* (Ramonville Saint-Agne: Érès, 2004).

Scheu, Henriette and Nathalie Fraoli (eds), *Lieux d'accueil enfants-parents et socialisation(s)* (Strasbourg: Le Furet, 2011).

Schmidt, Blandine, 'La Radio de tous les maux', *Recherches en communication*, 37 (2012), 99–109.

Schneider, William H., *Quality and Quantity: The Quest for Biological Regeneration in Twentieth-Century France* (Cambridge: Cambridge University Press, 1990).

Schultheiss, Katrin, *Bodies and Souls: Politics and the Professionalization of Nursing in France, 1880–1922* (Cambridge, MA: Harvard University Press, 2001).

Scott, Joan Wallach, *Only Paradoxes to Offer: French Feminists and the Rights of Man* (Cambridge, MA: Harvard University Press, 1996).

Sevegrand, Martine, *Les Enfants du bon Dieu: Les catholiques français et la procréation au XX siècle* (Paris: Albin Michel, 1995).

Shapira, Michal, *The War Inside: Psychoanalysis, Total War, and the Making of the Democratic Self in Postwar Britain* (Cambridge: Cambridge University Press, 2013).

———, 'Psychoanalytic Criminology, Childhood and the Democratic Self', in Matt Ffytche and Daniel Pick (eds), *Psychoanalysis in the Age of Totalitarianism* (Abingdon: Routledge, 2016), pp. 73–86.

Sheffer, Edith, *Asperger's Children: The Origins of Autism in Nazi Vienna* (New York: W. W. Norton, 2018).

Silberman, Steve, *Neurotribes: The Legacy of Autism and How to Think Smarter about People Who Think Differently* (London: Allen & Unwin, 2015).

Silverman, Chloe, *Understanding Autism: Parents, Doctors, and the History of a Disorder* (Princeton, NJ: Princeton University Press, 2011).

Singh, Ilina, 'Bad Boys, Good Mothers, and the "Miracle" of Ritalin', *Science in Context*, 15:4 (2002), 577–603.

Smith, Paul, *Feminism and the Third Republic: Women's Political and Civil Rights in France 1918–1945* (Oxford: Clarendon, 1996).

Sohn, Anne-Marie, 'Les Individus-femmes entre négation du moi et narcissisme. Les auditrices de Ménie Grégoire (1967–1968)', in Geneviève Dreyfus-Armand, Robert Frank, Marie-Françoise Lévy and Michèle Zancarini-Fournel (eds), *Les Années 68: le temps de la contestation* (Brussels: Éditions Complexe, 2008), pp. 179–97.

Spock, Benjamin, *The Common Sense Book of Baby and Child Care* (New York: Duell, Sloan & Pearce, 1946).

Steel, David, 'Les Débuts de la psychanalyse dans les lettres françaises: 1914–1922. Apollinaire, Cendrars, "Le Mercure de France", "La Revue de l'Époque", Morand, Bourget, Lenormand', *Revue d'histoire littéraire de la France*, 79:1 (1979), 62–89.

Stefanatos, Gerry A., 'Regression in Autistic Spectrum Disorders', *Neuropsychology Review*, 18:4 (2008), 305–19.

Surkis, Judith, *Sexing the Citizen: Morality and Masculinity in France, 1870–1920* (Ithaca, NY: Cornell University Press, 2006).

Sutton, Nina, *Bettelheim, A Life and Legacy* (Boulder, CO: Westview, 1997).

Szasz, Thomas, *The Myth of Mental Illness: Foundations of a Theory of Personal Conduct* (New York: Hoeber-Harper, 1961).

Texier, Ophélie, *Jean a deux mamans* (Paris: École des loisirs, 2004).

Thomson, Mathew, *Psychological Subjects: Identity, Culture, and Health in Twentieth-Century Britain* (Oxford: Oxford University Press, 2006).

———, *Lost Freedom: The Landscape of the Child and the British Post-war Settlement* (Oxford: Oxford University Press, 2013).

Tinker, Chris, *Mixed Messages: Youth Magazine Discourse and Sociocultural Shifts in Salut les copains (1962–1976)* (Oxford: Peter Lang, 2010).

Tumblety, Joan, *Remaking the Male Body: Masculinity and the Uses of Physical Culture in Interwar and Vichy France* (Oxford: Oxford University Press, 2012).

Turkle, Sherry, 'French Anti-Psychiatry', in David Ingleby (ed.), *Critical Psychiatry: The Politics of Mental Health* (Harmondsworth: Penguin, 1981), pp. 150–83.

———, *Psychoanalytic Politics: Freud's French Revolution* (New York: Guilford Press, 1992).

Vatin, François, 'Octave Mannoni (1899–1989) et sa *Psychologie de la colonisation.* Contextualisation et décontextualisation', *Revue du MAUSS*, 37:1 (2011), 137–78.

Vérine, Madame (Marguérite Lebrun), *La Mère initiatrice* (Paris: Spes, 1929).

———, 'La famille', in André Bellessort and Raymond Postal (eds), *France 1941: La Révolution nationale constructive, un bilan et un programme* (Paris: Alsatia, 1941).

Wallon, Henri, *L'Enfant turbulent. Étude sur les retards et les anomalies du développement moteur et mental* (Paris: Alcan, 1925).

———, 'Comment se développe chez l'enfant la notion du corps propre', *Journal de Psychologie* (1931), 705–48.

Weber, Eugen, *Action Française: Royalism and Reaction in Twentieth-Century France* (Stanford, CA: Stanford University Press, 1962).

Weil, Patrick, 'Georges Mauco, Expert en Immigration: Ethnoracisme pratique et antisémitisme fielleux', in Pierre-André Taguieff (ed.), *L'Antisémitisme de plume, 1940–1944: Études et documents* (Paris: Berg, 1999), pp. 267–76.

Weiner, Susan, *Enfants Terribles: Youth and Femininity in the Mass Media in France, 1945–1968* (Baltimore, MD: Johns Hopkins University Press, 2001).

Weisman, Richard, 'Reflections on the Oak Ridge Experiment with Mentally Disordered Offenders, 1965–1968', *International Journal of Law and Psychiatry*, 18:3 (1995), 265–90.

Winter, Sarah, *Freud and the Institution of Psychoanalytic Knowledge* (Stanford, CA: Stanford University Press, 1999).

Zahra, Tara, *The Lost Children: Reconstructing Europe's Families After World War II* (Cambridge, MA: Harvard University Press, 2011).

Zaretsky, Eli, *Secrets of the Soul: A Social and Cultural History of Psychoanalysis* (New York: Vintage, 2005).

———, *Political Freud: A History* (New York: Columbia University Press, 2015).

Index

Note: Page numbers in *italic* refer to illustrations.

EU authorised representative for GPSR:
Easy Access System Europe, Mustamäe tee 50,
10621 Tallinn, Estonia
gpsr.requests@easproject.com

www.ingramcontent.com/pod-product-compliance
Ingram Content Group UK Ltd.
Pitfield, Milton Keynes, MK11 3LW, UK
UKHW021834100926
8556IPUK00004B/331
* 9 7 8 1 5 2 6 1 5 9 6 2 5 *